Career Longevity

The Bodywork Practitioner's Guide to Wellness and Body Mechanics

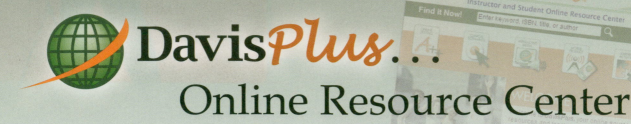

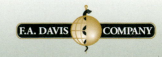

Career Longevity

The Bodywork Practitioner's Guide to Wellness and Body Mechanics

Jean'e E. Freeman, BS, AAS, NCTMB, LMT, CFT, RMT
Owner, Total Body Fitness
Instructor/Educator, Cortiva Institute
Tucson, AZ

Sandra K. Anderson, BA, NCTMB, LMT, ABT
Co-owner and Practitioner, Tucson Touch Therapies Treatment Center
Tucson, AZ

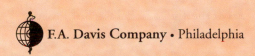

F.A. Davis Company • Philadelphia

F. A. Davis Company
1915 Arch Street
Philadelphia, PA 19103
www.fadavis.com

Copyright © 2012 by F. A. Davis Company

Printed in the United States of America

Last digit indicates print number: 10 9 8 7 6 5 4 3 2 1

Senior Acquisitions Editor: Christa A. Fratantoro
Manager of Content Development: George W. Lang
Developmental Editor: Stephanie Kelly
Art and Design Manager: Carolyn O'Brien

As new scientific information becomes available through basic and clinical research, recommended treatments and drug therapies undergo changes. The author(s) and publisher have done everything possible to make this book accurate, up to date, and in accord with accepted standards at the time of publication. The author(s), editors, and publisher are not responsible for errors or omissions or for consequences from application of the book, and make no warranty, expressed or implied, in regard to the contents of the book. Any practice described in this book should be applied by the reader in accordance with professional standards of care used in regard to the unique circumstances that may apply in each situation. The reader is advised always to check product information (package inserts) for changes and new information regarding dose and contraindications before administering any drug. Caution is especially urged when using new or infrequently ordered drugs.

Library of Congress Cataloging-in-Publication Data

Freeman, Jean'e E.
 Career longevity : the bodywork practitioner's guide to wellness and body mechanics / Jean'e E. Freeman, Sandra K. Anderson. — 1st ed.
    p. ; cm.
Includes bibliographical references and index.

ISBN 978-0-8036-2567-9

I. Anderson, Sandra K. II. Title.
[DNLM: 1. Occupational Diseases—prevention & control. 2. Allied Health Personnel. 3. Body Composition—physiology. 4. Massage—methods. 5. Mind-Body Therapies—methods. WA 440]
 LC classification   not assigned
 615.8'515—dc23

                                                          2011033511

To David Kent Anderson, my husband and my best friend. Without his love and support, this book would never have been written. To Jean'e Freeman, whose knowledge and expertise is crucial to writing this book.

Sandra K. Anderson

To my precious mother and guardian angel, life's free spirit (if love could have saved her, she would have lived forever). To my father, the best dad one could ask for, and without him, I would be lost. To my family for their patience and support during this book-writing process. To my students and peers who have inspired me to write this book, all of you have fueled my soul. To Sandy Anderson for this awesome opportunity and for believing in me.

Jean'e E. Freeman

Preface

> "It's not the load that breaks you down; it's the way you carry it."
>
> — Lena Horne

While the bodywork profession can be tremendously rewarding, there are many problems and issues student and professional practitioners may face. Often, bodywork practitioners leave the field because of injury, muscle strain, fatigue, and burnout. In order to have a long and successful career, it is important that practitioners have appropriate body mechanics, efficient breathing, strength, and stamina. Additionally, the choices practitioners make about self-care, health, and wellness impact their ability to perform their treatments, which, in turn, directly correlates to their career success.

The purpose of *Career Longevity: The Bodywork Practitioner's Guide to Wellness and Body Mechanics* is to help bodywork students and professionals develop lifetime tools that foster their ease of movement, decrease their chance of injury, and enhance their career longevity. These tools include doing honest self-assessments; recognizing the impact of lifestyle choices; developing body awareness and mindful movement; maintaining balanced posture; cultivating efficient breathing; using proper body mechanics when performing bodywork techniques; implementing self-care habits such as hydrotherapy, injury prevention, hydration, stretching, strengthening, and good nutrition; and integrating wellness and self-care into their bodywork practices and everyday lives.

Real-life examples of issues and dilemmas that students and professionals have faced are used to illustrate points. There is an emphasis in creative problem-solving. This is done through activities that encourage readers to discover personal beliefs and restrictions and challenge them to reframe views that are limiting their health and wellness. Other activities stimulate research and the creation of individual health and wellness plans for optimal strength, flexibility, and well-being. Guidance is given for tracking these self-growth tools.

The more wellness skills practitioners have, the more clients and practitioners themselves will benefit. Having a clear sense of oneself as a healthy and strong bodywork professional will be translated into effective treatments, greater stamina, and the ability to educate clients about their own health and wellness. In turn, this will lead to greater client satisfaction and a successful bodywork practice.

Career Longevity: The Bodywork Practitioner's Guide to Wellness and Body Mechanics is easy to read and offers numerous pedagogical features that encourage learning and information retention and increase interest in the subject matter. The enclosed DVD provides additional support by demonstrating good body mechanics when working on the table and on the floor, and by showing proper execution of stretching and strengthening techniques to help prevent injuries. Readers are encouraged to make the information their own through various activities and are supported in integrating the subject matter into their own experience.

ORGANIZATION

This book is divided into ten chapters that reflect the various aspects of the practitioner's health and wellness as a bodywork professional.

Chapter 1 **Bodywork and the Bodywork Practitioner's Wellness** This chapter focuses on the connection between the bodywork practitioner's wellness and his or her career longevity. The major components of career longevity are mental, emotional, and physical preparation, which includes proper body mechanics and injury prevention and management. Topics covered include how lifestyle, wellness, and professional appearance impact career longevity. A Wellness Profile is included in a special section. This is an assessment tool that students and professionals can use to determine, among other things, their levels of fitness, emotional and psychological stressors, posture, general and repetitive movement habits, health, nutrition, overall satisfaction with their lives, and how all of these intertwine to impact their well-being. It also includes ways to create positive health and wellness strategies and methods to check their progress. A series of questions help the reader perform a self-assessment on these topics and assist them in determining the areas in which they would like to improve. Support and tools for improvement are given throughout the rest of the text, and the Wellness Profile is used as a continual reference point.

Chapter 2 **Body Awareness and Mindful Movement** Movement and body awareness are discussed in depth. Proprioception is explained with clear illustrations. Mindfulness of the body and its parts as it moves are correlated with efficient, healthy movement and proper body mechanics. Ways to develop conscientious body movement are covered, such as through exercise, tai chi, and qigong. In addition, there are grounding, also known as centering or focusing, exercises.

Chapter 3 **Posture and Its Impact on the Body** Balanced posture is defined and illustrated. The muscles and muscle groups involved in maintaining posture are also illustrated. The benefits of balanced posture are discussed, as well as postural habits and how they impact the body. Balanced posture during the performance of bodywork on a massage table, a massage chair, and a futon on the floor are demonstrated. Also included is balanced posture during activities of daily living, such as working on the computer, exercising, playing sports, talking on the phone, doing laundry, and sleeping. Ways to improve posture and balance are presented, such as through specific exercises.

Chapter 4 **Breathing for Best Practice, Health, and Wellness** This chapter covers the importance of breathing properly, not just when performing bodywork treatments but also throughout activities of daily living. The anatomy and physiology of breathing is illustrated, along with types of breathing and how to breathe efficiently. Emphasis is placed on the proper rhythm of breathing during bodywork, both with delivery of technique and the practitioner's own internal rhythm. Breathing exercises to improve respiratory function, increase endurance and stamina, and clear and center the mind are included.

Chapter 5 **Body Mechanics** Using proper body mechanics is the foundation of efficient and effective bodywork. The difference between using muscular strength and using body weight to apply pressure is highlighted. The core of the body and the body's center of gravity are explained and illustrated. The importance of proper body positions and awareness of neutral wrists, joint alignment, head-to-tail connection, and positions for the head, shoulder, arm, hand, wrist, thumb, fingers, hips, knees, and feet is clarified and demonstrated through photos. Appropriate posture for the bodywork practitioner to have while stretching clients and themselves is incorporated into this chapter, as well as a description of how environmental factors and considerations impact body mechanics. These factors and considerations include table height, lighting, room space, clothing, shoes, hair, nails, music, and hygiene.

Chapter 6 **Injury Prevention and Management** Most injuries bodywork practitioners experience are due to poor body mechanics. Illustrations of the joints and body parts that are subject to common overuse injuries and repetitive use injuries are included, along with causes, prevention, and treatment of these injuries. Proper lifting of bodywork equipment and proper lifting in everyday life is explained and demonstrated in photos. Environmental factors, such as performing activities of daily living, reaching, bending, sleeping habits, and so forth, that can be involved in injury prevention and management are also included.

Chapter 7 **Stretching: Why, How, When, and Where?** Types of stretching and its benefits are defined, and the effects on muscle tissue, connective tissue, proprioceptors, and joints are explained and illustrated. Different types of stretches and protocols for flexibility are shown, and when to stretch—in between clients, during and after performing a bodywork treatment, and as part of a daily routine—is discussed. Stretches, and their modifications, are shown for each section of the body.

Chapter 8 **Strengthening: Why, How, When, and Where?** Types of strengthening and their benefits are defined. The effects on muscle tissue, connective tissue, proprioceptors, and joints are explained and illustrated. How to strengthen using body weight and using equipment, such as exercise balls, exercise tubing, and dumbbells, is shown. While ways to strengthen the entire body are presented, emphasis is placed on how to strengthen the core of the body and the legs. Included is an overall strengthening routine, as well as how to modify strengthening techniques for various levels of fitness.

Chapter 9 **Basic Nutritional Principles for Self-Care** The role of basic proper nutrition in the health of the body is explained. An in-depth discussion of water and its importance is incorporated, along with the functions of proteins, carbohydrates, fats, vitamins, and minerals in the body. Sources of these nutrients, including good and bad fats, is presented. There is also a section on common supplements, such as glucosamine and coenzyme Q10. Readers will be able to calculate their personal nutrient requirements by analyzing their daily energy needs. They will also be given tools to determine the best food sources for them and when, what, and how often they should eat.

Chapter 10 **Additional Support for Wellness and Self-Care** This chapter discusses additional factors that impact career longevity. These include the practitioner's attitude, preparation, motivation, and stress-relief methods, and how these can be used to prevent burnout. Determining how many treatments is too many, when to take a break, and when to take a vacation are discussed. Knowing when to refer clients and when to diversify the treatments offered are also features in career longevity in professional bodywork. Additional self-care methods are presented, such as leg and foot care, sleeping in healthy positions, propping, using splints if necessary, using bodywork hand tools, and receiving regular bodywork.

FEATURES

Each chapter has several pedagogical features designed to help generate readers' interest in the material and help them retain information and integrate this knowledge into their own experience. What follows is a list of the features and how readers can use them as signposts as they negotiate each chapter.

CHAPTER LEARNING OBJECTIVES

Each chapter-opening page contains measurable objectives for readers. These objectives help them identify key goals and what information should be studied thoroughly. Readers can use these as a checklist to help recall important information. Those readers who are students can use the objectives to help prepare for exams.

KEY TERMS

When key terms are initially introduced and defined within the text, they are boldfaced to highlight their importance. Readers can watch for these bolded key terms, knowing that these point to useful pieces of information.

WHAT DO YOU THINK?

"What Do You Think?" boxes are found throughout each chapter. These valuable self-reflection areas are for readers to identify personal thoughts, emotions, and behaviors that can affect various aspects of their career longevity. Readers are encouraged to use critical-thinking skills in determining the impact on their bodywork careers.

VOICE OF EXPERIENCE

"Voice of Experience" boxes contain advice from experienced bodywork practitioners about career longevity. This advice is based on challenges they have faced and how they have dealt with them, and they talk about their successes. They freely offer what they have learned throughout their careers.

FIELD NOTES

"Field Notes" boxes contain field interviews with experienced bodywork practitioners on body mechanics challenges or injuries they have faced, how they have dealt with them, and what they have learned from them.

CASE PROFILES

A case profile, drawn from professional bodywork practitioners' real-life experiences, is in each chapter. These case profiles illustrate situations readers are likely to encounter. Critical-thinking skills are enhanced as readers answer the questions posed in the case profiles.

WELLNESS PROFILE CHECK-IN

A section on checking in with the Wellness Profile completed in Chapter 1 helps readers track self-growth and awareness about their health and wellness. This is an opportunity to implement plans to improve areas in which they are challenged, based on the topics presented in the chapter.

CHAPTER SUMMARIES

Summaries at the end of each chapter provide an overview of major topics and information discussed. Readers can use these as quick references and for quick searches of the material presented in the chapter.

Reviewers

David Fazzino, MS, BS, LMT, NCBMT, AZ Lic MT
Instructor
Apollo College
Department of Massage Therapy
Tucson, Arizona

Karen Mitchell Jackson, LMT, NCTMB
Lead Instructor, Massage Therapy
St. Louis College of Health Careers
St. Louis, Missouri

Norman L. Johnson, PT, DPT, DEd, MSS, MBA
Director, Physical Therapist Assistant
    Programs
Community College of Allegheny County/Boyce
    Campus
Monroeville, Pennsylvania

Stacie Larkin, PT, DPT, MEd, DCE
Director of Clinical Education
University of Delaware
Department of Physical Therapy
Newark, Delaware

Maria Claire Leonard, CMT, MBA
Dean of Massage Therapy Programs
Minnesota School of Business/Globe University/
    Broadview University
Brooklyn Center, Minnesota

Lisa Mertz, PhD, LMT
Program Coordinator, Massage Therapy and
    Assistant Professor
Queensborough Community College/City
    University of New York
Department of Health, Physical Education,
    and Dance
Bayside, New York

Jean E. Middleswarth, MSW, LMBT
Clinical Coordinator, Instructor
Forsyth Technical Community College
Department of Therapeutic Massage
Winston-Salem, North Carolina

Odette Oliver, RMT
Director, School of Massage Therapy
ICT Northumberland College
Halifax, Nova Scotia

Dianne Polseno, LPN, LMT
Campus President
Cortiva Institute-Boston
Watertown, Massachusetts

Melissa W. Ramos, BA, NCTMB
Instructor, Massage for Wellness
Dover Business College
Clifton, New Jersey

Judy Smith, NCTMB
Formerly Chair, Massage for Wellness
Dover Business College
Clifton, New Jersey

Julie Smith, LMT
Chapter President
AMTA—New Hampshire
Hampton, New Hampshire

Eric Matthew Stephenson, LMT, NCTMB
Director, Massage Education
imassage, Inc.
Lexington, Kentucky

Janet K. Vizard, MA, LMT, NCTMB
Faculty and Director, Therapeutic Massage
    Wellness Education
Pima Community College, NW Campus
Tucson, Arizona

Sharon Weil, PTA, M.Ed.
Former Clinical Education Coordinator and
    Assistant Professor
Indian River State College
Physical Therapist Assistant Program
Health Science Division
Fort Pierce, Florida

Acknowledgments

Christa Fratantoro, Senior Acquisitions Editor, Health Professions & Medicine, for her faith in our abilities, attention to detail, wonderful sense of humor, and generous dining events.

Stephanie Kelly, one of the best developmental editors on the planet. She kept us going even when we thought we couldn't.

All of our colleagues who generously contributed their Voice of Experience and Field Notes: **Jill Bielawski, David Blum, Ginger Castle, Nancy Gamboian, Beverley Giroud, Julie Goodwin, Laura Key, Kathy Lee, Robert Litman, Whitney Lowe, Eric Mackey, Jesseca Maglothin, Aaron Mattes, Ann Mihina, Kathy Rinn, Becky Rosenthal, Jerry Weinert,** and **Christiane Testa-Rekemeier**

Sue Kauffman, Sandra's sister and one of her best friends. She is truly a love and a delight.

Annie Gordon, Carol Davis, and **Patricia Holland,** Sandra's friends who keep her laughing, keep her sane, and manage to pry her away from the computer once in a while.

The practitioners and staff of Tucson Touch Therapies, who are friends as well as dedicated professionals. Sandra wouldn't be anywhere without all of them.

James Freeman, Jean'e's husband and confidant. Thank you for your patience and support over the years, and letting me just "be myself."

Paris Freeman, Jean'e's daughter. My baby and a beautiful woman. You'll never know how much I admire you for your courage, strength, and determination. Thank you for being a part of this project.

Asia Freeman, Jean'e's daughter and a beautiful woman. Thank you for your laughter and giving me the best present in the whole world—a beautiful grandson, Julian. Remember, the world is at your fingertips.

Jesseca Macglothin, Jean'e's best friend, who always knows the right time to call. Thanks for all your years of friendship and support, you rock—holler!

All the instructors we have had the pleasure to work with through the years; we are standing on the shoulders of giants.

All the students we have taught through the years; they may never know how much they taught us in return.

Jason Torres, an extraordinarily gifted photographer. He made what could have been a grueling photo shoot into a fun and rewarding experience.

All the models in the photos and DVD, **Jessica Courtney, Ashley Earnest, Paris Freeman, Paul Gonzales, Sara Harders, Cora Jacobson, Dave Nelson, Luis Garcia Ramos, Alyssa Robertson, Andrew Rodriguez, Tara Srinivas,** and **Christiane Testa-Rekemeier**

Yvonne Gillam and **Key Robbins,** for their help with the script and logistics during the DVD shoot.

The director and crew at Center City Film and Video in Philadelphia for a relaxed yet professional atmosphere during the DVD shoot. Everything went so smoothly because of them.

Carolyn O'Brien, Art and Design Manager, for how wonderful all the artwork turned out.

Marsha Hall, Project Manager, Progressive Publishing Alternatives, for her excellent copyediting.

Contents in Brief

Contents

Bodywork and the Bodywork Practitioner's Wellness

Key Terms

Activities of daily living (ADL)
Anchoring
Assessment
Body mechanics
Boundaries
Burnout
Client-centered treatments
Client retention
Core
Ethics
Neurons
Neuropeptides
Neurotransmitters
Nonverbal communication
Presence
Psychoneuroimmunology (PNI)
Synapses

Learning Objectives

After studying this chapter, the reader will have the information to:

1. Discuss the connection between wellness and career longevity.
2. Explain the impact professional appearance, verbal and nonverbal communication, and mental and emotional preparation have on the practitioner's career longevity.
3. Explain the importance of setting and maintaining boundaries in the bodywork profession.
4. Discuss how the mind and body connection can be used by practitioners to make changes for career success.
5. Explain the importance of physical preparation for a career in bodywork.
6. Describe why efficient body mechanics contributes to career longevity.
7. Evaluate how the Wellness Profile can be used to create positive health and wellness strategies.

> "What lies behind us and what lies before us are tiny matters compared to what lies within us."
> — Ralph Waldo Emerson

CONNECTION BETWEEN WELLNESS AND CAREER LONGEVITY

The bodywork profession can be both tremendously rewarding and challenging. It gives practitioners the opportunity to make a difference in clients' lives by helping them recover from and prevent injuries as well as helping them maintain health and wellness by providing respite from the stresses and fast pace of everyday life. By using their knowledge and skills, bodywork practitioners work, on one level, with the body's tissues to effect change. On another level, they work with clients' emotional states and perceptions. Therefore, two of the challenges for practitioners are maintaining a balance between the physical and emotional aspects of bodywork, and maintaining appropriate boundaries with clients. All of these can affect longevity in the field.

There is no doubt that bodywork is a physical profession, putting practitioners at risk for work-related injuries. This is usually due to less-than-optimal body mechanics and, possibly, poor or inefficient posture. There are other physical reasons as well, such as lack of proper nutrition and regular exercise (both weight-bearing and cardiovascular), not sleeping enough or not sleeping well, and always being on the

1

go instead of taking time out to relax and rejuvenate. In fact, the U.S. Bureau of Labor Statistics (BLS), *Occupational Outlook Handbook*, 2008–2009 edition, states that, "Because massage is physically demanding, massage therapists can succumb to injury if the proper technique is not used. Repetitive motion problems and fatigue from standing for extended periods of time are most common. This risk can be limited by use of good technique, proper spacing between sessions, exercise, and in many cases, by the therapists themselves receiving a massage on a regular basis."

According to a survey conducted by Associated Bodywork & Massage Professionals (ABMP) and originally published in *Massage & Bodywork* magazine (December/January 2006), almost one out of every five practitioners surveyed had considered leaving the profession due to symptoms or injuries; this same number said they had to reduce the number of massages they perform because of symptoms experienced or injuries. One in ten respondents even had to stop practicing for a while. Common changes the practitioners made were the following:

- Modify the massage techniques they used
- Modify their body mechanics
- Increase their self-care
- Space treatments further apart
- Use different body parts to apply pressure (e.g., use their elbows more and their thumbs less)
- Alter the height of their massage table
- Sit more often during the treatment

Although most massage therapists know what they must do to stay healthy and avoid injury, most do not do strength-building and aerobic exercise, even though both of these help prevent injury. Finally, while 56% of those surveyed who had symptoms chose to make changes, a surprisingly large percentage (41%) of those with symptoms chose not to change the way they practice, even though most of them believed it was massage-related activities that caused or aggravated their symptoms. It is thought that this problem is more widespread than the survey indicates, since those suffering the worst symptoms may have already left the profession (Greene and Goggins, 2006).

Additionally, there are nonphysical factors that impact career longevity for bodyworkers. For example, lack of effective communication skills, lack of appropriate boundaries, and nonprofessional dress and demeanor can be reasons why a practitioner does not have a successful career. And even if everything else is in place, having a negative mental attitude can be yet another reason for failure.

How often do practitioners think about the connection between wellness and their career longevity? Ideally it would be every moment of every day, but this is not always the case. For some, it could be because during their entry-level training, learning how to perform the techniques to help facilitate health and wellness in clients was emphasized more than the practitioners' own health and wellness. For others, it could be a shortage of continuing education courses centered on body mechanics and other self-wellness topics. Or if these courses are available, practitioners who have limited funds may choose to take technique courses instead because of the more obvious, short-term return on their investment. Of course, long-term investment would be in courses in self-care and body mechanics, but many practitioners have busy daily lives and may think about wellness and career longevity only when a problem arises. This may be in the form of physical, mental, or even emotional issues that often seem to occur quite suddenly, even though the seeds could have been planted long ago. Not focusing on wellness as a significant contributor to career longevity could also be a combination of all of these factors.

Life is ever-changing. By keeping their bodies and minds fit through good health practices, practitioners will be better able to keep up with the changes and enjoy life to the fullest, as well as be examples to clients and others on how to better maintain their bodies. It is important for practitioners to remember that even the subtlest of changes can result in significant benefits.

This chapter introduces how having a professional appearance; using effective verbal and nonverbal communication; being mentally and emotionally prepared; performing regular exercise; having a good diet; using proper body mechanics, including injury management and prevention; having a balanced lifestyle; and having personal wellness increase the chances that practitioners will have career longevity. The rest of the chapters are devoted to presenting this information in more detail.

What Do You Think?

What does *wellness* mean to you? How do you think it affects your career longevity as a bodywork practitioner? Why do you think this?

PREPARATION FOR BODYWORK CAREERS

It is never too early to start planning for longevity in the massage and bodywork profession, nor is it ever too late to make changes if your career is not proceeding the way you want it to. In order to perform bodywork, practitioners need to be models for wellness and be physically capable of performing treatments.

WHAT IS WELLNESS?

What is wellness, and how is it different from health? *Health* is defined as "the condition of being sound in body, mind, or spirit." While there is no universally accepted definition of wellness, it can be thought of as being in good health. Wellness is pursued by people recovering from illness or those interested in optimizing their state of health. It involves a healthy balance of the mind, body, and spirit, which results in an overall feeling of well-being. Wellness is an active process of making choices toward a healthy and fulfilling life. True wellness is more than the absence of disease. It is a way of appreciating and positively experiencing life. It involves the process of living, growing, and achieving the life that expresses one's maximum potential as a human being. In short, wellness is about living life to the fullest.

There are many different aspects to wellness. These include wellness on the physical, mental, emotional, spiritual, social, occupational, and environmental levels. When considering wellness, it is useful to look at diet, exercise, lifestyle, and behavior patterns. Greater awareness of, and satisfaction from, all aspects of life, including fitness, good nutrition, relationships, stress-management methods, and an overall commitment to self-care are the cornerstones of health and wellness. A wellness wheel can assist in achieving this awareness (Fig. 1-1).

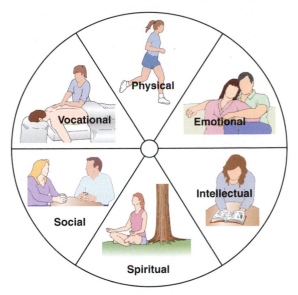

FIGURE 1-1 Wellness wheel.

On the wellness wheel, the sections represent six dimensions of life:

- Social
- Vocational
- Physical
- Emotional
- Intellectual
- Spiritual

Each dimension is important, and all are interconnected. The relative degree of balance within these dimensions helps define levels of wellness. You can look at the following list of suggestions for each wellness wheel dimension, then color in how much of each section represents that area for you. If you so choose, you can subdivide the sections further. For example, the Social section can be divided into family and friends. This exercise is designed to give you a picture of how balanced your life is now and what areas you need to work on to feel more balanced. You are encouraged to make copies of the wellness wheel and fill out new ones periodically throughout your life to see how effective the changes you are making are and to identify areas you need to keep working on.

These lists of suggestions are not meant to be complete, nor should you think you can color in a section completely only if all the suggestions in each section apply to you. Instead, the suggestions serve to stimulate thinking about how each of the areas look for you in your current life, and how you feel each of the sections are balanced in your life.

Social

- I take regular breaks from watching or reading the news.
- I have some close friends.
- I enjoy being with my family or certain family members.
- I enjoy some social situations in which I can connect with people.
- I have people in my life who can offer support when I need it.
- I am a good listener.
- I sit down to eat and enjoy leisurely meals.
- I am able to set clear boundaries.

Vocational

- I enjoy my job (either paid or volunteer job).
- I have a clear career path.
- I have future goals in mind.
- I enjoy acting on my ideas.
- I enjoy what I learn "on the job."
- I can think on my feet.
- I know what type of risk-taker I am.
- I am punctual and prepared.

Physical

- I am a nonsmoker.
- I drink no more than one cup/can/glass of a caffeinated beverage a day.
- I drink alcohol only in moderation.
- I get sick no more than once a year and recover within 3 to 4 days.
- I do a program of flexibility training regularly.
- I know the benefits of strength training and do a strengthening program regularly.
- I do cardiovascular exercises for 20 to 30 minutes at least three times a week.
- I get a good night's sleep most nights.
- I pay attention to how I use my body and practice good body mechanics in all situations.
- I pay attention to what I eat, and my diet is balanced.
- I drink the right amount of water for me each day (either six to eight glasses, or 1 ounce of water for every pound of body weight).

Emotional

- I feel as though I am in charge of my life.
- I have ways to manage or relieve stress, and I use them regularly.
- I accept praise well.

- I feel good telling the truth and consider myself as having integrity.
- I respect other people, yet I do not feel responsible for their happiness.
- I receive and give healthy touch regularly.
- I never eat to entertain myself, to ease emotions, or to alleviate boredom.
- I like to take care of my personal living environment.
- I learn from situations that do not go as planned.
- Life is interesting to me.
- I am able to set clear boundaries.

Intellectual

- I like to have new experiences.
- I have an open mind.
- I ask questions in all learning or unknown situations.
- I enjoy acting on my ideas when appropriate.
- It is easy for me to accept feedback.
- I am able to give clear, concise feedback.
- I read for enjoyment and to advance my knowledge base.
- I know my learning style; however, I can adapt to other learning styles.
- I know the best environment for me to study.

Spiritual

- I have made a conscious commitment to my own well-being.
- I learn from difficult or even crisis situations.
- I regularly spend time in natural environments.
- I think of myself as part of, not separate from, nature.
- I believe in some power higher than myself.
- I regularly worship in a way that is comfortable to me.
- I am comfortable with myself.
- I sometimes experience a feeling of not being aware of the time or being outside of time when doing something.
- I keep some kind of record of my life such as a journal, progress in some pursuit, written goals and plans, marking on a calendar, and so forth.
- I give myself time to think.

Figure 1-2 shows an example of how a wellness wheel can be filled out. Jorge is a full-time student enrolled in a massage therapy school. His wife, Amelia, is working to support the family while Jorge pursues his dream. Since they also have two young daughters, Jorge and Amelia are under a lot of stress

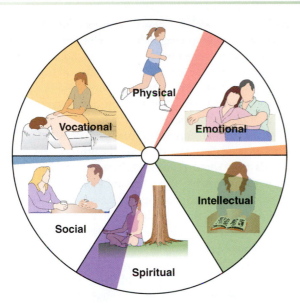

FIGURE 1-2 Jorge's wellness wheel.

to make sure they are taken care of as well. Recently, Jorge's father died. They were very close, and Jorge misses him greatly. Lately he has noticed he has been gaining weight. After filling out his wellness wheel, Jorge realizes he eats every time he thinks about his father. He does not think he can take the time to mourn him because he has to study for school. He has also stopped exercising because he just cannot seem to fit it in between attending school, caring for his daughters, and spending at least a little time with his wife. The wellness wheel activity has shown Jorge the areas he needs to focus on to improve his quality of life, which would also improve the quality of life for his wife and daughters.

PROFESSIONAL APPEARANCE

First impressions are just that—the split-second impression made when first looking at someone. Practitioners need to be aware of how others first perceive them and recognize the value of presenting themselves professionally. Clients, colleagues, potential employers, and business contacts, to name a few, make judgments about the practitioner's appearance. Many times the client's decision on whether to receive a treatment from a particular practitioner, or another professional deciding whether to do business with the practitioner, is based on a first impression.

When meeting someone for the first time, a visual **assessment**, or evaluation, is usually the first measure

taken. In this case, the assessment takes in clothes, hygiene, hairstyle, makeup, skin art (tattoos and piercings), jewelry, complexion, the eyes (color of the whites and clarity, whether they look watery or bloodshot), posture, gait, body size, and level of fitness (such as whether the muscles look toned). If a potential client or business partner finds any of these questionable, it could mean lost opportunities. Practitioners must be able to really see themselves through the eyes of a client or associate.

Professional Dress

In current Western culture, especially the United States, the latest fashions do not depict professional dress for bodywork practitioners. For women, this includes tight tops that show cleavage (in varying amounts), stomachs, and low backs. Pants and shorts tend to ride low on the hips, with the shorts being very short. For men, the trend includes loose, baggy pants and shorts that ride low on the hips or even lower. Some fashionable shirts are really baggy, some are tight, and some are cut so that the underarms and the chest are exposed upon movement.

Some professional practitioners argue that since this type of clothing is currently in fashion, it is fine to wear while performing bodywork. These practitioners view fashion as being the same as professional, which is not always the case.

Many bodywork schools have dress codes that reflect professional dress for their students. Even so, some students choose not to follow it, follow it marginally, or wear appropriate clothing only while on campus and not while performing bodywork treatments elsewhere. They are surprised to learn that how they dress as a student is unacceptable in professional bodywork settings.

In any profession, a major part of being taken seriously is through being professionally dressed. Being dressed unprofessionally invites uncomfortable situations and outcomes, because certain clients may think that it means it is okay to make suggestive remarks or that sexual services are available. It may also make certain clients think the practitioner lacks bodywork skills. They may think, "If she's dressed like *that*, did she even learn anything in bodywork school? I don't want to get a treatment from her." These messages may not be what the practitioners intended to communicate and may, in fact, be very far from how these practitioners perceive themselves and their skill levels. They may indeed have a high level of skill, but unless they present themselves as professionals, and dress accordingly, they can lose prospective clients.

The following are guidelines for professional appearance:

- Clothes should fit; match; be clean and odor-free; be free of advertising, writing, or logos that are offensive; look neat (e.g., wrinkle-free); and be appropriate for the work setting.
- Undergarments should be worn so that attention is not drawn to the genitalia and breasts. Clothing fabrics should be thick enough so that undergarments cannot be seen through them.
- Footwear and socks should be clean and well kept.
- Personal hygiene should be such that the practitioner is clean and odor-free.
- Fingernails should be short and preferably unpolished (cracked nail polish provides crevices for bacterial growth).
- Hair should be clean and combed or brushed, kept out of the practitioner's eyes, and tied back if it is long.

As is discussed in greater detail in later chapters, clothing, shoes, and hygiene all can also impact the bodywork practitioner's body mechanics. For instance, if a practitioner is wearing shoes that have a high heel on them, it will affect how she moves around a treatment table while performing techniques, whether she is able to lunge appropriately while applying deeper pressure, and/or whether she is able to set the table to the correct height for the treatment. The practitioner is also setting the stage for injuries to the feet, ankles, legs, and so forth.

If a practitioner has bad breath, it may cause him to avoid talking to or breathing toward the client, which means his head could be held in awkward positions, placing strain on the upper back and neck muscles.

Tattoos and piercings are not acceptable by many bodywork employers. Depending on the placement of the body art, practitioners may not be hired because of them, or, if hired, be required to conceal them while working.

To ensure that all their bodyworkers look professional, some bodywork businesses, such as clinics and wellness centers, and most spas require their staff to wear a uniform or follow a specific dress code. In these settings, practitioners who do not initially have an understanding of professional dress quickly learn what it is. Work environments that do not have specific dress codes but have practitioners who dress professionally can serve as models for new practitioners who do not know what appropriate bodywork clothing is. In all these instances, practitioners who still choose not to dress professionally are likely to find themselves with unsuccessful practices or out of a job.

Your appearance, wherever you are, always must be a priority. You never know when or where you might encounter current clients, prospective clients, employers, colleagues, or other health-care professionals who could be in a position to network and make client referrals. If you are not looking your best, always, chances are you will not leave a good lasting impression, and this can directly impact your career longevity and success in the bodywork profession.

Ultimately, practitioners would like clients to listen to their recommendations. If you do not exude professionalism at all times, why would clients take what you have to say seriously? Creating and maintaining a professional image is one of the most important things a practitioner can do to build repeat clientele, thus affecting the success of the practitioner.

VERBAL COMMUNICATION

American English contains a great deal of slang, so much so that those who learn it as a second language sometimes have difficulty truly understanding what Americans are saying. Since America is a country built on immigrants who have come from all around the world, words from their languages have been incorporated into American English lexicon. Couple that with the American fascination with and desire for ingenuity, and it is easy to see how new words and phrases are constantly being added and created, and old ones are being discarded.

Since the use of slang has become so commonplace in everyday language, it often makes its way into professional communications. Depending on how current the slang may be, it may be all right to use it every now and then, but to rely on this type of communication instead of using more formal language sends the message of being unable to communicate professionally.

The challenge facing practitioners is to be sure that the language matches the image they want to project to their clients. The level of a person's professionalism is measured by the ability to filter out slang and use proper English. Also, the higher the level of professionalism, the more awareness the practitioner has on how diverse types of people will respond to slang.

Since younger members of the bodywork community tend to be more immersed in the latest trends, they have a greater responsibility to review their use of language, or increase their "language intelligence," so to speak, to meet the professional needs of the community.

Sometimes practitioners may think the use of slang makes them more "cool" and accessible to the clients, but the reality is that it often does the opposite. Perhaps a practitioner who uses these types of words thinks the message he is sending is one of welcome to clients, but the message received could be, "He doesn't even know how to speak like a grownup. Maybe he just goofed off in school and didn't learn anything. I don't think I want a treatment from him." If clients are going to trust their bodies to a practitioner, they want to have a good impression of the practitioner's ability to communicate the needs of the session.

Contemporary American culture is also filled with sexual innuendo and sexual images, so much so that people may not be aware of how harmful sexualized language can be. This is particularly true of the bodywork profession, especially massage therapy, as it is still often "joked" about as being part of the sex industry. When practitioners do not address the raised eyebrow or the worn-out jokes about providing happy endings, or if practitioners use sexualized language themselves, they are connecting bodywork with sexual acts. While this may not be their intention, the result could be that they are, at the very least, not taken seriously as a bodywork professional or, at the very most, viewed as available for sexual services. In either case, it does not promote career longevity.

Successful practitioners who have enjoyed long careers in bodywork know they have the right to be treated with dignity and respect. They should think of addressing the remarks as an opportunity to educate the people making them since many times people are unaware of how what they are saying can be perceived as offensive. Some of the methods they use to educate include:

- talking about how massage and bodywork are part of the health-care profession.
- talking about the education and licensing necessary to become a bodywork practitioner.
- bringing up the past connection of massage and bodywork to the sex industry, and mentioning how it is still perceived that way, then letting the people know that by making these remarks, they are applying them to every bodyworker, including the one they are talking to.

- trusting that most people will get the message the first time. If not, take the risk of being a broken record or limiting contact until the person or people can show respect and understanding for the profession.

NONVERBAL COMMUNICATION

Nonverbal communication means communicating without spoken words. It includes body language, sign language, touch, and eye contact. According to research, 55% of impact is determined by body language (postures, gestures, and eye contact), 38% by the tone of voice, and 7% by the actual words used in the communication process; however, the exact percentage of influence may differ from person to person, depending on such things as family upbringing and cultural background (Mehrabian and Ferris, 1967). What this means is that 93% of communication is nonverbal, and only 7% has to do with the words used.

Keeping this in mind, be aware that you can make your first impression without saying a word. This is done by the way you carry yourself, how you approach the client, and your facial expressions. Having good posture and a confident bearing can inspire confidence in clients. A confident bearing means that you stand up tall, with shoulders back, and have a stable stance. This body language is considered open, which indicates that you are welcoming interaction with the client. In Western culture, a firm handshake, but not one in which the hand is gripped painfully, is also regarded as open body language and is an appropriate greeting.

Facial expressions are extremely important when interacting with clients. Warm, welcoming expressions in which you look the client in the eye (if culturally appropriate) while smiling will greatly increase the chances of a positive interaction between you and the client, more so than a practitioner who looks bored, disinterested, angry, or preoccupied.

Just as important as all of these is the energetic aspect of the practitioner. This may also be thought of as your **presence**. More than just poise and how you carry yourself, presence is the quality of staying focused and centered. It is most often used to describe how the practitioner should be during client interactions and treatments (as in being present), but it is also an important attribute during any interchange.

Nonverbal first impressions quite often mean the difference between whether clients are comfortable or uncomfortable receiving a treatment from a particular practitioner. Positive nonverbal impressions mean that clients are receptive to you, and if your skills meet client expectations, these clients are much more likely to continue seeing you for treatments and are willing to follow your recommendations for increased health and wellness. This means a stable client base for you, and thus career success.

Refining Professional Image

The process of refining professional image is ongoing and requires practitioners to stay constantly aware of the verbal and nonverbal messages they are sending. Sometimes it is difficult to change behavior, because it is what is familiar and so it feels safe. Also, sometimes it never occurs to people that changes are necessary or possible. You can do some self-inquiry to assess what image you are projecting and determine if it matches your intended professional image. Here are some questions you can ask yourself:

- What am I wearing and what image does it project? Is it the image I want to project?
- How do I talk with my clients? Does it sound professional, or does it include curse words, slang, gossip? Am I letting the client speak, or am I interrupting him? Are the topics and the amount of talking I do during the treatment appropriate, or am I talking to draw attention to myself?
- Did I take enough time to prepare for the session so that I look graceful and confident rather than rushed and hurried?
- Is there anything else that could be influencing how others react to me?

Seeking information on self-presentation from others can help you get an objective viewpoint. These can include peers or someone you respect and consider a mentor. Practitioners who do this must be willing to ask direct questions about their behavior and image and must be willing to hear the answers. Doing so can be a huge step toward professional

development. Some examples of questions you may ask of peers and mentors include the following:

- What has your experience been of my professional behavior, attire, and language?
- What have you noticed about how others react to me?
- What information do you have for me that would enhance my professionalism?

Paying attention to how clients respond is another cue for needing to assess what image is being projected. For example, if a practitioner is often asked out for dates or drinks by clients or experiences inappropriate behavior from clients, the practitioner may want to consider what messages he or she is sending. If the practitioner is wearing professional dress and uses appropriate professional language and is still getting unwelcome advances from certain clients, then the practitioner must be willing to find out what else could be prompting such a reaction. This inquiry is best done with trusted friends, peers, supervisors, or clients who can be objective. Choosing to take responsibility for your professional image is a major component in your career longevity.

MENTAL AND EMOTIONAL PREPARATION

Many people are drawn to the bodywork profession by a genuine desire to help others heal and maintain their health. However, some practitioners may see bodywork as a career that is easy to receive training for, because many educational programs are a year or less in length, and that is lucrative, since the fee for an hour treatment is approximately $60 (depending on the region). What these practitioners may not even consider is the amount of person-to-person contact involved in performing bodywork, contact that goes far beyond simply applying techniques to the client's body.

The contact with the client begins in the initial greeting, whether it is on the telephone booking the client or greeting the client in person for the treatment. The contact continues throughout the treatment, afterward during the post-treatment interview, and sometimes even after clients leave if the practitioner makes phone calls to check in with clients to see how they are feeling and to receive updates about the effects of the treatment. To stay present and focused with the client during all of this means to give **client-centered treatments**. The

What Do You Think?

Look at the practitioners in Figures 1-3A and 1-3B. Which one would you rather receive a treatment from? What specifically about each of these practitioners makes you answer the way you did?

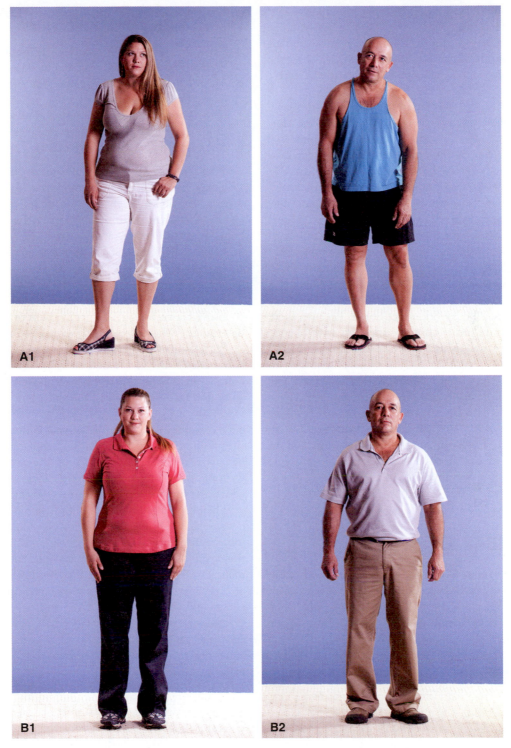

FIGURE 1-3 (A) Inappropriate practitioner. **(B)** Appropriate practitioner.

client should be your first priority, and the client should feel this. Most clients instinctively know when the practitioner is not focused on them. This is the foundation of **client retention**, which is the repeat business of clients, and is part of career longevity.

Practitioners who are not prepared for this level of connection and interaction with clients may experience considerable mental and emotional drain. It may never have occurred to them how much client interaction is required in bodywork. Some practitioners may become complacent in their practices and forget how important client communication and connection are, and some practitioners may not want to be bothered with this aspect of bodywork. Perhaps they have an "assembly-line" approach to their work, are not confident about their abilities to communicate, or simply think it is a waste of time and effort. This can severely hinder success as a bodywork practitioner, because there will likely be no genuine connection with clients, leaving clients to feel they are not special or that they are just another body for the practitioner to work on. These clients probably will not come back, which can have a major impact on the practitioner's practice. It also limits possibilities for employment in companies where practitioners are expected to have high levels of communication skills and to generate repeat clients. As can be seen, then, mental and emotional preparation are just as important as the physical side of bodywork.

BOUNDARIES

Part of the preparation for a career in bodywork is the ability to set **boundaries**. Simply put, boundaries are limits. They are about a person's actions, what they choose to reveal about themselves, and what behavior

What Do You Think?

A client arrives late for her appointment. She is flustered and talking a mile a minute. How would you respond? What would you need to do to center yourself before the treatment starts? What would you say to the client, and how would you say it? Why would you say this, and why would you say it in this way?

and information they will accept from others. Some types of boundaries include the following:

- *Physical:* people determine for themselves how their bodies will be touched and by whom
- *Mental and emotional:* people determine how much they think and feel about various topics, choose how much they disclose about what they think and feel, and decide how much to mentally and emotionally engage with others

There are personal and professional boundaries. Personal boundaries are those that, through their life experiences, upbringing, and education, people have chosen to govern their words and actions. These boundaries also create safety and provide structure. Some personal boundaries are consciously chosen and some are not, but all are dependent on the person's personal **ethics**. Ethics are a system or set of principles that people use as a framework for choosing between right and wrong behavior and for determining what is good and what is bad.

Professional boundaries differ from personal boundaries in the nature of their intent. Professional boundaries govern the conduct of people in their work life. In the bodywork profession, the intention is to provide professional and quality treatments. In a professional setting, well-defined boundaries on the part of the practitioner assure clients that they do not have to be concerned about the practitioner wanting or needing anything from them. This, then, allows the therapeutic relationship to form.

The purpose of boundaries in the bodywork field is to create safety for all parties involved and to promote transparency so that the client and the practitioner are clear about each other's expectations and requests within the therapeutic relationship. The goal is to find the balance between being open to all clients and yet not set boundaries so firmly that the practitioner is viewed as detached. If practitioners are clear about their professional boundaries, it is easier to remain warm and friendly with clients while tactfully deflecting or redirecting as needed.

Professional boundaries can include the following:

- Staying within the defined treatment lengths
- Performing treatments within the practitioner's designated work schedule
- Requiring payment when services are rendered
- Maintaining professional relationships with clients but not crossing the line into personal relationships with them

- Performing only those techniques the practitioner is qualified to perform, even when requested otherwise by clients

Practitioners who know their boundaries, communicate them clearly to others, and are not willing to step outside them even when pressured to do so are generally much happier in their work. These limits give the practitioner an understandable framework to work within and help them maintain their integrity. They are much less likely to feel taken advantage of because they will not be pushed beyond their limits. Clients will respect them for it as well. Also, these practitioners are much more able to deal with difficult client behaviors, leading to greater job satisfaction, which factors into career longevity.

DIFFICULT CLIENT BEHAVIORS

Practitioners may encounter the following examples of difficult client behavior from clients who:

- have needs that are hard to satisfy no matter what the practitioner does. For example, there is always something that did not feel quite right as techniques are applied, muscle tension was not relieved enough, the music was not right, and so forth.
- tend to push the boundaries or limits of the business policy statements. For example, being late on a regular basis, canceling at the last minute, not having their payment with them at the time of treatment, calling to request a change in the appointment time to accommodate their schedule without regard for the practitioner's schedule, or even smoking within 20 feet of the entrance to the bodywork business.
- attempt to become friends with the practitioner even when they have been told that the practitioner does not socialize with clients.
- try to get extra treatment time for free or consistently request more work at the end of the treatment.
- have a negative outlook on life and tend to be draining on the practitioner.
- are "silent clients." These are the clients who do not say a word of feedback during the session when asked if there is anything they need. But once the treatment is over, the clients have a litany of complaints for which there is no time to make changes.
- are not sure what they want, take a long time to describe what they are feeling or needing from the practitioner, and so forth.

The last can be especially frustrating for practitioners, as it is difficult for them to come up with an appropriate treatment plan that the client can agree upon. This can also result in the client putting faith in and expectations on the practitioner to "fix" him rather than having a mutual working relationship.

Other behaviors that can be categorized as "difficult" are the nonverbal behaviors a client may display such as heavy sighing, fidgeting on the table, not being communicative in the intake process, and so forth. Any behavior from a client that prevents the practitioner from connecting in a real and authentic way is difficult behavior. Another hallmark of difficult clients is when the practitioner begins to dread seeing the client, makes up excuses not to book the client on a regular basis, or feels resentment due to being drained by the client's behavior. It is important to pay attention to these feelings of resentment so you can explore them and determine if there is a way to either resolve the feeling or refer the client to another practitioner.

USING THE MIND AND BODY CONNECTION

Practitioners can make considerable use of the connection between the mind and the body when choosing to implement changes in their lives to enhance their health and well-being. The brain is, of course, a complex organ whose functions are not all completely understood yet. There is a certain amount of understanding of how it interacts with and regulates the rest of the body on structural and functional levels, and how the rest of the body can affect the brain. However, there is not much information on the more esoteric connections, such as how thoughts can

What Do You Think?

Choose three of the difficult client behaviors described. How would you handle each of them? Why would you handle them this way? Do you think your methods will contribute to your career success? Why or why not?

create changes in body tissues or how changing patterns of body movements can cause the person to think in new ways. But whether or not the exact mechanisms of how the body affects the mind and how the mind affects the body are ever discovered, what is important is that there is a connection between the mind and the body.

Traditional Eastern medical theories such as Chinese medicine and Ayurveda, the ancient medical system of India, have been around for at least 5,000 years. These medical theories are based on the connection between the body and the mind, as well as processes and rhythms found in nature. These connections play important roles in physical, mental, and spiritual health and wellness. Western culture and medical interest in these connections is relatively recent, starting in the 1960s and continuing to present day.

In 1975, Dr. Robert Ader, a psychologist, and Dr. Nicholas Cohen, an immunologist, conducted research into the connection between the brain and the immune system. They coined the term **psychoneuroimmunology (PNI)**. It is the study of the relationships between psychological processes and the nervous and immune systems of the body. In 1981, they, along with researcher Dr. David Felten, edited the groundbreaking book *Psychoneuroimmunology*, which discusses the premise that the brain and immune system represent a single, integrated system of defense. (An updated, fourth edition was released in 2006.) Continuing research in PNI may explain the relationship between peoples' thoughts, emotions, and actions.

Dr. Candace Pert is an American neuroscientist and pharmacologist who discovered the opiate receptor, the cellular binding site for endorphins in the brain. She has held a variety of research positions with the National Institute of Mental Health, founded and directed a private biotech laboratory, and was a research professor in the Department of Physiology and Biophysics at Georgetown University School of Medicine in Washington, DC.

She appeared as one of the experts in Bill Moyers's 1993 PBS video production *Healing and the Mind*. In this landmark PBS documentary, Bill Moyers talked with physicians, scientists, therapists, and patients who were taking a new look at the meaning of sickness and health. Dr. Pert also appeared in the 2004 film *What the #$*! Do We Know!?* This film combined documentary-style interviews, computer-animated graphics, and a narrative that suggests a spiritual connection between quantum physics (a mathematical description of the interactions of energy and matter) and consciousness. Dr. Pert has published over 250 scientific articles on **neuropeptides**—chemical messengers that the brain sends into the body in response to thoughts—and the role they play in the immune system.

It is believed that every thought, idea, or belief has a neurochemical response in the body. Science and medicine are confirming that a clear link exists between thoughts and what happens in response to thoughts, both in the person's body and in his behavior. These provide practical tools practitioners can use to enhance their mental and emotional preparation, as well as their physical preparation and techniques, for successful bodywork careers.

FOCUS ON WHAT IS WANTED

When a person's thoughts, emotions, and actions are in alignment with each other, most aspects of the person's life seem to flow naturally. When these are not in alignment, there is generally a feeling of resistance or struggle. For example, if someone wants to bring more money into his life, but focuses on his lack of money and financial stresses such as bills, debts, things needing repair, and so forth, rather than working to achieve financial success, he is most likely to feel he is struggling.

Another example are those people who say they want to feel healthy and full of energy, but instead talk constantly about how tired, stressed out, and sleepy they are. Instead of choosing to take steps to increase their health and energy levels, such as seeing a dietitian to create a better food plan and increasing their levels of activity through exercise, some may choose to focus on what is going wrong in their lives. These people are also likely to feel they are struggling through life.

Thoughts that contradict themselves create a life or a lifestyle that is more than a little out of alignment. These can lead to people spending much time wondering why they are where they are in life. Sometimes this even leads to blaming other people and life circumstances for making life challenging, instead of choosing to look at personal thinking patterns and deciding to make changes starting there.

Focusing on what is wanted rather than what is not wanted is sometimes easier said than done. Most people know precisely what is wrong with their lives and what needs improvement. They may have a list of what is not working and what needs to happen before they will be happy. This means they are focused on their present realities instead of what they want their futures to become.

If, however, a person's present situation is the culmination of what has happened in his life prior to this moment, it makes sense for him to shift his thoughts to what he wants to have, instead of creating more of what he currently has. The following are activities designed to assist practitioners in doing this.

Dreaming Big

Dreaming big means the sky is the limit. There are no boundaries placed on what you can envision. These activities are meant to stimulate creativity and create excitement. The excitement releases brain chemicals associated with pleasure, resulting in a greater sense of well-being and a decrease in stress levels. It can also give you ideas of steps that would help make some or all of the "big dreams" come true. The following ideas will help get you started on dreaming big:

1. Write down your appreciation for all that has happened in your life. Imagine that you have everything that you have always dreamed of, and you are writing about the ideal day you just had. Imagine and write about the clothes you are wearing, the food you are eating, and the activities you are doing. Make it as real and detailed as possible, and involve all of your senses. For example, when describing the ideal meal, make sure you include what the food looks like, smells like, and tastes like. Have fun with this!

2. Create a vision board, also known as a *dream board.* Purchase an inexpensive corkboard and keep it in an area that is readily visible, such as your office. Make a collage by putting on the board all pictures, drawings, and writings that symbolize the life you desire. Look at your board at least twice a day, imagining your life with these items or activities. It is not the specific item that is as important as the way you feel when you think about your vision board. This way, you are aligning your thoughts, emotions, and behavior with an improved life.

3. Begin and end your day with a 5- to 10-minute focus session. In the morning, imagine your day going exactly as you plan. In the evening, imagine sleeping easily and deeply before waking up feeling refreshed.

DISCARDING UNPRODUCTIVE THOUGHT PATTERNS

One of the biggest drawbacks to achieving change and reaching goals is having unproductive thought patterns. These are sometimes so ingrained that people may not be aware they have them. For example, if a person makes a mistake, she may automatically think, "I'm a failure," rather than accepting that she simply made a mistake and can learn from it. When choosing a goal, achieving it needs to be the primary focus, with mistakes considered temporary setbacks or learning experiences.

Sometimes practitioners focus on what is wrong with their technique performance or what is wrong with their bodies or health. They may define themselves by saying things like, "I'm not a good student. I'll never be able to do this technique or know all those muscles." The reality is that most have the ability to be successful bodywork practitioners, but they will not achieve this until they let go of their unproductive thought patterns.

It can sometimes be a huge challenge to change ingrained ways of thinking. One way to do this is through **anchoring**. Anchoring is when a person connects a word, a touch, or a visual cue to a desired state. In everyday life, people create anchors, or strong associations with objects, words, and feelings. For example, children tend to become attached to a favorite blanket or toy. Another example is a song that reminds someone of her first love, and she flashes back to the romantic feelings she had with the person. Some athletes will wear only specific items of clothing, such as a certain pair of socks, during a competition because of the power they feel when they have them on.

Anchoring can be either positive or negative. An example of negative anchoring could be the scent of the perfume a particularly mean aunt wore. Every time the person smells the perfume, she may experience feelings of dread. Another way anchoring can be negative is if people have feelings so firmly anchored to an object that they think they cannot possibly succeed without it. Instead of being an assistance to success, the object becomes the focus of success.

The brain is made up of approximately 100 billion tiny nerve cells called **neurons** (Fig. 1-4A). A typical neuron has branches reaching outward. There are small gaps between neurons called **synapses**. Neurons produce chemicals called **neurotransmitters** that cross the gaps, which is how neurons communicate with each other. This is how thoughts are created.

According to neuroscience, if a person says or does something once, a loose collection of neurons will form a network, as shown in Figure 1-4B. When something is practiced over and over again, such as a movement, behavior, or thought pattern, the associated neurons release their neurotransmitters more readily, the communication among them becomes strong, and the network pathway becomes reinforced. This is shown by the arrows in Figure 1-4B. The mind and body connection becomes stronger as well. In fact, it will become more familiar, automatic, and easy until it is almost subconscious. This does not happen if the movement, behavior, or thought is done only once.

An example of this is learning to ride a bike. It starts with the thought, "I want to learn how to ride a bike." If this thought is followed up with focus, practice, and determination, over time the person will be successful at riding a bike. The neurons that send nerve impulses to the muscles needed to ride a bike while maintaining balance form a network that becomes stronger every time the person practices riding the bike. Other neurons in the network are involved in the feeling of pleasure that goes along with riding a bike and the sense of satisfaction in accomplishing this feat.

Most people are not successful the first time they try riding a bike, but if their desire is strong, then it outweighs the initial lack of success. It takes mental focus and emotional desire along with the physical practice to achieve success in bike riding. The success also means that the person no longer has to think about how to maintain balance and what muscles to use to pedal; all of that is now subconscious because the network of neurons is so strong.

This principle applies not only to learning to ride a bike but also to learning bodywork techniques, creating methods to successfully manage stress, and developing a successful bodywork practice. In other words, it applies to ensuring career longevity as a bodywork practitioner.

Consciously choosing an anchor can help with deliberately forming new neuron networks. Recall that anchoring means connecting a stimulus to a response. The following is an exercise you can use to shift out of procrastination, depression, or frustration and bring yourself quickly into a more balanced state of being. The goal is to anchor the feeling of confidence to a small movement of the hand.

Anchoring Exercise

Since awareness is the key to unlocking unproductive habits, it is helpful for practitioners to realize what it is they are focusing on. They may find it helpful to keep a notebook for a few days in which they jot down as many of their thinking patterns as they can. For example, how often during the course of a day are they thinking thoughts like, "I don't have any money," or "I'm not any good at doing bodywork," or "I'll never lose weight."

Once they begin to find the dominant themes in their thinking, they can create anchors to shift themselves out of those unproductive thought patterns. This activity is a template for creating any anchors they would like:

- Close one of your hands lightly into a fist. Now close it more tightly and squeeze your fist once as you say, "Yes!" The motion does not have to be big and may, in fact, be almost invisible to others.
- The next step is to anchor the motion to the feeling of confidence. To make your anchor more effective, squeeze your fist and say "Yes!" at the peak of intense emotion. To do this, close your eyes and remember a time when you were powerfully confident in yourself and in complete control of a situation. You knew exactly what to do at the time, and how to do it. Feel your enthusiasm and energy and confidence.
- If you are having trouble remembering such a time, then simply imagine how good it will feel to be confident, on top of the world, and buzzing with excitement. Feel the energy in your body as being strong, and focused, and sure.
- As you continue to envision being powerfully confident, say to yourself, "The better it gets, the better it gets," then squeeze your fist and say, "Yes!"
- Keeping this focus in your mind, feel your confidence as you sit or stand. Say to yourself either out loud or in your head, "I choose to take charge of my life!" Squeeze your fist again and say, "Yes!"
- Take a deep breath and bring in more vitality and enthusiasm than you ever thought possible, and squeeze your fist and say, "Yes!" once more, then open your eyes.

Repeat this exercise periodically to develop it into a reliable anchor. Keep in mind that you are combining a strong emotion with a word and an action to create a strong neuron network. Keep doing this until you reach the point where you feel calmer and more confident just by imagining yourself squeezing your fist and saying "Yes!" whenever you want.

Practice using it before a treatment, before class, or when you need to make an important decision. Know that you have a powerful tool for success at

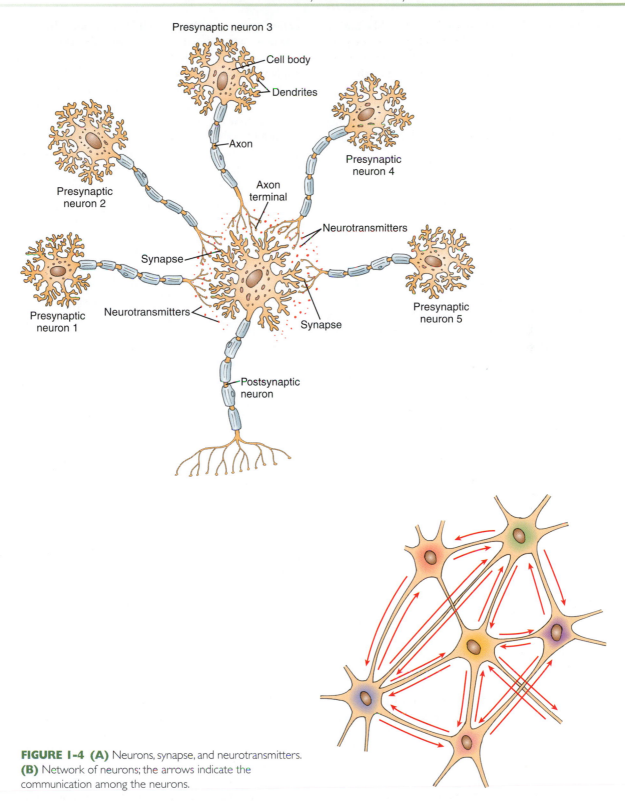

FIGURE 1-4 (A) Neurons, synapse, and neurotransmitters.
(B) Network of neurons; the arrows indicate the communication among the neurons.

your disposal that you can tweak as you like until it feels right. For example, other options are to press your thumb against your first finger, lightly press two fingers together, clasp your hands together, or squeezing your thigh instead of making a fist. Words or phrases other than "Yes!" can be used, such as "Right!" or "I feel confident!" The important things are to use the same tone in your voice and the same pressure with your hand each time.

ACT AS IF ...

Another useful mind and body connection technique to help replace unproductive behaviors with ones that promote health and wellness is to act as if they have already happened.

In her book *Molecules of Emotion*, Dr. Candace Pert first coined the phrase *molecules of emotions* to describe the fact that emotions are not just elusive thoughts. Instead, they are chemical responses experienced within the body at the cellular level. Every thought produces a chemical response. Happy thoughts cause the brain to manufacture chemicals that are sent throughout the body, making the person feel happy, joyful, and physically good. Negative or angry thoughts mean the brain is producing chemicals that are sent throughout the body, making the body feel physically bad. When the same chemical response happens over and over, it creates an emotional history. This history becomes hardwired in the brain the same way that thoughts repeated over time create a stronger neurological response until the response becomes almost automatic.

It is not the thoughts or words themselves that trigger the release of chemicals as molecules of emotion. Instead, it is the interpretation of the thoughts or words. Feelings and perceptions come from the person's unique interpretation of these thoughts and words. "Acting as if " the goal has been accomplished, along with focusing on how it will feel once the goal has been achieved, triggers the release of positive emotional chemicals.

Waiting for all the circumstances to come into perfect alignment before feeling good and believing change is possible can sometimes make for a long wait. "Acting as if " is a way to stop waiting and start taking action. For example, if a practitioner thinks that she would like to work for a particular spa but also thinks it will not be possible because there are so many other bodywork practitioners who have more experience than she does, then she is already

defeating herself. "Acting as if " means she tells herself that she is already hired, she is already feeling the good emotions of being hired, and then she can apply to the spa with confidence.

The confidence would also come through in the way she carries herself and conducts herself in the job interview. While there is no guarantee she will be hired, she at least took steps toward achieving that goal, rather than not even bothering to apply. Or if she did apply but told herself there was no way she would get the position, she would be less likely to present herself in a confident and professional manner, which would decrease her chances of being hired.

Note that there is a difference between confidence and arrogance. "Acting as if " is designed to assist practitioners in motivating themselves to take the steps necessary to achieve their goals. "Acting as if " does not mean that you will reach your goals by simply thinking the thoughts and not putting any other effort into it. Nor does it mean that you should be thinking of yourself as better than everyone else. Interviewers tend to pick up on those whose conceit does not make them good team members.

In practicing "acting as if," think of something you would like, such as greater income, a larger client base, or a position at a company for which you would like to work. Then, for at least 3 days, say to yourself, "Even though I don't know how it will happen, I choose to be delighted and surprised at how easily _____ (whatever goal you have chosen) comes into my life." Notice how you felt about achieving the goal before you start the exercise, how you feel while doing the exercise, and how you feel after 3 days of doing the exercise. Then ask yourself the following:

- How do I feel about achieving my goal now?
- Does it seem possible to achieve the goal now?
- What steps am I willing and able to take to make this goal happen?
- How and where should I start?

Based on that, you can decide whether you want to continue doing the exercise and continue working toward your goal.

My Perfect Day Exercise

- Take 10 or 15 minutes and write your description of an ideal day. Use as many descriptive words as possible, making sure you include all your senses. What would you see, taste, hear, smell, and feel?

- Allow yourself to fully indulge in the pleasure of imagining this day as you are writing about it.
- Store your document in a place that is easy for you to retrieve it.
- Read over the description of your perfect day whenever you are feeling less than optimal and begin to "act as if" you are in your ideal day.

ADAPTABILITY

People who have adaptability are willing to change thinking, feeling, or behavioral patterns that are no longer serving them well. Some may think that having reached a certain age or time in their lives, it is too difficult to learn new things. This is not necessarily true. Recall that the brain has the natural ability to form new neuron connections in response to new ideas, thoughts, and movements. Its ability to respond to new stimuli is so fast because it needs to quickly figure out how to deal with the new situation and respond accordingly. This happens throughout a person's entire life.

In fact, while there is no cure or absolute prevention for Alzheimer disease, mental stimulation, exercise, and a balanced diet are often recommended, as both a possible prevention and a sensible way of managing the disease. According to www.alzcommunity.com, an online resource devoted to helping Alzheimer patients, their families, and their caregivers, those who stimulate their minds through working on puzzles, learning a new language, or finding new ways to move their bodies such as dancing or exercising have decreased chances of developing dementia.

The following are suggestions of new things you can try to stimulate your brain. The focus is on making a conscious choice to shift your normal patterns every now and then and see what happens:

- Have something for breakfast that is totally different from what you normally eat.
- Read your e-mail at the end of the day if you usually read it at the beginning of the day, or vice versa.
- If you normally watch television before going to bed, read a book instead.
- If you like having the television on or the radio playing during your day, try a day of silence. If you normally like your day to be silent, try playing music.

You can use your imagination for what you would like to try differently. Sometimes even the smallest shifts can wake up your mind and senses.

VISUALIZE THE STEPS

Because making changes and reaching goals can sometimes seem daunting, it is usually best to think of these in terms of the steps necessary to reach them. While it is important to keep the overall goal in mind, it is equally important to make each step in reaching the goal as clear and as doable as possible. Instead of seeing the goal as a huge staircase that will take forever to climb, focus on reaching the next stair step, and how to do it. Step by step, the staircase is climbed, until the goal is reached. Instead of having one goal that is potentially overwhelming, have a series of individual goals that are quite reachable.

This process involves envisioning exactly what you want to happen before you do it. The visualizing should be as clear and detailed as possible. That way, you know exactly what you want and need to have happen. You can then expend energy on just those things you need to do, rather than waste your time and energy. Also, the focus is on personal responsibility and accountability for thought patterns, emotional responses, and the consequences of those thoughts and feelings. It is not on external circumstances, or blaming others if things do not turn out like you imagine. Instead, by being flexible, you merely choose new ways to meet the challenges and accomplish the goals.

Visualize the Steps Exercise

Try the following as a way to practice visualizing the steps:

- Choose a day in which you will be particularly busy.
- The evening of the day before your busy day, visualize the day. Go through each part of the day in sequence, starting with when you get up in the morning. You can either visualize it in your mind or write it out if that helps you.
- Be very specific about what you will be wearing, what you will be doing, what you will need to do it, how you will be doing it, and how you will feel while you are doing it.
- Take a deep breath before you visualize each section of the day; this will help you remain calm and focused. If you start feeling stressed about anything you need to do during the day, take a deep breath and return to a calm state of mind.
- When your busy day is actually over, think about how you felt when you went through each part and did what you needed to do. Did visualizing the steps help you remain calm and focused? Why or why not?

Myth: If the practitioner is having a bad day, her body and her treatments will not be affected.

FACT: The ability to maintain a positive mental attitude, which helps keep the practitioner's "head in the game," helps her maintain perspective. She is more able to communicate effectively with her clients, pay better attention to her own body and body mechanics, and focus on giving client-centered treatments. Everyone has bad days, of course, but practitioners must be able to set aside personal issues when working in order to have a successful practice.

PHYSICAL PREPARATION

When considering a career in bodywork, sometimes thought is not given to just how physically demanding the profession is. Those who do it well make it look effortless. Most people drawn to bodywork are those who prefer to work with their hands, but what they may not consider is that they actually use their entire bodies to do the work. For example, the strength for applying pressure comes up through the practitioner's legs, through the torso, and then out the arms. Thus, leg strength and **core** strength are just as important as shoulder, arm, and hand strength. Core strength comes from muscles in the center of the body, specifically the rectus abdominis, external and internal abdominis oblique, and transverse abdominis. In fact, external and internal abdominis oblique and transverse abdominis wrap around the anterior and lateral aspects of the trunk to attach to the spine (Fig. 1-5). Weight-bearing exercise is a must to develop and maintain the muscular strength and stability needed to perform any type of bodywork.

Being able to breathe efficiently is important. Practitioners who are out of breath during a treatment are not performing bodywork optimally, are not centered within themselves, and are not connected well with the client. Cardiac efficiency is also important. The blood needs to be pumped out to the muscles to ensure they receive the oxygen and nutrients they need to function properly. Therefore, cardiovascular health is necessary; to achieve this, regular cardiovascular exercise is a must. These topics are covered in more detail in Chapters 4 and 8.

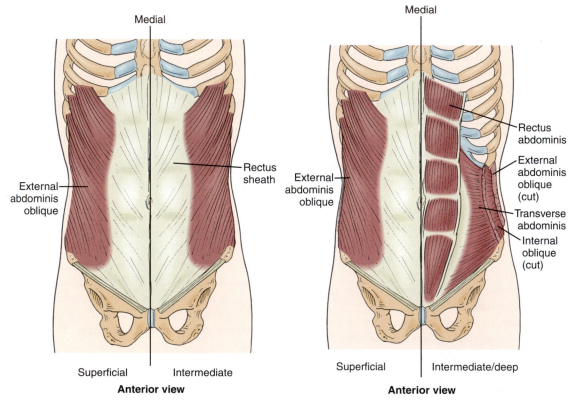

FIGURE 1-5 Core muscles.

Other factors that are part of physical preparation include ensuring that the body is getting the proper nutrients through a well-balanced diet and the proper amount of water intake. Sometimes practitioners think that because they have a hectic bodywork schedule (and perhaps their lives in general are hectic), they do not have time to eat like they know they should. This will eventually affect the body—physically, mentally, or both. Energy input and output should be as close to equal as possible, and that balance can best be maintained through a proper diet, rather than reliance on quick energy foods (such as candy bars), which, while providing an initial surge of energy, end up causing a "crash" in energy once the body has finished metabolizing it. At that point, the person likely feels tired and the body physically accommodates that fatigue by relaxing, not maintaining proper posture, and, possibly, leaving the practitioner open to injury. Good nutritional choices need to be made to maintain energy and keep the body working at optimal levels. This is discussed in more detail in Chapter 9.

Practitioners should also make sure they get plenty of rest, have effective stress management techniques, and take time out for themselves. More information can be found in Chapter 10.

BODY MECHANICS

One of the major aspects of career longevity is **body mechanics**. Body mechanics involves practitioners using their bodies in a careful, efficient, safe, and deliberate way to perform bodywork. It involves good posture, balance, leverage, and use of the strongest and largest muscles to perform the work. There are three main elements to proper body mechanics:

- *Keeping the back straight.* Efficient posture, alignment, and use of the body while performing bodywork will help prevent fatigue, muscle strain, and injury. A properly aligned skeleton will provide the body support necessary for you to perform bodywork techniques without injury to your soft tissues. Proper posture and alignment keep the abdomen and chest open so you can take deep, efficient breaths.
- *Using body weight and larger muscles to do the work.* Larger muscles are stronger and less prone to injury than smaller muscles. Smaller muscles tend to fatigue more quickly than larger muscles.
- *Remembering to breathe.* Deep, relaxed breathing puts the body in parasympathetic mode and helps practitioners have clear, focused thoughts. Overall, breathing should be done slowly and mindfully.

Case Profile

Patel and Grace graduated from the same bodywork program. While they were not close friends in school, they did share classes, lunches, and study sessions. During that time, Patel formed the opinion that Grace was not a dedicated student and would probably not stay in the profession long after graduation. He was uncomfortable with the inappropriateness of her conversations, as they were often laced with swear words, and she liked to discuss her weekend exploits with her dates. She wore tight, revealing clothes and sometimes seemed like she had not showered before coming to school. Often, she fell asleep during class, even though she always had a huge container of coffee with her as well as candy bars. She said she needed those to keep her energy up.

About a year after graduation, Patel runs into Grace at a bodywork convention. Grace looks exactly like she did while in school. She is excited to see Patel because the business she opened 6 months ago has not been very successful, and she wants to get Patel's opinion as to why not. She has heard through the grapevine that Patel's bodywork business has been growing since he started it right out of school. In fact, he is looking for a larger office and came to the convention to network with other practitioners because he needs more staff to provide treatments.

Grace describes her business as an on-location service. She has networked with the owners of several bars and sports clubs. Still, few of her clients come back for additional treatments, and she has no idea why.

- *What is your impression of Grace?*

- *What do you think are the issues Grace is struggling with?*

- *How do you think these issues are impacting Grace's career longevity?*

- *What advice do you think Patel should give Grace?*

It should not be done too fast or too deeply because of the chance of hyperventilating. You must be able to breathe smoothly and evenly throughout the treatment to ensure you have enough oxygen to do the work. Running out of breath during the treatment or breathing shallowly can be an indication that you are not focused.

Chapter 5 is devoted to body mechanics and contains a great deal of detailed information on this topic.

BURNOUT

Feeling drained by clients can also lead to a decrease in career longevity because it can cause **burnout**. Burnout is a psychological term for experiencing long-term exhaustion and diminished interest in aspects of life, especially in one's career. It is a gradual process that occurs over an extended period of time. While it does not happen overnight, it can creep up if the person is not paying attention to the warning signals. The signs and symptoms are subtle at first, and then get worse as time goes on if the causes are not addressed and managed.

According to HELPGUIDE.org, an online resource that provides information and encouragement for people to take charge of their health and well-being and make healthy choices, warning signs and symptoms of burnout include:

Physical:
- Feeling tired and drained most of the time
- Frequent headaches, back pain, muscle aches
- Change in appetite or sleep habits
- Lowered immunity, feeling sick a lot

Emotional:
- Sense of failure and self-doubt
- Loss of motivation

- Feeling helpless, trapped, and defeated
- Increasingly cynical and negative outlook
- Decreased satisfaction and sense of accomplishment
- Detachment, feeling alone in the world

Behavioral:
- Withdrawing from responsibilities
- Isolating self from others
- Using food, drugs, or alcohol to cope
- Procrastinating, taking longer to get things done
- Taking frustrations out on others
- Skipping work or coming in late and leaving early

It is crucial that practitioners continually assess their feelings about their work and their life in general, and make changes before a mental, emotional, or physical crisis occurs. Having the ability to cope with the stresses that come along with the bodywork profession enables practitioners to remain healthy and have the career longevity they desire. The early symptoms of burnout are warning signs or red flags that something is wrong. If practitioners pay attention to these early warning signs, they can prevent a major breakdown. If they ignore them, then it is likely they will eventually experience burnout.

It cannot be emphasized enough that it is important for practitioners to take care of themselves. They must understand the foundations of wellness in order to have a clear sense of their own wellness, challenges to their wellness, and methods to make changes. This information can assist in facilitating health and wellness not only in practitioners but in their clients as well.

WELLNESS PROFILE

Since there are so many different aspects of wellness, it may be difficult for practitioners to know where to start when thinking about how to maintain

---

Body Awareness

Take a moment and focus on your breathing right now. Is it shallow? Is it deep? How do you think you breathe when you are performing treatments? Next time you perform a treatment, pay attention to how efficient your breath is.

Voice of Experience

Be sure to diversify. I've lasted 25 years in the profession because I taught massage part-time and did bodywork part-time. My body and my interest didn't burn out because of this. Know who you can trust for support and sound advice. And don't give your bodywork away. It's how you make your living and it has value.

Kathy Rinn, NCTMB, licensed massage therapist since 1984. Owner of the Right Touch Massage Therapy in Tucson, Arizona

or enhance their well-being and career longevity. Emotional and psychological stressors, posture, general and repetitive movement habits, health, nutrition, and overall satisfaction with life all intertwine to impact how much the practitioner and the practitioner's career are thriving. Even the practitioner's lifestyle is a factor. This is an area that is probably not thought about in terms of career longevity. However, it does play a key role. Through filling out the wellness profile at the end of this chapter, it will become evident how much lifestyle choices impact your career.

Ultimately, wellness is different for everyone. However, the benefits for each person include wide-ranging effects, not just within the bodywork profession but in other areas as well. These benefits include reducing the risk of medical problems, decreasing costs for medical care, increasing mental concentration and alertness, creating emotional stability, forming a better outcome on life, increasing self-confidence, and decreasing stress levels.

To assist you, the following is a profile that can be used as an assessment tool to determine how various factors influence your health and wellness. Also included are ways to develop positive strategies and methods to check progress. You are encouraged to use this assessment tool as a continual reference point throughout your career.

I. SELF-ANALYSIS

This first section lists potential problem areas. Take your time and be honest and detailed in your self-analysis.

- Physical History. This information will provide you with a general estimation of possible problem areas.
  - Overall physical condition (e.g., cardiovascular ability, muscular strength, age, exercise, etc.) _____
    _____
    _____
    _____
  - Previous injuries (e.g., old volleyball injury on your shoulder) _____
    _____
    _____
    _____

- Medical conditions and their effects (e.g., recent pregnancy causing your joints to loosen, diabetes impairing your blood flow) _____
  _____
  _____
  _____

- Medications you are currently taking and their effects on your body (e.g., anticoagulants causing you to bruise easily, antidepressants causing mental fatigue) _____
  _____
  _____
  _____

- Activities you participate in regularly. Consider how these affect you physically, mentally, and emotionally. (For example, staying up late at night makes you tired the next day; when you are tired, your posture becomes worse; mountain biking jars your shoulder and wrist joints; crocheting or knitting involves repetitive wrist and hand movements; reading with a book in your lap causes muscle strain in your posterior neck, shoulders, and back.) _____
  _____
  _____
  _____
  _____

- Emotional or psychological stressors in your life (e.g., unpaid bills are piling up; family is visiting for several weeks) _____
  _____
  _____
  _____

- Posture. Look at yourself in the mirror while standing naturally:
  - What does your posture look like to you? (Think of how you conduct a postural assessment on your client, except you are assessing yourself.)
    _____
    _____
    _____
  - What have people told you about your posture? (For example, do your coworkers mention that you are hunched over your computer?)
    _____
    _____
    _____

- What postural tendencies do you have while exercising? Do you use proper form?

  _____
  _____
  _____
  _____

- In what position do you usually sleep—on your back, side, or stomach?

  _____

- How aware are you of your posture while doing **activities of daily living (ADL)**—brushing your teeth, sleeping, reading, watching TV, and so forth?

  _____

- What movements do you habitually perform? For example, if you have a baby, do you always carry the baby on the same hip? If you have a heavy shoulder bag, do you always carry it on the same side of your body? Do you always cradle the phone between your ear and shoulder?

  _____
  _____
  _____
  _____
  _____
  _____

- How many bodywork treatments do you perform:
  - Daily? _____
  - Weekly? _____
  - Monthly? _____
  - How long of a break do you have between treatments? _____
  - How many days in a row do you work? _____
- Factors affecting your delivery of treatments:
  - If you use a massage table, is it at the appropriate height for you?

    _____

  - Is your treatment space arranged so that you can use it efficiently, or are there, for example, items you need in hard-to-reach places? _____

    _____
    _____

  - What type of clothing and shoes do you wear? _____

    _____
    _____

- What is your posture while doing bodywork? For example, when you work on the client's neck, does your head drop down? Think about the following regions of your body:
  - Feet/ankles: _____
  - Knees/legs: _____

- Hips/pelvis: _____
- Back/trunk: _____
- Shoulders: _____
- Head/neck: _____
- Arms/forearms: _____
- Wrist/hands: _____
- Fingers/thumbs: _____
- How is your breathing? Is it shallow, using just your intercostal muscles, or is it deep, using your abdominal muscles?

  _____

- Movements while performing bodywork:
  - How much do you move your joints while doing bodywork?
  - How do you move them?
  - Do you often use particular strokes or body positions? Which ones and how much? For example, do you like to use the heel of your hand or your fingers much of the time? What percentage would you estimate you use each area of your body while performing bodywork (e.g., when massaging, you use your forearm for 20% of your strokes)?

    _____
    _____
    _____
    _____
    _____

- Pressure while performing bodywork:
  - What parts of your body do you use when you apply pressure?

    _____
    _____

  - What parts of your body do you feel strain or stiffen when applying pressure? For example, when using your elbows, do you feel your back muscles tighten and your shoulders elevate?

    _____
    _____
    _____
    _____

- Where do you feel pain in your body when performing bodywork? List the areas of your body that get tight, sore, stiff, or achy while doing bodywork.

  _____
  _____
  _____
  _____

- List injuries you have experienced since you started your bodywork career. For example, have you had painful knees, sore thumbs, or carpal tunnel syndrome?

  _____
  _____
  _____
  _____
  _____

- List anything else that has physically affected your ability to perform bodywork.

  _____
  _____
  _____
  _____
  _____

II. FOCUS YOUR ANSWERS

Relist or highlight anything in your answers that you think has either greater importance or a negative impact on your ability to perform bodywork. Rank the items in your list from the most serious to the least serious.

III. CREATE POSITIVE STRATEGIES

Go through each item you have in Section II and write down solutions. If warranted, consult with your health-care provider. Focus on specific actions to take. Each chapter has useful guidelines for addressing specific conditions and situations related to your career longevity.

IV. CHECK YOUR PROGRESS

Make a short- and long-term check-in list. An example for a short-term check-in is 2 weeks; a long-term check-in could be 2 months. Mark the dates in your calendar or day planner. At your check-in, write down

- if you are continuing with your plan;
- what your results are;
- any adjustments that need to be made to your positive strategies.

Focus on Wellness

Journal writing is one of the most beneficial and powerful things you can do in your day-to-day life. The journaling process has several distinct benefits:

- Provides an outlet for feelings and emotions (e.g., fear, anxiety, confusion, doubt, anger, inadequacy, guilt, worry, and so forth)
- Provides valid feedback on your hopes, expectations, and goal-setting results, and heightens your insights and awareness on how to expand your achievements
- Is a tool for logging your experiences, personal goals, and goal-setting activities. You can use this to analyze your progress and your achievements.
- Helps you tap into and bring into your awareness a rich source of information and ideas from both your conscious and subconscious mind.

Learning how to journal is one of the biggest steps you can take toward self-empowerment, since what you discover can only reinforce that your ideas and solutions have come from you alone. This can help you build your levels of self-trust, self-belief, and self-reliance.

The words *journal* and *journaling* hold different meanings for different people. There is no right way or wrong way to journal. If you are unclear as to how to begin, though, you can use the following suggestions.

What You Will Need

To record your journal entries, all you need is a notebook or a binder with loose-leaf paper and a pen. If you prefer, you can purchase a book specifically for this purpose, although any writing material will suffice. You can also use a diary, but the limited number of pages may inhibit the amount you write.

Just as books often have a table of contents for easy navigation, you might also want to set aside several pages at the beginning of your journal with a list of dates and topics. This can help you locate your entries more easily later on.

When you want to journal, find a quiet corner where you will not be disturbed or interrupted. Make sure you have an environment that will help you relax and feel centered. For example, use lighting that you find soothing, play music that you

Continued

like, use aromatherapy, have a glass of water or snacks available, and so forth.

Journal Writing

Journal writing is a process of expressing your feelings and experiences, thus creating movement within you. This movement will stimulate your creative thinking and open windows of ideas, notions, and insights as to how to overcome challenges to your goals.

Journaling is not meant to be a difficult process. Being a good writer or having good writing skills are not prerequisites for journal writing. Since the journal is meant for only you to read, there is no need to worry about your grammar, spelling, or use of punctuation. What is important is that you develop a style that suits you and that you are comfortable with. As you progress with your writing, your journaling skills will also develop.

You can enhance your journal writing by following these basic guidelines:

- Date each of your journal entries
- Include the time, the place, the emotions you are experiencing, your mood, and so forth. These can help you later as you review your entries and see the progress you are making.
- Write down the first thoughts, ideas, feelings, and emotions that pop into your head. This information is fresh and is more likely to contain the most truthful information about how you are feeling. (When you take your time writing down your thoughts or actively think about what you are writing, you may be filtering out some of what you are honestly thinking, feeling, and experiencing.) It is also brainstorming and may contain solutions to challenges you are struggling with.
- If you find yourself hesitating or wanting to erase or edit your journal writing, this could mean you are feeling uncomfortable about something you might subconsciously want to avoid. It is best to leave the entry alone and start a new paragraph or entry. Later, you can return to the entry that you wanted to change, and see if there is an issue you are avoiding and, if so, how to best deal with it.

Journaling Techniques

There are numerous techniques for writing a journal. What follows are several you can consider. You might even find that you have your own personal style already. Either way, the following journaling techniques are meant to be guides.

Reflection

The aim of this style of journal writing is to record from an observer perspective. This is written in the third person, replacing *I* with *she*. By taking yourself out of the situation, you can become more objective in your journal writing. For example, instead of starting an entry with, "I decided this wasn't a good move for me to make," write it as if you are commenting on an observation you have made: "It looks like her decision wasn't the best one to make." Continue your personal journaling with a detailed account of events, including recollection of scents, sounds, sights, emotions, feelings, and so forth.

Clustering

Personal journaling using the clustering approach is very effective when you experience writer's block or find that your thoughts do not flow well enough for you to record them. Start by writing the subject of your recording in the middle of the page. Circle it to make it stand out, then immediately make associations with the subject. As each idea emerges, write it down, draw a circle around it, and link it with a line to the main subject. This simple yet effective method can present an array of ideas that may surprise you. You can even later develop each circle into expanded ideas, or simply leave them as they are.

Another technique for writer's block is recording how you are presently feeling, or simply describing an event or even a conversation you have had. Once you start, you may find your writing naturally continues to flow.

Unsent Letter

This is an empowering technique that will help you freely express what you are experiencing, and how you are experiencing it. Whether it be an event, a situation, another person, or even yourself, writing a letter provides a way for you to speak out, especially if you are uncomfortable with, or it is not possible to have, a more direct, face-to-face approach. Your unsent letter is just for you.

You might find this technique useful when learning how to assert yourself and improve your communication skills. For example, you might have a goal to build your assertiveness with your partner or an employer. By writing to him about how his actions or behavior impact you, you bring to your attention your responses and how you would like to change and develop them more appropriately for you.

Start the letter in exactly the same way as you would any other letter, which is by addressing the person or situation by name. Follow with an uncensored outpouring of what you are thinking and feeling. You may be amazed by the amount and quality of what you communicate on paper.

Catharsis

A catharsis is a purging of emotions. Having the security of a safe and trusting environment in which you can truly express all your deepest fears and concerns is not always easy to come by. However, your personal journaling will always provide you with this much-needed space. Journaling strong emotions such as anger, frustration, pain, fear, and worry is a very liberating experience. Furthermore, your personal journal is not subject to others' judgment, disapproval, and criticism. Writing a journal allows you to express your thoughts and emotions freely.

You may want to start with a sentence such as, "I am presently feeling ..." Then allow your writing to flow without limit. When you review your journal later, you may find that having put it all down on paper, you now do not want to hold on to these particular entries. Discreetly disposing of the pages can be symbolic of letting go of the emotions once and for all.

Journaling Goal-Setting Activities

Learning how to journal your goals involves developing a relationship with your journal, specifically one that is tailored to your needs and aims. Treat your journal or diary as your personal coach.

First, determine your goals and what actions you are willing and able to take to meet them. Your journal will act as your coach and will help you formulate ideas and insights to help you achieve your goals. By being creative with the journaling techniques you use, and being clear with why you are using them, your journal will be a great support in your efforts.

Journaling Attentively

Being attentive means journaling your goal-setting activities with thoughtfulness—that is, noting the ideas, notions, and strategies that emerge out of your journaling, then acting upon them. This will help you to explore how you think, what your areas of strength are, and where and how to develop your challenge areas. Another important aspect of journaling your goal-setting activities is to take yourself, your aims, your experiences, and your unconscious resourcefulness seriously. This means setting aside time to write in your journal on a regular basis. This will help you get the most out of your efforts.

For example, rather than feeling overwhelmed by one of your more ambitious goals, journaling can help you break down larger, long-term goals into smaller, short-term achievable steps. You can start by writing about where you would ideally be in any aspect of your life in 5 years. Then write down the steps you would need to achieve in 4 years, then 3 years, then 2 years, then 1 year to achieve this goal. After that, write down what you would need to do each month to achieve your first-year goal.

Journaling Using Images

The different ways to journal is limited only by your imagination. Once you have set your goals, use your journal to scrapbook images—pictures you have cut out from magazines, drawings you have made, and so forth—to reinforce and strengthen your motivation toward achieving your goals.

Take, for example, the goal of losing weight. You have already journaled your feelings and thoughts about what it will mean to you to attain a certain weight or to look a certain way. Cut out images from magazines on your ideal look, or use old photos of yourself when you were thinner. Then every time you open your journal, you will be greeted by these images that are positive statements of intent of where you want to be. Another possibility is promising yourself a special gift, such as a world cruise, once you have reached your target weight. If every time you open your journal you see a beautiful cruise liner surrounded by endless blue sea and skies, that may be enough to keep you going.

Journaling Progress Toward Goals

You can note down your thoughts, fears, concerns, and mistakes you feel you might have made in relation to progress toward your goals. This will give you valuable feedback on what changes you can make and will provide insights into the root causes of fears you may be experiencing.

When you journal, it is quite normal to feel very deeply moved. Keep in mind that this is normal and healthy when working on issues you may be having. Think of it as releasing emotions that could otherwise cause you more harm if you kept them to yourself.

Should you feel the need for outside help to work through certain thoughts and emotions, consult with trusted mentors, colleagues and friends, or a qualified counselor.

Reviewing Your Journal

Once you have finished writing an entry, take a short break before reading it. When you do read it, be kind to yourself and avoid being critical. After all, what you have put on paper is a valid account of

Continued

your reality, the objective being to gain insights into how you are experiencing it and what you can now do to positively change or build on it.

After reading the entry, write a few lines about any insights or ideas you have gained, as well as what you've learned from your writing. Sometimes you might find your writing very revealing. Other times, you might not get such instant clarity and might get very little, if anything, from rereading.

It is important to at least get into the practice of rereading your entries in the coming days or even weeks. At some point, you may find that some of your insights seem to appear out of nowhere. You will find answers within yourself and can journal this effect.

A Few More Tips

- Keep your journal safe, private, and confidential. If you think that it is not secure or that other people might read it, you might not write as freely as you would otherwise, and your journaling could be hampered. Just as you keep your best friend's secrets private, do the same with your journal.
- Treat your journal as you would a good friend and, again, as your coach.
- Write a welcoming message or inspirational quote that greets you every time you open your journal.
- Journal anything and everything that gives you cause for celebration, not just any frustrations you are experiencing. Journaling should not be strictly reserved for when you are under stress or having difficulties. You will learn just as much from journaling when you are feeling happiness, gratitude, joy, and success.
- Make your journal exciting and a place you want to visit on a daily basis. In addition to journaling thoughts, ideas, and feelings, you can jot down inspirational quotes, short stories, or anything else that will make it interesting and meaningful.

Journaling is not set in stone. Use a technique that best suits you and your personal style of writing. You, more than anyone else, know how to journal correctly and effectively for you.

SUMMARY

In order to perform bodywork, practitioners need to be models for wellness and be physically capable of performing treatments. Having a professional appearance; using effective verbal and nonverbal communication; being mentally and emotionally prepared; doing regular exercise; having a good diet; using proper body mechanics, including injury management and prevention; having a balanced lifestyle; and having personal wellness all increase the chances that practitioners will have career longevity.

Practitioners can use the connection between the mind and the body when choosing to implement changes in their lives to enhance their health and well-being. Ways to do this include focusing on what is wanted, discarding unproductive thought patterns, acting as if the change has already occurred, being adaptable, and visualizing the steps necessary to create change before actually doing the steps.

Boundaries are also important for success in the bodywork profession. The purpose of boundaries in the bodywork field is to create safety for all parties involved and to promote transparency so that the client and the practitioner are clear about each other's expectations and requests within the therapeutic relationship.

Practitioners should also be aware of the signs and symptoms of burnout, which can limit or end a bodywork career. While it does not happen overnight, it can creep up if the person does not have a balanced lifestyle and does not pay attention to the warning signals.

When considering a career in bodywork, some people don't think about how physically demanding the profession is. Practitioners use their entire bodies to do the work. Leg and core strength are just as important as shoulder, arm, and hand strength. Weight-bearing exercise is a must to develop and maintain the muscular strength and stability needed to perform any type of bodywork. Being able to breathe efficiently is important to ensure that the body's cells are getting the oxygen they need. Cardiac efficiency is also necessary, because blood needs to be pumped out to the muscles to ensure they are receiving the oxygen and nutrients they need to function properly. Other factors that are part of physical preparation include ensuring that the body is getting the proper nutrients through a well-balanced diet and the proper amount of water intake.

Body mechanics involves practitioners using their bodies in a careful, efficient, safe, and deliberate way to perform bodywork. This includes good posture, balance, leverage, and use of the strongest and largest muscles to perform the work. The three main elements to proper body mechanics are keeping the back straight, using body weight and larger muscles to do the work, and remembering to breathe.

Since there are so many different aspects of wellness, it may be difficult to know where to start when thinking about how to maintain or enhance your well-being and career longevity. To assist you, the Wellness Profile can be used as an assessment tool to determine how various factors influence your health and wellness. These factors are emotional and psychological stressors, posture, general and repetitive movement habits, health, nutrition, and overall satisfaction with life. All of these intertwine to your wellness and career longevity.

Review Questions

MULTIPLE CHOICE

1. The energetic aspect of the practitioner is referred to as the practitioner's
   a. dress code.
   b. verbal communication.
   c. presence.
   d. boundary.

2. The repeat business of clients is called
   a. client-centered treatment.
   b. retention.
   c. preparation.
   d. verbal communication.

3. When a person connects a word, a touch, or a visual cue to a desired state, this is called
   a. psychoneuroimmunology.
   b. anchoring.
   c. burnout.
   d. clustering.

4. The gaps between neurons are called
   a. synapses.
   b. neurotransmitters.
   c. boundaries.
   d. neuropeptides.

5. Being willing to change thinking, feeling, or behavioral patterns that are no longer productive is called
   a. anchoring.
   b. burnout.
   c. health.
   d. adaptability.

6. Which of the following is a sign of burnout?
   a. Change in appetite or sleep habits
   b. Increasingly cynical and negative outlook
   c. Isolating from others
   d. All of the above

7. Which of the following is essential to proper body mechanics?
   a. A straight back
   b. Using larger muscles to do the work
   c. Breathing efficiently
   d. All of the above

FILL-IN-THE-BLANK

1. When meeting someone for the first time, a visual _____ is usually the first measure taken.

2. Neuropeptides are _____ _____ that the brain sends into the body in response to thoughts.

3. _____ are about a person's actions, what they choose to reveal about themselves, and what behavior and information they will accept from others.

4. A system or set of principles that people use as a framework for choosing between right and wrong behavior and for determining what is good and what is bad is referred to as _____ .

5. Using the body in a careful, efficient, safe, and deliberate way to perform bodywork is referred to as _____ _____ .

6. The muscles in the center of the body are referred to as _____ muscles.

7. Bathing, dressing, brushing the teeth, driving, and sleeping are all referred to as activities of _____ _____ .

SHORT ANSWER

1. List and describe at least five guidelines for professional dress.

2. Explain at least three ways the mind and body connection can be used to help practitioners change behaviors to ensure career longevity.

3. Explain at least four reasons boundaries are important to maintain in the bodywork profession.

4. Describe at least four difficult client behaviors.

5. Describe the three major factors involved in having good body mechanics.

6. Briefly explain the purpose of filling out the Wellness Profile.

7. Explain at least five benefits that journaling can provide.

Activities

1. Make an appointment to visit a professional bodywork office. Write down what you notice about the practitioners'
   - dress.
   - hygiene.
   - verbal language.
   - nonverbal language.
   - Would you want to get a treatment from the practitioners? Why or why not?

2. With another student or practitioner, role-play each of the difficult client behaviors described in this chapter and how to address them. One student can be the client and the other the practitioner; then switch roles. How did you feel while you were the client, and how did you feel while you were the practitioner? Did you have a successful outcome to the role-play?

3. Go to a place where you are likely to see a large number of people walking around, such as a mall, a park, or other recreational area. Observe how people dress and what their posture is. List the conclusions you draw about what people wear and how they hold themselves.

4. Choose one of the activities described in the section "Using the Mind and Body Connection." Perform it at least once a day for 3 weeks. How did you feel before you started the activity? How did you feel after doing it for 1 week? Two weeks? Three weeks? Did it give you the results you wanted? Why or why not?

5. Start a journal using one of the journaling methods described in the Focus on Wellness box.

REFERENCES

Bureau of Labor Statistics. *Occupational Outlook Handbook,* 2008–2009 edition. Retrieved October 2010 from www.bls.gov/oco/ocos295.htm.

Greene, Lauriann, and Rick Goggins, Musculoskeletal Symptoms and Injuries Among Experienced Massage and Bodywork Professionals, Survey Results (2006). Retrieved May 2011 from www.massagetherapy.com/articles/index.php/article_id/1130.

Mehrabian, Albert, and Susan R. Ferris. Inference of attitude from nonverbal communication in two channels. *Journal of Counseling Psychology* 31;1967: 248–252.

Body Awareness and Mindful Movement

Key Terms

Agonist
Antagonist
Articulations (arthroses)
Appendicular skeleton
Axial skeleton
Body awareness
Centering
Fixator
Grounding
Ideokinesis
Kinesthesia
Kinesthetic awareness
Mindful (intentional)
  movement
Meditation
Muscle spindle
Muscle tone
Musculotendinous junction
Prime mover
Proprioception
Proprioceptors
Qi
Range of motion (ROM)
Reflex
Stillness
Synergist
Synovial joints (diarthroses)
Tendon organ
Thermogenesis

Learning Objectives

After studying this chapter, the reader will have the information to:

1. Explain the importance of body awareness.
2. Explain the factors involved in the mechanics of movement.
3. Evaluate the connection between stillness and mindful movement.
4. Identify, describe, and integrate the principles for effective mindful movement.
5. Analyze and describe awareness of personal patterns during both rest and movement.
6. Describe and incorporate options for developing mindful movement into a bodywork practice and everyday life.

"The Body Beautiful: It is highly dishonorable for a Reasonable Soul to live in so Divinely built a Mansion as the Body she resides in, altogether unacquainted with the exquisite structure of it."

—Robert Boyle

THE IMPORTANCE OF BODY AWARENESS

At its simplest, **body awareness** is a person's ability to be aware of what his body is doing—how it is moving; what sensations he is feeling; what physical, emotional, and mental responses he is having; where his body is in relation to other people and nearby objects; how stable and balanced he feels; and what his posture is. Good body awareness can also enhance the person's sense of integrity and wholeness, and it helps promote good mental and emotional health. This is because body awareness is a connection between the mind and the body. The stronger the connection, the better a person feels on all levels.

Body awareness is crucial to performing bodywork. The level of body awareness practitioners have can make a difference in how much they learn about performing techniques, how fluid their treatments are, whether they will be prone to injuries, and even how much they enjoy doing bodywork. All these factors play significant roles in how long a career in bodywork practitioners have.

Dr. Moshe Feldenkrais (1904–1984) had a perfect quote, summing up awareness: "Awareness is the part of the consciousness which involves knowledge." He was an engineer, physicist, and judo master, and he developed a system of movement reeducation when working to heal from a knee injury. The Feldenkrais Method is a type of bodywork in which the practitioner communicates new sensory movement patterns to a client through performing passive movements. The sensory and motor aspects of the nervous system are then reeducated through repeated movements. Another type of Feldenkrais work is Awareness Through Movement in which a group leader guides participants through structured movement sequences performed on the floor. More information can be found through the Feldenkrais Educational Foundation of North America and the Feldenkrais Guild of North American at their website www.feldenkrais.com.

Through continual body awareness, practitioners learn to sense where and how they can use their bodies without unnecessary tension, when they should stop in order not to tense up against movements, and focus and refocus as needed. Practitioners can experience their own bodies as guides, both in terms of how they use them, how to use them more efficiently, and in knowing what their limits are. They can develop **mindful movement**, or **intentional movement**, which is focused and deliberate movement performed in the most efficient and healthy ways possible.

All bodywork students are encouraged to have a "beginner's mind," which means being open and receptive to new ideas and new ways of doing things. There is something to learn in every situation. Being flexible not only helps students adapt to the demands that school places on their lives, but it also helps them adapt to the changes necessary to have a successful bodywork practice.

There are some bodywork students who learn the techniques, proper body mechanics, and application of pressure quite easily. They are naturals at performing bodywork. They may not have had any training in developing body awareness and mindful movement but just have an innate sense of it. Yet other students can have a difficult time at first. Some of them may struggle throughout their bodywork programs, and some may make steady progress in their skills. The difference between these two types of students is an ability and willingness to develop body awareness and to take it to the next level, which is mindful movement.

In addition to performing techniques on clients, practitioners also serve as educators for them. They do this through recommendations for stretching and strengthening, water intake, stress management, and more efficient movements and postures while working and doing activities of daily living. Therefore, practitioners need to be in tune with their own bodies so that they can assist clients in being in tune with theirs.

No matter what background or natural ability students have, they need to cultivate their body awareness, develop mindful movement, and integrate these with the techniques they are learning. Integrating body awareness with techniques they have learned comes only through students practicing on as many clients as possible and by receiving treatments. Research has shown that one of the benefits of receiving bodywork is an increase in body awareness (Menehan, 2009). It is also the only way that bodywork students can gain a sense of how the techniques are supposed to feel (when done correctly) or are not supposed to feel (when done incorrectly).

The development of mindful movement depends on three main factors. The first is an understanding of the body's structure and how these structures function to create movement. This is covered in the next section, "The Mechanics of Movement." The second factor is an understanding of **stillness**, which is a place of no movement. It can be thought of as a baseline against which movement is compared. Stillness is also the absolute starting point of cultivating body awareness. The third factor is having a sense of how one's own body feels, which, as has been discussed, is body awareness. This is covered under the section "Cultivating Body Awareness." How all of these concepts work together for mindful movement is covered under the section "Mindful Movement."

THE MECHANICS OF MOVEMENT

Movement depends on the interaction of the nervous, muscular, and skeletal systems. Bones are like levers, and when muscles contract, they pull on these levers, creating movement in the spaces between the bones, or joints (Fig. 2-1). A muscle will contract only if a nerve impulse stimulates it (Fig. 2-2).

However, very rarely does just one muscle contract, creating one movement. Instead, the nervous system coordinates the contraction and relaxation of the muscles to create the smooth, integrated movements of activities such as walking, playing the piano, bicycling, and petting a cat. When first learning how to do these movements, people had to concentrate and do them over and over until they mastered them; for instance, a baby learning how to walk, a young child learning to write, someone learning to draw, and a student learning how to perform bodywork. The concentration and repetition involved in mastering these movements is, on a physiological level, the brain figuring out how many nerve impulses to send to which muscles and when, to ensure the proper amount of muscle contraction necessary to pull on the bones to create just the right movement in the joints. The brain is also figuring out when to stop sending nerve impulses to stop muscle

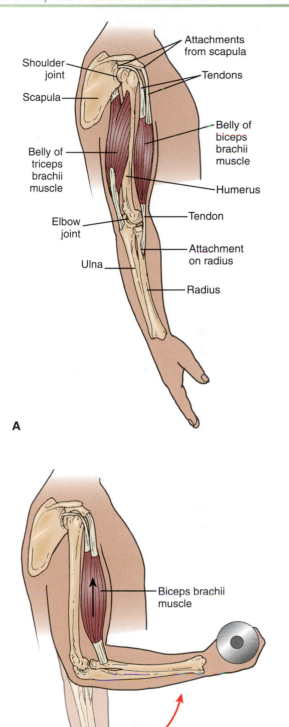

A

B

FIGURE 2-1 Muscles contract and pull on levers (bones). **(A)** Biceps brachii crosses the elbow joint **(B)** Biceps brachii contracts and moves the forearm

What Do You Think?

Think of someone who struck you as not being in tune with his or her body. What made you think that about this person? How comfortable were you around this person? Did being around this person make you think about how in tune you are with your body?

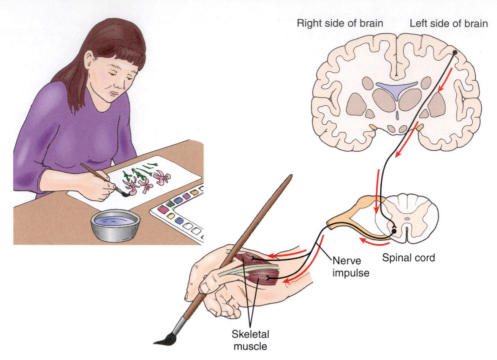

Right side of brain   Left side of brain

Nerve impulse

Spinal cord

Skeletal muscle

FIGURE 2-2 Connection between the nervous and muscular systems.

contractions to stop the movements at the joints when movement is no longer needed.

Over time, most movements become easier and easier to control until most people become unaware of their movements as they are doing them. Since the body developed the sense of what is needed for coordinated movement, the person no longer had to consciously focus on refining movement. This is known as **proprioception**, which is the sense of knowing where one's head and limbs are located in relative position to each other, and how they are moving even if the person is not looking at them. Because of proprioception, people can walk, type, dress themselves, and perform bodywork without using their eyes. **Kinesthesia**, an aspect of proprioception, is the perception of body movements. When the perception of body movements is coupled with body awareness as a whole, this can be thought of as **kinesthetic awareness**.

NERVOUS SYSTEM

The spinal cord and brain make up the central nervous system (CNS). All the nerves that communicate with the brain and spinal cord make up the peripheral nervous system (PNS). Cranial nerves

communicate directly with the brain; spinal nerves communicate directly with the spinal cord. The spinal cord and brain also communicate with each other. This communication encompasses detecting sensations from the body and the external environment via *receptors*. Receptors are specialized nervous tissue that responds to certain stimuli by creating nerve impulses. The nerve impulses are sent into the CNS, which assesses and integrates the information. If the CNS decides a response to the initial stimulus is needed, the CNS transmits nerve impulses out to *effectors* that respond to the nerve impulses. These effectors are muscle tissue, which can respond by contracting or relaxing, and glands, which can respond by secreting or stop secreting certain substances such as hormones.

The peripheral nerves that send nerve impulses into the CNS are called *sensory* nerves because they detect sensations. Another term for them is *afferent* nerves; *afferent* is from Latin and means "to bring to." The peripheral nerves that carry nerve impulses away from the CNS to effectors are called *motor* nerves because they send impulses out to muscle tissue to make it contract or relax, or to glands to make them increase or decrease their secretions. Another term for motor nerves is *efferent* nerves; *efferent* is from

Latin and means "to carry outward." Most peripheral nerves contain both sensory and motor nerves.

The PNS is further divided into the somatic nervous system (SNS), which controls skeletal muscles and voluntary movements (*soma* is from Greek and means "of, relating to, or affecting the body"), and the autonomic nervous system (ANS), which controls the cardiac muscle of the heart, the muscle in organs, and glandular secretions. The ANS has two divisions: the parasympathetic branch, which is responsible for maintaining the body's daily functions, and the sympathetic branch, which overrides the parasympathetic branch during emergencies and exercise. See Figure 2-3 for a visual representation of the full nervous system.

Emergencies and exercise place stress on the body, and the body responds by readying itself for action. Some of these responses are noticeable, such as an increased heart rate and tensed muscles. Other body responses that are equally important but not noticed are pupil dilation (to see better), increased transport of blood glucose to cells (for energy), and increased blood pressure (to better facilitate substance exchange between the blood and the cells).

Thirty-one pairs of spinal nerves emerge from between the vertebrae on both sides of the spinal column, and from the sacrum and coccyx. Each section of the spinal cord from which a pair of spinal nerves arises is called a *segment* (Fig. 2-4). There are eight pairs of cervical nerves (C1 to C8), 12 pairs of thoracic nerves (T1 to T12), five pairs of lumbar nerves (L1 to L5), five pairs of sacral nerves (S1 to S5), and one pair of coccygeal nerves (Co1). Twelve pairs of cranial nerves emerge from the brain, and they are labeled cranial nerve (CN) I through CN XII.

The brain consists of four major parts: brainstem, cerebellum, diencephalon, and cerebrum (Fig. 2-5). The brainstem, made up of the medulla oblongata, pons, and midbrain, is continuous with the spinal cord, and it functions to relay sensory input and motor output between other parts of the brain and spinal cord. It also has vital centers that regulate heartbeat, blood vessel diameter, and breathing. The cerebellum compares intended movements with what the person is actually doing to make complex, skilled movements smooth and coordinated. The diencephalon consists of two parts. The thalamus relays almost all sensory input to the appropriate parts of the cerebrum. The hypothalamus controls and integrates activities of the ANS and the pituitary glands, and regulates certain emotional and behavioral patterns. The cerebrum has sensory areas that are involved in translating sensory information, motor areas that control voluntary

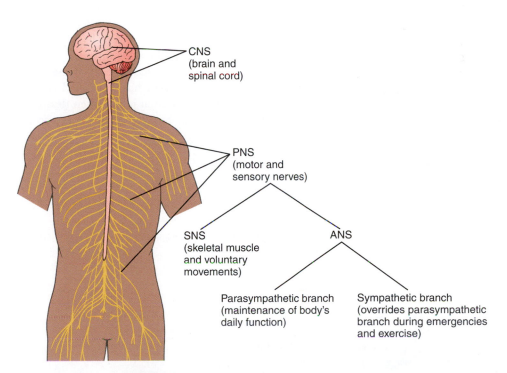

FIGURE 2-3 Organization of the nervous system.

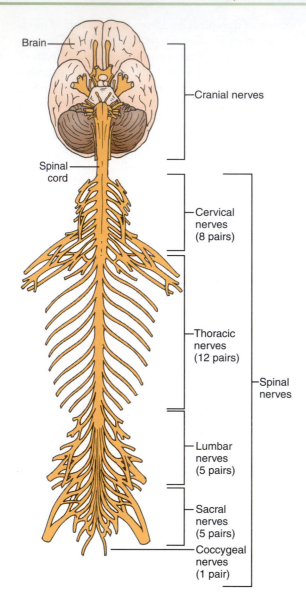

Brain

Cranial nerves

Spinal cord

Cervical nerves (8 pairs)

Thoracic nerves (12 pairs)

Spinal nerves

Lumbar nerves (5 pairs)

Sacral nerves (5 pairs)

Coccygeal nerves (1 pair)

FIGURE 2-4 Cranial and spinal nerves.

muscular movement, and association areas that are involved in sophisticated integrative functions such as memory and intelligence.

SKELETAL SYSTEM

The skeletal system consists of the bones, joints (also called **articulations**, or **arthroses**), and associated cartilage. There are two main divisions to the skeletal system: the **axial skeleton**, which are the bones forming the trunk and the skull, and the **appendicular skeleton**, which are the bones forming the upper and lower extremities. These can be seen in Figure 2-6.

Joints are formed between two bones, between bone and cartilage, and between bone and teeth. Flexible connective tissues form joints that hold bones together while still allowing either a small amount of movement or a great deal of movement. Generally, ligaments attach bones to bones, but other types of connective tissues may be present. The joints that provide the most amount of movement in the body are called **synovial joints** or **diarthroses** (from Greek "to fasten by a joint"). They have a space between the bones called a *synovial cavity*. This gap allows quite a bit of movement at the joint; joints that do not have this gap have very little or no movement. The bones in a synovial joint are joined by an articular capsule made of dense irregular connective tissue, and they often have accessory ligaments surrounding them for support.

The largest movements of the body occur at the shoulder, elbow, hip, knee, and ankle joints and at the intervertebral joints when flexing and extending the trunk. Smaller movements occur at the wrist,

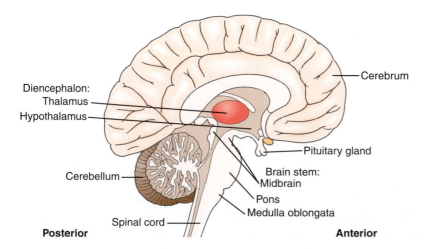

Diencephalon:
Thalamus
Hypothalamus

Cerebrum

Cerebellum

Pituitary gland

Brain stem:
Midbrain
Pons
Medulla oblongata

Spinal cord

Posterior

Anterior

FIGURE 2-5 The brain.

Division of the skeleton	Structure	Number of bones
Axial skeleton 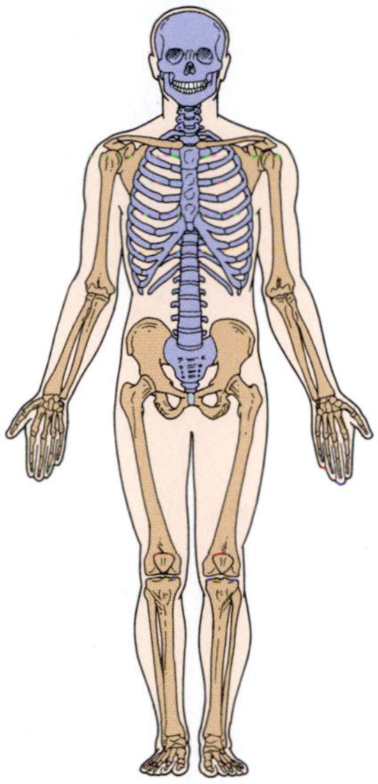	Skull	
	Cranium	8
	Face	14
	Hyoid	1
	Auditory ossicles	6
	Vetebral column	26
	Thorax	
	Sternum	1
	Ribs	24
		Subtotal = 80
Appendicular skeleton 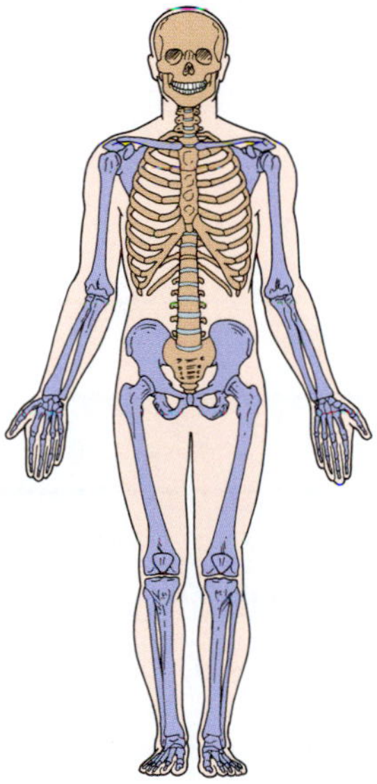	Pectoral (shoulder) girdles	
	Clavicle	2
	Scapula	2
	Upper limbs (extremities)	
	Humerus	2
	Ulna	2
	Radius	2
	Carpals	16
	Metacarpals	10
	Phalanges	28
	Pelvic (hip) girdle	
	Hip, pelvic, or coxal bone	2
	Lower limbs (extremities)	
	Femur	2
	Patella	2
	Fibula	2
	Tibia	2
	Tarsals	14
	Metatarsals	10
	Phalanges	28
		Subtotal = 126
		Total = 206

FIGURE 2-6 Divisions of the skeletal system.

fingers, toes, and the intervertebral joints of the neck, and between the vertebrae and the skull.

Figure 2-7 shows the major joints of the body. Table 2.1 defines standard directional terms used when locating parts of the body; this makes the information in Tables 2.2 and 2.3 more clear. Table 2.2 shows the different types of synovial joints in the body, and Table 2.3 lists the movements that occur at joints.

Flexibility refers to the degree of **range of motion (ROM)** in a joint. Range of motion is the range, measured in degrees of a circle, through which the bones of a joint can be moved. Optimal ROM is achieved when the bones are in proper alignment and the tissues surrounding the joints are healthy, pliable, and relaxed. Proper body alignment is necessary for optimal function of the skeletal system.

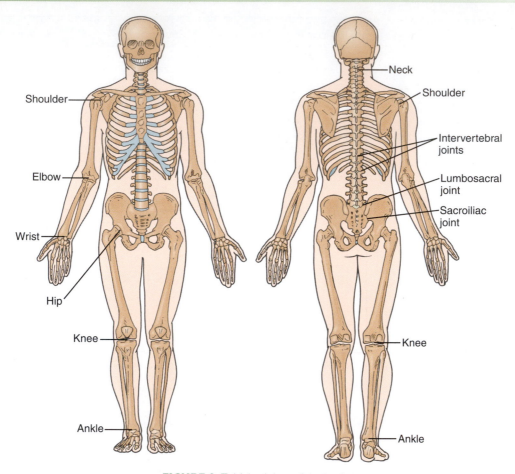

FIGURE 2-7 Major Joints of the body.

TABLE 2.1 Directional Terms

Direction	Meaning
Superficial	Toward or on the surface of the body
Deep	Away from the surface of the body
Superior	Toward the head, or upper part of a structure
Inferior	Away from the head, or the lower part of a structure
Anterior	Nearer to or at the front of the body
Posterior	Nearer to or at the back of the body
Medial	Nearer to the midline of the body
Lateral	Farther from the midline of the body
Intermediate	Between two structures

TABLE 2.1 Directional Terms—cont'd

Ipsilateral	On the same side of the body as another structure
Contralateral	On the opposite side of the body as another structure
Proximal	Nearer to the attachment of a limb to the trunk
Distal	Farther from the attachment of a limb to the trunk

TABLE 2.2 Types of Synovial Joints in the Body

Joint	**Description**
Planar joint 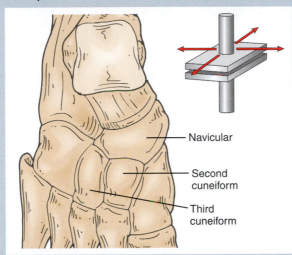 Navicular / Second cuneiform / Third cuneiform	The articulating surfaces are flat or slightly curved. Examples of planar joints include intercarpal and intertarsal joints.
Pivot joint 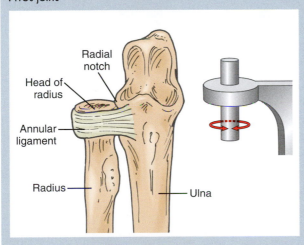 Radial notch / Head of radius / Annular ligament / Radius / Ulna	The rounded or pointed surface of one bone articulates with a ring formed by part of another bone and a ligament. An example is the proximal radioulnar joint—the radius pivots around the ulna.

Continued

TABLE 2.2 Types of Synovial Joints in the Body—cont'd

Joint	Description
Condyloid joint 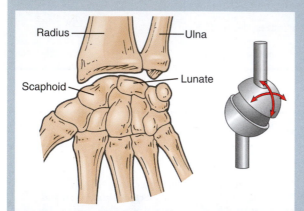	The rounded, oval-shaped part of one bone fits into the oval-shaped depression of another bone. An example is the wrist joint.
Saddle joint 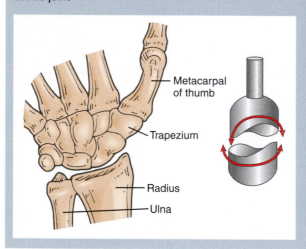	The surface of one bone is saddle-shaped, and the articular surface of the other bone fits into the saddle, just as a rider sits in a saddle. An example is the carpometacarpal joint of the thumb.

TABLE 2.2 Types of Synovial Joints in the Body—cont'd

Joint	Description
Hinge joint 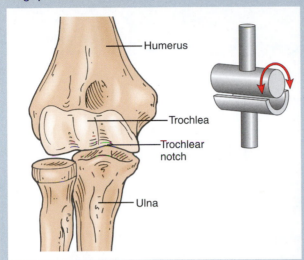 Humerus / Trochlea / Trochlear notch / Ulna	The rounded surface of one bone fits into a depression in the articulating surface of the other bone just like a hinge. Examples include the elbow, knee, and interphalangeal joints.
Ball-and-socket joint 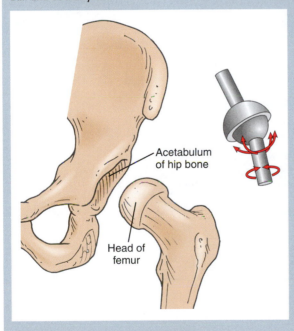 Acetabulum of hip bone / Head of femur	The ball-shaped surface of one bone fits into the cup-shaped depression in the articulating surface of the other bone. Ball-and-socket joints have the most freedom of movement. Examples include the shoulder and hip joints.

TABLE 2.3 Movements That Occur at Joints

Movement	Description
Flexion	Decrease in the angle of a joint
Extension	Increase in the angle of a joint
Lateral flexion	Decrease in the angle of a joint to the lateral side of the body
Abduction	Movement away from the midline of the body
Adduction	Movement toward the midline of the body
Horizontal abduction	Movement away from the midline of the body in a horizontal plane
Horizontal adduction	Movement toward the midline of the body in a horizontal plane
Circumduction	Movement of the distal end of a body part in a circle
Medial (internal) rotation	Movement around a longitudinal axis toward the midline of the body
Lateral (external) rotation	Movement around a longitudinal axis away from the midline of the body
Downward (medial) rotation	Movement of the scapula so that the inferior angle turns medially and downward
Upward (lateral) rotation	Movement of the scapula so that the inferior angle turns laterally and upward
Elevation	Upward movement
Depression	Downward movement
Protraction (abduction)	Forward movement of the mandible and scapula
Retraction (adduction)	Backward movement of the mandible and scapula
Supination	Movement of the forearm in which the palm is turned anteriorly
Pronation	Movement of the forearm in which the palm is turned posteriorly
Inversion	Movement of the soles of the feet inward so they face each other
Eversion	Movement of the soles of the feet outward so they face away from each other
Dorsiflexion	Flexing the ankle so the foot moves upward
Plantarflexion	Extending the ankle so the foot moves downward

MUSCULAR SYSTEM

The muscular system plays a very important role in the health of the body. In addition to movement, it provides many other benefits, such as assisting in blood circulation, generating body heat, playing a role in metabolism, and, of course, creating kinesthetic awareness.

There are three types of muscle tissue. Cardiac muscle is found only in the heart and functions to contract and pump blood out of the heart. It is involuntary, which means it cannot be consciously controlled. Smooth muscle is located in the walls of hollow internal structures such as blood vessels, airways, and the digestive tract. It functions to store and move substances within the body. Like cardiac muscle, it is involuntary.

The third type of muscle is skeletal, and it is so named because most of it functions to move the bones of the skeleton. Some skeletal muscles, though, attach to and move the skin or other skeletal muscles. The muscular system (Fig. 2-8A, B) is made up of skeletal muscles, which are attached to bones by tendons. The attachment area is referred as the **musculotendinous junction**.

The functions of skeletal muscles are to

- produce body movements, including movement of the whole body such as walking and running, and localized movements such as grasping a pencil or nodding the head. Body movements involve the bones, joints, and skeletal muscles working together.
- stabilize body positions by contracting to stabilize joints and help maintain body positions such as

standing or sitting. Postural muscles contract continuously when awake, as is shown by contractions of the posterior neck muscles to hold the head upright.

- generate heat as they contract. This process is called **thermogenesis**. Much of the heat generated by muscles is used to maintain normal body temperature. Involuntary contraction of skeletal muscle is called *shivering*, which can greatly increase the rate of heat production.

Muscle Length and Tension

Muscles function by shortening or lengthening and by increasing or decreasing in tension. As discussed previously, they do so in response to increased or decreased nerve impulses. Muscles can increase in tension without having a change in length. An example of this is when holding something steady in an outstretched hand, such as a heavy book. The elbow

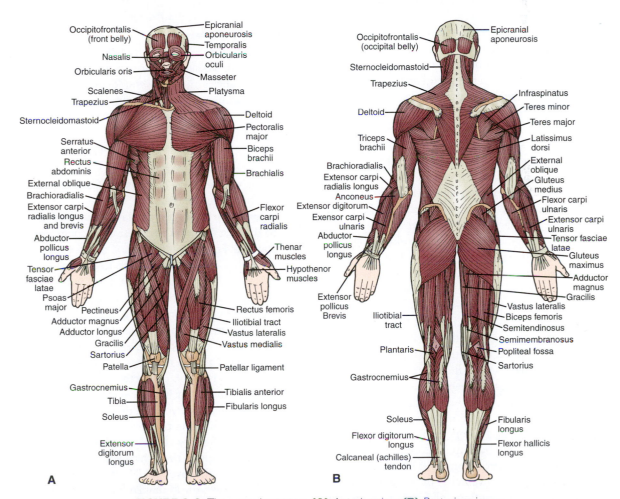

FIGURE 2-8 The muscular system. **(A)** Anterior view. **(B)** Posterior view.

joint stays extended, which means that no movement is occurring there. Triceps brachii is staying contracted, and biceps brachii is staying in a lengthened position. However, biceps brachii will increase in tension to keep from dropping the item.

Skeletal muscles also have **muscle tone**, which is a small amount of tension in the muscle. Muscle tone keeps skeletal muscles firm but does not result in movement. For example, when the posterior neck muscles are in tonic contraction, they keep the head from falling forward onto the chest.

When muscles change in length, a movement occurs at the joints that the muscles are crossing. Movements are often the result of several muscles working together in a group. Most muscles are arranged in opposing pairs at joints, which means they perform opposite actions. When a muscle action opposes another muscle's action, the muscles are said to be **antagonists**. For example, there are flexors and extensors, abductors and adductors, and so forth. Within opposing pairs, one muscle is the main one contracting and is referred to as the **prime mover** or **agonist**. Its antagonist will lengthen, or stretch, and yield to the movement of the prime mover. The roles of the prime mover and the antagonist can switch for different movements. For example, when biceps brachii shortens, the elbow joint flexes. At the same time, triceps brachii is lengthening. However, when triceps brachii shortens, the elbow joint extends and biceps brachii lengthens. If the prime mover and its antagonist contract at the same time with equal force, there will be no movement. The prime mover and the antagonist are usually located on opposite sides of the associated bones or joints.

Within the group of muscles working together, some are called **synergists**. These aid in the movement of the prime mover. Also, sometimes the prime mover actually crosses other joints before it reaches the joint where its primary action occurs. Synergists contract and stabilize the intermediate joints. For example, muscles that flex the fingers also cross the wrist joint. If synergists did not stabilize the wrist joint, then the wrist would flex every time the fingers flexed. Some muscles in the group also act as **fixators**. They stabilize one of the bony attachments of the prime mover so that it can provide a more efficient action. For example, fixators stabilize the proximal end of a limb while movements occur at the distal end (Tortora and Derrickson, 2009).

As can be seen, movements of the body are due to the complex interactions of many muscles, the nervous system, and the joints. When smooth movements occur, it is because certain muscles contract at just the right time and for just the right amount of time, while other muscles are relaxing and stretching at just the right time and for just the right amount of time. People are born with the ability to create the choreography necessary for synchronized, coordinated movements, but the actual creation of movement comes through practicing, reevaluating, and practicing again. When learning how to do something new, having body awareness and doing mindful movement can be invaluable to the process. This is certainly true of learning to perform bodywork.

Body Awareness

How stable and balanced on your feet are you? Try the following yoga pose to find out.

Mountain Pose

Mountain Pose is designed to help you feel the strength, solidity, and power of a great mountain. It helps stabilize the body and focus the mind. It teaches proper posture and puts the mind into an alert state. The following describes how to perform Mountain Pose:

- Stand with both feet parallel and close together, hands hanging by your sides.
- Focus your eyes on an object in front of you and try to remain still.
- Imagine you are strong and tall like a mountain so that not even the strongest wind could blow you over. Feel how it is to stand on your feet, and notice how stable and balanced you feel.
- For more fun: If you do this activity with someone, one of you can test the other's concentration by pretending to be a bird flying around the mountain, or take a blanket and shake it to make wind against the mountain. This will challenge you to keep focused and not be distracted.
- For even more fun: If you live near a mountain or even a hill, or if you can drive to one easily, hike with someone to the top and sit for a while. Together, try to feel the energy of the mountain. Notice everything you can about it—the ground cover, wildlife, its shape, slopes, and dips. Even try Mountain Pose up there.

PROPRIOCEPTION

Developing proprioception involves enhancing an awareness of the body and the positions of various joints relative to each other. Proprioceptive sensations arise in specialized nerve cells or receptors called **proprioceptors**. These are embedded in muscles, especially postural muscles, and in tendons, and they provide the nervous systems with information about the degree to which muscles are contracted, the amount of tension on tendons, and the positions of joints. Hair cells of the inner ear monitor the orientation of the head in relation to the ground, and monitor head position during movements. Thus they also provide information for maintaining balance and equilibrium.

The brain continually receives nerve impulses related to the position of different body parts and makes adjustments, through the cerebellum and parts of the cerebrum, to ensure coordination of movements. In fact, the majority (60%) of incoming sensory information is from proprioceptors. Proprioceptive sensations also allow a person to estimate the weight of objects and determine how much muscular effort is necessary to perform a task. For example, most people automatically know to use more muscle strength to pick up a carton of books than to pick up a carton of Styrofoam peanuts (Tortora and Derrickson, 2009).

Proprioception also allows a person to perform certain movements without using the eyes. When climbing stairs, just by placing the foot on the first step, most people can contract the hip and leg muscles the right amount to climb the stairs smoothly and without thinking. This is further evidenced when there is one less step than anticipated, and the person falls forward. It is startling because the leg and foot are already in position and the muscles are contracting in anticipation of pushing up off another stair step.

Reflexes

A **reflex** is a quick, automatic, involuntary sequence of actions that occurs in response to a particular stimulus. Reflexes serve to protect the body. They occur so quickly that the person is usually either unaware of them, such as the sequence that occurs to increase heart rate just before and during exercise, or becomes aware of them after the reflex has happened. For example, an innate reflex is pulling the hand away from a hot surface. Only after the hand has been pulled away does the person realize that the surface is hot and that his hand is no longer in danger. Other reflexes are learned, such as those used while driving. Most drivers automatically check their rearview mirrors before changing lanes, and slam on the brakes to keep from hitting an unexpected object.

There are certain reflexes that involve skeletal muscle movements. These are referred to as *somatic reflexes* because they involve the somatic nervous system. These reflexes serve to smooth and coordinate movements but are protective as well.

Stretch Reflex

The proprioceptors involved in stretch reflexes are called **muscle spindles**. These are found in the belly of skeletal muscle fibers. They have sensory neurons wrapped around intrafusal muscle fibers (*intrafusal* means "within the spindle"; Fig. 2-9). The monitor changes in length of skeletal muscle fibers. When a muscle has stretched far enough during a particular movement, it is stimulated to contract, relieving the stretch. This is the stretch reflex. It prevents injury by not allowing muscle tissue to overstretch or possibly tear (Tortora and Derrickson, 2009).

Tendon Reflex

The proprioceptors involved in tendon reflexes are called **tendon organs**. They are found in the musculotendinous junction and consist of sensory nerve receptors entwined in collagen fibers that are enclosed in a connective tissue capsule. The receptors measure tension applied to tendons from muscle contraction. The tendon reflex protects tendons and associated muscles from damage by causing muscle relaxation in response to excessive tension on tendons by muscle contraction (Tortora and Derrickson, 2009).

Joint Kinesthetic Receptors

Joint kinesthetic receptors are found in and around the articular capsules of synovial joints. There are several types. Free nerve endings and type II cutaneous mechanoreceptors (Ruffini corpuscles) respond to pressure; lamellated (pacinian) corpuscles in connective tissue around joint capsules respond to acceleration and deceleration of joints. Articular ligaments contain receptors similar to tendon organs that adjust reflex inhibition of the adjacent muscles when excessive strain is placed on the joint (Tortora and Derrickson, 2009).

Overall, then, muscles, tendons, and joints have sensory cells that indicate the degree of movement, contraction, stretch, and tension placed on them. The result is awareness, on some level, of the relative

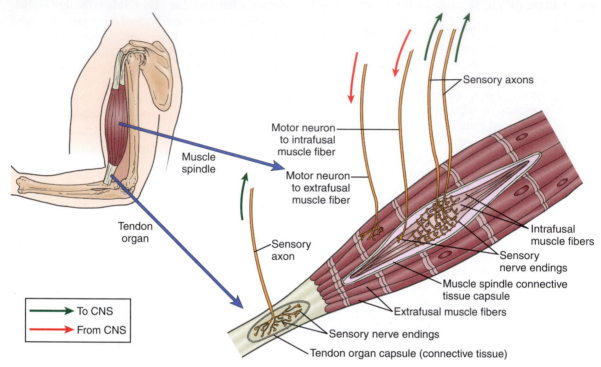

FIGURE 2-9 Muscle spindle and tendon organ.

position of those body areas. The awareness could be subconscious, such as for habitual postures, or conscious, such as focusing on the body movements required when learning how to swing a bat.

A person's state of mind affects the level of his muscular reactions as well. Nervousness, anxiety, anger, or pain often cause a person to react with increased tension in the muscles, so many people automatically tense up against even small amounts of pressure. However, with the development of body awareness, practitioners can decrease the amount of tension and resistance in their muscles. Body awareness is also the gateway to practicing mindful movement. This reduces wear and tear on the body, makes the body function more efficiently, decreases the chances of injury, and promotes career longevity.

STILLNESS

Before practitioners can understand what mindful movement is, they need to understand what stillness is. There is a great deal to be said about turning off technology and "tuning out" the noise of modern

life. Current American culture promotes being on the go all the time and having a continual onslaught of information, especially through electronic means, such as televisions, computers, cell phones, or portable media players such as iPods and MP3 players.

However, being still and quiet allows for the development of internal awareness. If practitioners do not know what it feels like to be still and quiet, there is a good chance they cannot focus inward to really sense what it is like to be in their bodies or what their movements actually feel like. Unless they

Body Awareness

Have you ever received a treatment from a practitioner who did not vary his or her application of pressure for any of the techniques used? How did that feel? How do you think that connects to the practitioner's personal body awareness?

have been part of activities that focus on the connection between body and mind, such as athletics, dance, or martial arts, they may only focus on what they are seeing, hearing, smelling, tasting, touching, and thinking, and not on what they are feeling, both internally and externally.

Stillness is a crucial aspect of bodywork treatments as well. Just the stillness involved in a practitioner resting her hands on a client can be tremendously therapeutic. It is an invitation to the client to leave the busy outside world and join the practitioner in the same quiet, motionless space. This space allows the client to relax the body, let the mind go, and be receptive to the treatment.

Some practitioners may think that just being still with clients is not doing anything at all. It may be a totally new concept for them. There may be the idea that bodywork is performing all the techniques the practitioner possibly can or that talking with the client through the whole treatment is the only way to engage in the therapeutic process. While it is true that some clients want and need this, it is equally true that simply being with a client with therapeutic intent can be valuable to the client's health and well-being.

ACHIEVING STILLNESS

Stillness is just what it sounds like—that is, not moving and tuning out all the internal and external "noise" of life. It is a state of being in which the body is relaxed, thoughts are let go, and the focus is on being receptive to what the body is experiencing. Without stillness, movement cannot be appreciated. Without movement, stillness cannot be appreciated. Movement and stillness work together to create a centered and whole person.

Another way to think of stillness is in terms of relaxation and the benefits relaxation give the mind and body. According to the University of Pittsburgh Healthy Lifestyle Program, it is possible to quiet the mind and reduce the effects of stress by practicing relaxation techniques. These techniques encourage the mind to free itself of mental chatter, and the person experiences serenity, peacefulness, and a greater sense of clarity. The mind becomes less responsive to stress and readjusts so that a baseline level of stress is lower. Practicing relaxation techniques enables people to maintain throughout their day the calm and peaceful feelings gained during a relaxation exercise. The person

becomes more efficient in everyday life and better equipped to deal with life's stresses and challenges (UPMC, 2011).

Once practitioners become comfortable with being still, the stillness can be brought into other aspects of life and work, such as keeping cool under the pressure of deadlines, having more patience with children, taking time to make decisions instead of choosing quickly what seems best in the moment, and having greater degrees of clarity about situations.

Stillness can also become a valuable component of performing bodywork. In addition to resting the hands quietly on a client, the practitioner can wait until a sense of connection with the client happens before moving into the more active parts of the treatment. It is in this connection that the true therapeutic work can happen, because the connection means that the client trusts the practitioner, and the practitioner trusts the client. This is achieved because, through stillness, the practitioner is able to truly listen to the client. Even during the movements of performing treatments, practitioners can maintain a still frame of mind by focusing on only the client and the client's needs and not allowing extraneous thoughts to intrude.

One way to achieve stillness is through **meditation**. This is a mental discipline by which one attempts to get beyond the "thinking" mind and into a deeper state of relaxation or awareness. Meditation often involves sitting comfortably, turning attention to a single point of reference, and letting thoughts flutter through the mind like birds, without stopping and building nests. Throughout history, it has been part of various religions, such as Buddhism, Christianity, Hinduism, Islam, Judaism, and Taoism.

The exercises in the Focus on Wellness box are designed to guide practitioners through simple meditation exercises. Exercise A incorporates the crown chakra into the meditation. More information about chakras can be found in the Body Awareness box about chakras.

CENTERING AND GROUNDING

Much like meditation, **centering** and **grounding** are terms used to describe other ways to achieve stillness. Centering is defined as bringing all mental processes into the center of the person's mind in order to have the focus necessary to meditate,

Focus on *Wellness*

Meditation Exercises

Exercise A

I place my body in a comfortable position . . . I am neither too warm nor too cold . . . I let my jaw relax and fall slightly open . . . I feel the muscles in my face soften and let go . . . I pay attention to my breathing . . . My breath is always with me . . . As I breathe in, I breathe in light . . . As I breathe out, I breathe out anything that I do not want or need . . . I let each breath take me deeper and deeper within . . . I let my breath take me to the silent place within, to the depth, to the core of my being . . .

As I move to the silent place within, I let go of distractions from the outer world, from today's experiences. As thoughts float through my head, I acknowledge and release them . . . As noises in my environment remind me of the outside world, I acknowledge them with a moment's attention and then return to the inner, silent place . . . As feelings come up, I notice and acknowledge them and turn again to that inner place . . .

Again, I let my breathing help me. I breathe in light and breathe out heaviness . . . I breathe in clarity and breathe out confusion . . . I breathe in peace and breathe out disharmony . . . I breathe in and I breathe out, becoming more at peace and more relaxed . . .

I open "at the top." I open at the crown chakra just above the top of my head. I see or imagine that I see a ball of energy sitting above my head. I welcome this vibrant, healing, beautiful energy as it flows in and flows downward . . . It helps me to feel lighter and freer . . . As this energy moves into all the layers and levels of my being, I find it easier to give up dark density, to give up anything that is unkind or heavy or uncomfortable . . . I let go easily with each out-breath.

As I continue to bring this energy from the higher planes into my awareness, I bring it right down through my physical body, down to my heart space . . . down to my waist . . . down to my ankles . . . down to the bottoms of my feet . . . and down to the center of the earth. This establishes a flow of energy, a path, anchoring me to the earth . . .

As energy from above is anchored down deep into the center of the earth, I open "at the bottom"—at the bottoms of my feet and the base of my spine. Earth energy flows upward. This rich, dense earth energy replaces and even displaces dark density released because of the light from above. I feel (sense, see) this energy flowing through me.

Again, I turn my attention to breathing deeply, moving myself to a deeper state of consciousness

. . . deeper within . . . deeper into the silence . . . deep into the core of my being . . .

I begin to turn my attention to my next activity . . . I turn my attention there effortlessly, entrusting myself to the universe. I take three deep breaths. Each in-breath breathes in light, and each out-breath breathes out anything I do not need or want. On the third exhalation, I move into that next activity, feeling alert and refreshed.

Exercise B

Sit in a chair with your feet flat against the floor. Let your spine be straight and comfortable. If you want to lean against the back of the chair, do so. Take a moment to make yourself perfectly comfortable, and then close your eyes.

Gently let your attention come to your breathing. No need to change your breathing in any way, just become aware of it. Become aware of the air entering your nose and traveling down into your chest. Be aware of the slight pause before you breathe out. In, pause, and out. Be aware of the muscles that work as you draw in the air, and how they relax as you let the air out. Easily and effortlessly. Gradually your breathing becomes deeper and more even as you relax into it. Breathe in relaxation and let any concerns that you don't need to pay attention to now seep away with your out-breath. In, relaxing; out, releasing. Enjoy this rhythm for a few moments.

Now let your awareness feel where your body touches the chair. Feel where the weight is lighter and where it is heavier. And bring your awareness to the point where your gluteals are firmest on the chair. Feel that connection to the chair, and let your breathing focus on that spot, drawing your breath deep to that point of connection and feeling as if the out-breath seeps out through that spot. Breathe in a deep, deep breath right to the chair, then out, straight through your body and seeping through the chair and down below it toward the floor. In and out.

And as you breathe deep and deeper, let your connection to the floor deepen, so that some intangible part of you is sinking deep and deeper through the floor and the foundations to connect with the earth below your feet. Easily and effortlessly. Breathing deep, through this connection right down into the earth, and then push that air out, into the soil. Letting the connection grow farther and deeper. Feel the nourishing coolness of the soil. Sense the roots of the trees around your feet, and greet them if you wish.

Farther and deeper, through the soil, down through the rocks underneath, down through the bedrock as far down as you feel comfortable going. Feel that part of your being that you have extended deep into the earth go straight through to the core of the planet, to the heart of the earth. Feel the connection and enjoy it.

Be aware that energy can travel through this connection. Let the grounding flow up through the earth . . . and the floor . . . and into your body. Let it flood your whole being. Once you have felt this feeling, you can make the connection more quickly by focusing on your breathing to bring yourself into your body, and then extending your grounding through the floor and deep into the earth.

visualize, or do bodywork. Grounding means being stable and connected to the earth. Some people think that centering is necessary before grounding can happen; others suggest grounding needs to happen first. The reality is that if a person is hopelessly ungrounded, he probably will not be able to center very well, and if he cannot center himself, he most likely will not achieve a stable connection to the earth. Neither of these scenarios is helpful for achieving stillness.

Like a plant's root system, grounding stabilizes the person so that whatever happens in the world around her, she is not carried away. She remains stable in the calm steadiness of the earth. Being grounded also helps the person stay solid in her body, which helps her be more aware of the sensations and energy flows inside her body and aware of details of the world around her. This helps her respond to the world in a more immediate and appropriate way. She tends to stay in the present moment, letting the past be and trusting that the future will be even better. This skill is vital for personal healing, healthy living, and performing therapeutic treatments.

There are many different ways to become centered and grounded. The following are suggested methods designed to assist you in doing this:

- To center yourself, let your awareness come to a point in the very center of your head. Put one finger directly between your eyebrows and another at the base of your skull in the cleft at the top of your neck. Imagine a point halfway between your two fingers. See or feel a golden light glowing there. Breathe in and see or feel it glow a little brighter. Focus on the light, breathing quietly until your thoughts quiet and the light is all you are aware of. At any time during the exercise, if your thoughts seem to get scattered, you can quiet them and center yourself by taking a few deep breaths while focusing on this light in the middle of your head.

Body Awareness

Chakras are part of Ayurveda, which is the traditional medical system of India. Ayurveda is a Sanskrit word that means "science of life"—*ayus* meaning "life" or "living" and *veda* meaning "knowledge" or "science." Ayurveda is a holistic approach to life and health that encompasses nutrition, meditation, yoga, essential oils, medicinal herbs, positive thinking, breathing, and exercise. The Ayurvedic system dates back at least 5,000 years, making it one of the oldest medical systems in the world.

This complex medical system encompasses knowledge based on natural rhythms and life cycles. Ayurvedic theory believes that health results from harmony within oneself, which is harmony among the purpose for being, thoughts, feelings, and physical actions. Temperature, light, herbs, food, minerals, exercise, and meditation (to engage the mind and emotions) are the means by which health, or balance and harmony in the body, can be achieved. Emphasis is placed on preventing ill health.

Prana is one of the Ayurvedic concepts. Basically, prana is the life force or energy of the body (it is comparable to qi in traditional Chinese medicine), and its vehicle is the breath. Prana gives and maintains life and unifies the person as a whole. Prana travels throughout the body.

Chakras are centers of prana. They are located along the spinal column in the areas of certain glands and nerve plexuses (*plexus* means "braid" or "network"). Chakras are the link between the prana of the universe and the prana of the body. Chakra translates as "wheel," and they are indeed wheels of energy that govern the various physical organs and emotions. Table 2.4 describes the seven chakras of the body, and Figure 2-10 shows their locations.

TABLE 2.4 The Seven Chakras of the Body

Number	English Name	Indian Name	Associated Color	Location	Function
1	Root chakra	*Muladhara*	Red	Perineum (anal area)	Main foundation or support of chakras above it
2	Sacral chakra	*Svadhisthana*	Orange	Genital region	Controls reproduction, adrenal glands, and prostate
3	Solar plexus chakra	*Manipura*	Yellow	Navel areas	Controls the connection of the person to the universe
4	Heart chakra	*Anahata*	Green	Near the heart	Controls the sacred heart or the connection to pure consciousness
5	Throat chakra	*Vishuddha*	Blue	At the throat	Regulates the connection between mind and body
6	Brow chakra	*Ajna*	Indigo	Between the eyebrows	Also called the "third eye"; connected to the meditative process, insight and development of higher consciousness
7	Crown chakra	*Sahasrara*	Silver, gold, white, violet	Beyond the top of the head	Not exactly a chakra; activates all the brain centers; associated with the highest refinement of consciousness and the connection of individual Prana with universal Prana

(Douillard, 2004; Ninivaggi, 2008)

- If your strongest sense is hearing, try to find a note or a pitch that will resonate in the area of your head described above. Intone that note a few times, allowing the vibration to fill your head, and let it become all you are aware of.
- In Asian bodywork, the practitioner's center of gravity is down in her belly. Having the center of gravity here is so significant that practitioners are taught ways to focus on this area. One way to do this is by sitting comfortably on the floor, either cross-legged or with your gluteals resting on your heels. Focus your breath inward and downward into your belly. Imagine a glow of warmth in your belly to help expand awareness into it. The warmth can then be visualized as extending out through all your muscles and bones, and out to your fingers, toes, and top of your head. Visualize extending it beyond your body to connect with the sky, the ground, and all around you.
- Crawling is a movement natural to children and is something that adults generally "forget" how to do. Try practicing crawling until it becomes comfortable again. Feel your weight shift from hand to hand, knee to knee, and from hands to knees.

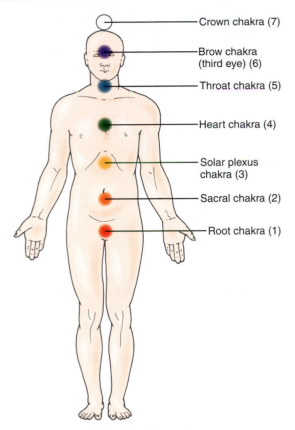

FIGURE 2-10 Chakras.

Crown chakra (7)

Brow chakra (third eye) (6)

Throat chakra (5)

Heart chakra (4)

Solar plexus chakra (3)

Sacral chakra (2)

Root chakra (1)

- Have a real good belly laugh.
- Sing the deepest note you can. Feel it vibrate deep in your belly and pelvis. Imagine the sound extending deep into the earth and see if you can sing a little deeper.
- Touch and hold stones such as obsidian, black tourmaline, or tiger-eye. If these are not available, any rock can help you reconnect with the earth.

Once you know how to ground, you can often do so in two to three deep breaths. There is a feeling of downward flow of energy as when breathing out, like a special type of gravity is pulling you into deep connection with the earth. On the in-breath, feel energy coming up to you. A quick way you can confirm whether you are grounded is to balance on one leg. If you are properly grounded, this should be easy, and you should be able to move the other leg around in the air without losing your balance.

CULTIVATING BODY AWARENESS

Body awareness means listening to one's body and paying attention to the signals it sends about feelings, sensations, and actions. The starting point for this process depends on the individual, but no matter the point at which the practitioner starts, the way he experiences his body can be improved and expanded. The more in tune he becomes with his body, the more he will realize all its patterns, like the position of his spine when sitting or sleeping, what foot he leads off with when walking, where he holds tension in his body when he is angry, and, of course, how he moves his body when performing bodywork.

Most people notice the obvious aspects of their bodies. They know, for example, when they are hungry or full, if their clothes are too tight, if they are experiencing pain, or if they are having an angry outburst. But to develop body awareness, you should ask

While crawling, use your belly as your center of gravity. Feel your connection to the earth, the sky, and all around you. In time, crawling will again be as effortless as walking.

- Take off your shoes and socks and stand on bare earth or grass. Feel the earth under your feet and feel your body sinking in. Breathe right down into the earth so that it begins to feel like an extension of your body.
- When it is too cold or wet for bare feet outdoors, take off your shoes and walk very slowly across a room. Concentrate on feeling all the shifting of the muscles, bones, and tendons in your feet and legs as you ever so slowly move and change your balance. It should take 3 to 5 minutes to walk across a 20-foot room. About halfway across, start focusing on the downward flow of your energy from your feet to the earth and on the upward energy flow supporting your weight. You will be grounded by the time you reach the other side.
- Pet an animal. Animals are always grounded, and by connecting with them, the feeling of being grounded is naturally transferred.

What Do You Think?

What does being centered and grounded mean to you? Think of a time when you have felt centered and grounded, and a time when you did not. How did each time feel to you? What caused you to feel centered and grounded, and what caused you to not feel that way?

yourself if you really notice the small details in how you are feeling. These details are as equally important as the more apparent features of your body, your movements, and your sensations. The small details can have just as big an impact as the more noticeable features.

Start by concentrating on what your body is feeling during various times of the day, including during all your activities of daily living (ADL). Then answer the following questions, either mentally or by writing them down as a journal entry you can reflect back on.

- When you wake up in the morning:
  - How are you lying? Do you feel comfortable, or could you loosen up your muscles or change the position in which you sleep?
  - Without using a lot of energy, try to stretch long and steadily on one side of your body at a time. How are you lying now and how do you feel?
  - How are you breathing? Is it shallow, just involving your intercostal muscles (muscles that expand and contract the rib cage), or is it deep, involving your abdomen?
- How does it feel when you walk down the street? Can you feel the mobility of your feet, that you have heels and toes?
- When you sit:
  - How are you resting on your gluteals? How do your thighs feel against the chair and your feet against the floor?
  - How do your spine and shoulders feel? If your back is not straight but rounded or slouched, that position often begins at the hip joints. Try repositioning yourself to sit on your ischial tuberosities. Does this make your spine become aligned? An aligned spine means your head and spine are lined up, natural curves are maintained, and you feel the least amount of stress in your back. An aligned spine gives your body maximum efficiency. Any deviation from this indicates, and may result in, an imbalance or dysfunction in your body, which can lead to injury. This is discussed in more detail in Chapter 3.
  - Try placing a phonebook under your feet. Does this change your alignment, as in bringing your ankles in alignment with your knees, and your knees in alignment with your hips? How does that feel?
  - Go through your entire body—your neck and head, shoulders, back, arms, hands, legs, and feet. Are you sitting well? Can you sit better by

moving a little? Do you feel that you need to fidget?
  - How are you breathing? Is it shallow, just involving your intercostal muscles, or is it deep, involving your abdomen?
- Stand up. Imagine you are standing somewhere for a length of time, such as waiting for a bus. Feel how you are standing. If your knees feel stiff, perhaps you are hyperextending them. Flex them a little so they become softer in the joints.
  - It may now feel as if the weight on your feet has shifted. Move your feet until you are comfortable. If one or both hips feel tight, move them as well. Continue shifting the rest of your body until all parts feel comfortable. Make sure you have an aligned spine.
  - How do your spine and shoulders feel? Is your back rounded or slouched? If so, try straightening your spine and pulling your shoulders back. Since keeping the back absolutely straight all the time can be exhausting, let your shoulders drop and relax your back while keeping your spine aligned.
  - How are you breathing? Is it shallow, just involving your intercostal muscles, or is it deep, involving your abdomen?

At this point, you may be becoming aware that all your muscles and joints are connected, either directly or through other muscles and joints. The change in the position of a joint will, through the muscles, affect the position of other joints. That is why tensing or hyperextending the knee joint can cause discomfort in the feet, hips, or back, and why loosening the tension in the knees by softening or flexing them slightly gives you the impulse to loosen up in other places in your body. This is the beginning of mindful movement.

The next step is to take the awareness of how your body feels while lying, sitting, and standing and bring it into other movements, both those for performing bodywork and ADL. For example, answer the following questions for yourself:

- How do I hold my shoulders when I am brushing my teeth? Carrying groceries? Performing bodywork? Do I feel discomfort in my body during these activities? How can I shift or change my movements to be more efficient and comfortable?
- Is my back straight when performing bodywork? Lifting items out of the car? Sitting down watching TV? Do I feel discomfort in my body during these activities? How can I shift or change my movements to be more efficient and comfortable?

- Am I using the strength in my legs to lift something heavy? To perform bodywork? Do I feel discomfort in my body during these activities? How can I shift or change my movements to be more efficient and comfortable?
- How are my feet placed while walking? Standing in line at a department store? When performing bodywork? Do I feel discomfort in my body during these activities? How can I shift or change my movements to be more efficient and comfortable?
- How often am I looking down? Do I look down while texting or talking on the cell phone? During the entire bodywork treatment? Do I feel discomfort in my body during these activities? How can I shift or change my movements to be more efficient and comfortable?

Changing habitual body movements may or may not feel comfortable. It involves changing muscular movement patterns, neurological patterns, and your view of yourself. But since there is a connection between the mind and what the body feels, this discomfort will decrease over time if you keep a positive frame of mind and are genuinely interested in developing body awareness and efficient movement. The "movement goal" is what you should focus on, and it can begin immediately with no further preparation than a desire to change.

> **Myth:** If the practitioner does not move much while performing treatments, he will have more energy.
>
> **FACT:** It takes more energy to remain in a static, or fixed, position than dynamic, or moving, positions. Remaining static for long periods is also harder on the body in general, as this decreases range of motion (ROM) and flexibility at the joints, and decreases muscle tone. Ultimately the body's strength and mobility will be compromised, and the body is more likely to become injured.

MINDFUL MOVEMENT

The ultimate goal of mindful movement is to learn what it feels like to be in efficient postures, where the joints are aligned; the muscles are in their strongest positions; and there is the least amount of stress on muscles, nerves, blood vessels, and connective tissues. Once practitioners have a good sense of what an efficient posture feels like, they can practice mindful movement patterns that keep them within comfortable ranges of motion of joints and that allows them to use their strongest muscle groups to perform the tasks of daily living and, of course, the movements involved in doing bodywork.

Mindful movement involves conscious awareness of how the nervous, skeletal, and muscular systems function, how they are interrelated, and how they influence each other. By working with what they experience, practitioners are taking part in an ongoing process that will coordinate their movements and will eventually improve their body's overall functioning. A mindful movement pattern is one that allows practitioners to use the least amount of effort and has the least amount of stress on the body.

Such movement and coordination is not necessarily automatic. While some people come by it naturally, it is usually developed through paying attention to many body awareness signals. The next step is to use the information from the signals the body is sending to change the way the body is used and moved. It may feel strange at first, but if continued for a long period of time, muscles and other tissues will change the signals they are sending. You will feel comfortable with these new ways of moving and will, in fact, experience mindful movement. Ultimately you increase not only your career longevity, but also your wellness.

Muscles work best when exercised and allowed to move freely. In fact, inaction is an unnatural state for living beings. When beings become hurt, ill, or stop moving for other reasons, the neural circuits that transmit sensory and motor information do not operate as effectively, and restrictive movement patterns may be the result. Mindful movement involves conscious decisions to reroute the neural-muscle pathways the person has become used to, pathways that are compensatory yet inefficient. The goal is to live without restrictive patterns.

When practitioners keep moving while performing bodywork, they do not get stuck in uncomfortable, stress-producing and potentially harmful stances and holds. When practitioners make it a habit to consciously and continually move during treatments, they will be less likely to form or stay in harmful holding patterns. The movements do not have to be large or forceful but rather should be whatever feels right for your body.

BECOMING MORE AWARE OF MOVEMENT STYLES

Whether practitioners have a slow and calm style of moving, a faster, more energetic style, or a combination of both, their movement styles make them unique and will draw to them a group of loyal clients who respond to their particular styles. By being aware of their own movement styles, practitioners can also take cues from their clients and adjust their movements in order to increase the chances of developing rapport. For example, if a client is moving slowly, making quick movements might put the client on guard. On the other hand, if a client is anxious and is moving quickly, moving slowly can possibly help calm the client. Practitioners can also match their movement styles to clients' needs to enhance the treatment.

Noticing a client's breathing pattern can also give you an idea of the client's movement style. If a client has a restrictive breathing pattern, you can visually assess the client to see if she or he has a restrictive movement pattern. If it is difficult to observe the breathing pattern, you could assess the client's movement pattern first since one affects the other.

To become more aware of your personal movement style, ask yourself the following questions:

- How do you physically greet your clients?
- What kind of hand gestures and body language do you use to explain your work?
- During your work with clients, what are some specific movements you make that physically feel good to you (e.g., slow and lengthening strokes, static pressure, grasping strokes, and so forth)?
- When you move, do you feel static and stuck or comfortable and flowing?

The next step for you to identify your movement style is realizing when your body mechanics feel natural, comfortable, and easy. Being unaware of movement style can lead to frustration, boredom, and burnout as you try to perform techniques or work in modalities that really are not suited to your style.

What Do You Think?

Think of a time when, while working with a client or fellow student, you felt as if your body had a certain flow, that your movements came naturally, and you felt yourself enjoying the sensations of your movements. Why do you think you felt that way? How often do you feel that way while performing bodywork? While doing your everyday activities?

DEVELOPING MINDFUL MOVEMENT

The following are methods practitioners can use to develop mindful movement. If these feel uncomfortable at first, you are encouraged to continue doing them until you are able to perform them with ease and confidence. By respecting what you feel and using what you feel to make changes, your experience will become integrated into your body and mind, and these new ways of moving will become a natural part of your daily life.

Mindful movement is not just dynamic movement. It also pertains to static movement, which, in fact, is where it begins. Visualizing a line of movement through the body while not moving can change the habitual patterns of messages being sent from the brain through nerve pathways to the muscles. As long as this new thinking pattern is activated during movement, a new pattern of muscle activity is automatically being used to decrease physical stress and maintain a more balanced alignment of the skeleton. Over a period of time during which there is continual daily attention to new patterns in thinking and action, the body's shape will be transformed. Previously overused muscles become more flexible and smoothed out, while previously underused muscles develop greater tone, strength, endurance, and contour.

PRINCIPLES OF MINDFUL MOVEMENT

Based on the previous development activity for development, there are several principles of mindful movement to keep in mind. These include the following:

- Conscious awareness
  - Listen to your body and its signals
  - Determine what you can do or not do
- Breathe
  - Focusing attention on something so simple as the movements of breathing can help quiet the mind.
  - Awareness of your breath can access the spiritual nature of bodywork. One way of thinking of this is that breath is a point of entry to deeper resources within yourself as well as to the greater world outside yourself.
  - Breath supports all other aspects of movement—balance, shifting body weight for efficient movement, and generating strength.
- Surroundings
  - Being aware of what is around you helps you navigate obstacles efficiently so that you can perform bodywork treatments smoothly.

- Creating calm surroundings greatly enhances the therapeutic aspects of bodywork treatments.
- Even if your surroundings are not optimal, if you have mindful movement, you will be able to maintain necessary calmness and focus.
- Emotions and feelings
  - Discover what unconscious thinking, emotional, and behavioral patterns you have that are not serving a useful purpose.
  - Be willing to let go of emotions and feelings that risk endangering your positive outlook on life and sense of calm. These are the basis of all that you have to offer.
  - Do not limit your possibilities. Instead, free yourself from the grooves of old habits, and reorient yourself to better understanding and feeling for your thoughts, emotions, and structural body.
- Reactions
  - These are influenced by external factors and can have a huge effect on both mind and movement, especially toward your attitudes and behaviors.
  - Anticipating your reactions will help you avoid certain situations that may affect your overall well-being, especially if you know that you will not respond to them well.
  - Thinking before you react helps promote the conscious use of your mind and body connection.
- Know your limits and respect them
  - When something feels painful, focus is usually drawn to the inevitable, which is that limits have been exceeded.
  - Ignoring body needs will eventually lead to some type of physical, mental, or emotional issue that may even escalate into something serious.
- Work slowly
  - This aids in body awareness and mindful movement, thus interrupting habitual patterns and allowing change for more efficient movements to occur.

METHODS OF ACHIEVING MINDFUL MOVEMENT

There are actually quite a few methods practitioners can use to achieve mindful movement. In addition to the activity discussed in the previous section, practitioners can explore exercise, meditation, tai chi, and

Body Awareness

Think of the room or space in which you usually perform your bodywork treatments. What does the environment look like? What kind of furniture is in there, and where are your pieces of treatment equipment placed? Is there a heating and cooling vent or a fan? Where is that in relation to where you perform the actual treatment? What about artwork? Where is it placed?

Now visualize yourself doing a treatment in your treatment space. Are you able to move around your client easily? Do you need to watch out for furniture or other objects in the room to make sure you do not bump into them? How do you move your body to compensate for how the space is set up? Have you noticed any places in your body that feel stressed, tight, or painful because of how you have to move in your treatment space?

qigong. Also, receiving bodywork on a regular basis is an excellent way to become more aware of your body and the signals it gives off.

Exercise promotes blood and lymphatic flow, increases and maintains lung function, increases muscle strength, increases stamina and strength, clears the mind, and increases focus. Exercise can take many different forms: yoga, Pilates, swimming, weight training, and walking, to name a few. The point is to do some sort of movement on a regular basis. It needs to be refreshing and invigorating. How much movement and how often the movement should be done will be different for everyone. Practitioners also need to spend time focusing inward to clear their minds and take time out from the demands of life. Meditation, whether the traditional sitting meditation, or a moving meditation, such as needlework or gardening, acts as a restorative for body, mind, and soul. It quiets the mental "noise" people may experience from the hustle and bustle of everyday life. When this noise is lessened, people are better able to listen to their bodies and may be more relaxed and willing to put in the effort necessary to change habitual movement patterns.

Tai Chi

The full name of this practice is tai chi chuan. It is actually a Chinese martial art that consists of fast forms and slow forms. The fast forms are more of the martial art aspects of the practice. The Mandarin term *t'ai chi ch'uan* literally translates as "supreme ultimate fist," "boundless fist," "great extremes boxing," or simply "the ultimate." Today, the studied, flowing movements of the slow forms of tai chi are most often recognized by Westerners (Fig. 2-11). Tai chi is practiced for health and longevity and has spread worldwide. Focusing the mind just on the movements of the form helps to bring about a state of mental calmness and clarity.

The physical techniques of tai chi chuan are described in the tai chi classics (a set of writings by traditional masters) as being characterized by the use of leverage through the joints based on coordination in relaxation, rather than muscular tension, in order to neutralize or initiate attacks.

Slow, repetitive work is involved in the process of learning how that leverage is generated gently and then increases measurably and opens the circulation of breath, body heat, blood, lymph, and digestive functions.

The study of tai chi chuan primarily involves three aspects:

- *Health:* An unhealthy or otherwise uncomfortable person may find it difficult to meditate to a state of calmness or to use tai chi as a martial art. Therefore, tai chi's health training concentrates on relieving the physical effects of stress on the body and mind. For those focused on tai chi's martial application, good physical fitness is an important step toward effective self-defense.
- *Meditation:* The focus and calmness cultivated by the meditative aspect of tai chi is seen as necessary in maintaining optimum health (in the sense of relieving stress and maintaining homeostasis) and in applying the form as a soft-style martial art.
- *Martial art:* The ability to use tai chi as a form of self-defense in combat is the test of a student's understanding of the art. Martially, tai chi chuan is the study of appropriate change in response to outside forces—the study of yielding and "sticking" to an incoming attack rather than attempting to meet it with opposing force.

Practitioners wear loose, comfortable clothing and flat-soled shoes. Basic tai chi training has two aspects. The first is the solo form, a slow sequence of movements that emphasize an aligned spine, abdominal breathing, and a natural range of motion. The solo form should take the students through a complete, natural ROM over their center of gravity. Accurate, repeated practice of the solo routine is said to retrain posture, encourage circulation throughout the students' bodies, maintain flexibility through their joints, and further familiarize students with the martial application sequences implied by the forms. The second aspect involves different styles of pushing hands as part of the soft martial arts form (Kit, 2002; Mayo Clinic staff, 2009).

Qigong

Qigong (also known as *Chi Gong* or *Chi Kung*) originated in China many thousands of years ago. **Qi** can be translated as "breath" or "energy." Here, breath does not simply mean taking air into and out of the lungs; it also includes the more subtle breath or energy in the body. Bioelectric energy is the energy of the body and of all living creatures. In a larger view, qi is the energy or force that keeps things coherent—from the subatomic particles that comprise atoms to the forces that permeate the cosmos. *Gong* translates as "practice" or "cultivation." *Gong* is a word used in reference to the cultivation of many

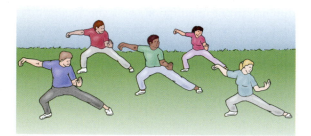

FIGURE 2-11 Tai chi.

things, from gardening to honing musical ability to continuing the practice of bodywork. The performance of qigong is an activity, while qi itself is a tangible, felt quality in the body.

People of any age can practice qigong. The ancient practice of qigong is performed specifically to help the practitioner focus on developing qi, breath, and awareness. It increases flexibility and stamina, improves strength, and is a form of moving meditation. In fact, by practicing this one type of movement, the practitioner can accomplish most of what is necessary to maintain heath.

The health benefits of qigong are many. They include improving balance, strengthening the legs, releasing the lower back, aligning the spine, improving body mechanics, improving internal organ function, increasing immunity, calming and centering the mind, increasing and organizing energetic reservoirs and pathways, becoming present, and releasing nonuseful energetic and physical patterns of movement. Overall, practicing qigong enhances consciousness of body, mind, and spirit while instilling an appreciation of relationship and connection with others, nature, and the universe.

The practice session involves three main actions: warming up, doing the qigong practice itself, and closing, although all three actions do not need to be performed every time. Practicing outside is considered more favorable because the air quality is generally fresher and the qi more abundant, though weather and urban conditions sometimes prevent this. Practicing in the wind, rain, or extreme cold is undesirable; excessive noise or odor also tends to disturb the qi.

Warming up can be as simple as taking a stroll or involve more complex body movements while walking. Warming up gently gets the blood moving, warms connective tissues, and generally helps loosen the tissues of the body. It also helps move the consciousness from the head into the body. The next step is the actual qigong practice itself. It involves specific stances for body alignment, efficient movement, focus on the channels of qi flow in the body, and exercises to feel the body's qi and to enhance it (Fig. 2-12). Since breathing is a major component of qigong, emphasis is on abdominal breathing. Closing involves techniques to close the person's energy fields (Friedman, 2009).

Yoga

Yoga is an ancient art originating in India (Fig. 2-13). It is based on a harmonizing system of development for the body, mind, and spirit. Yoga brings about emotional stability and clarity of mind. The word

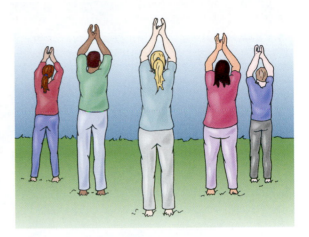

FIGURE 2-12 Qigong.

yoga means "union" in Sanskrit, the classical language of India. It is one of the oldest systems of physical and mental exercise ever created. People discovered that it made them feel good to go out into nature—into the forests and jungles, next to rivers, in view of mountains—and watch animals and the environment. These people became interested in their natural surroundings and kept inventing new poses to imitate things they saw. By watching closely and imitating how the animals moved and how the trees and mountains are structured, the people felt good, full of positive energy, and healthy.

Many people think that yoga is just stretching. While stretching is involved, yoga is actually about creating balance in the body through developing both strength and flexibility, and it is about focusing the mind. This is done by performing poses or postures, each of which has specific physical, mental, and spiritual benefits. The poses can be done quickly in succession, creating heat in the body through movement, or they can be done more slowly to increase stamina and perfect the alignment of the pose. The poses are a constant, but the approach to them varies depending on the tradition in which the teacher has trained.

The postures and exercises of yoga are not necessarily easy for the beginner. Some require difficult balances, and others require finding and working on the edge of the person's flexibility or strength. Some simply require much concentration to keep track of what arm and what leg goes where. However, yoga can yield quick results with consistent practice. For example, a person who cannot even touch his knees may be able to, a week later, reach his shins. The person who practices yoga regularly becomes more

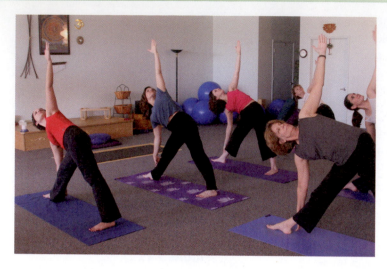

FIGURE 2-13 Yoga. *Photo courtesy of Yoga Rasa—Houston, TX. www.yogarasa.net/ home.php.*

self-aware and will notice even small gains in flexibility, strength, and mental clarity.

There are many different types of yoga:

- *Hatha*: This is a general term for many types of yoga. Hatha is actually two words in one: *ha*, meaning "sun" and *tha* meaning "moon." Hatha style is usually slow-paced and gentle and is a good introduction to basic yoga poses. Its purpose it is to balance mind and body through the poses and controlled breathing, and to calm the mind through relaxation and meditation.

- *Iyengar*: Based on the teachings of the yogi B. K. S. Iyengar, this style of practice is most concerned with bodily alignment. In yoga, the word *alignment* is used to describe the optimal positioning in each pose for maximum benefits and to avoid injury. Iyengar practice usually emphasizes holding poses over long periods rather than moving quickly from one pose to the next. This type of yoga encourages the use of props, such as yoga blankets, blocks, and straps, to bring the body into alignment: The purpose is to develop strength, stamina, flexibility, and balance, along with the mental aspects of concentration and clearing the mind through meditation.

- *Kundalini*: The emphasis in Kundalini is on the breath in conjunction with physical movement, with the purpose of freeing energy in the lower body and allowing it to move upward. All types of yoga involve controlling the breath. However, in Kundalini, exploring the effects of the breath on the postures is essential. Kundalini uses rapid, repetitive movements rather than poses held for a long time, and the teacher will often lead the class

in call-and-response chanting. Kundalini yoga is called *the yoga of awareness* because its practitioners believe that it directly affects consciousness, develops intuition, increases self-knowledge, and releases unlimited creative potential.

- *Kripalu*: This is associated both with a style of hatha yoga and a yoga and wellness center in Stockbridge, Massachusetts. Both were founded by yoga guru Amrit Desai, who came to the United States from India in 1960. This type of yoga emphasizes meditation, physical healing, and spiritual transformation. It focuses on finding answers by looking within.

- *Bikram/hot yoga*: Pioneered by Bikram Choudhury, this style is also referred to as *hot yoga*. It is practiced in a room that is 95° to 100°F. The classes are 90 minutes long and consist of a series of 26 postures and two breathing exercises. The goal is toward general wellness, and the heat facilitates deeper stretching and injury prevention while reducing stress and tension. The profuse sweating that occurs is thought to be cleansing (Pizer, 2010).

The practice of yoga makes the body strong and flexible, and retrains the entire body to position itself in a way that allows it to function more effectively. It also improves the functioning of the respiratory, circulatory, digestive, and hormonal systems. Some of the physical benefits include improved sleep; pain management; weight normalization; increased energy and endurance, strength, flexibility, coordination, and dexterity; better balance and stability; improved immune function; and better posture.

The mental and emotional benefits include improved concentration and attention, a decrease in feelings of depression and anxiety, increased memory retention, greater mental clarity. The vigorous yet calming effect of yoga helps improve sleep. Yoga cultivates mindfulness, which means being acutely aware of and present in each moment. Working the body can calm the mind and working the mind can calm the body.

Ideokinesis

Ideokinesis uses imagery to change neuromuscular pathways. It is the combination of the word *ideo*, meaning "idea" or "thought," and *kinesis*, meaning "movement." Thus, ideokinesis refers to movements based on focused thoughts, which is another way of describing mindful movement.

Mabel Elsworth Todd was a major contributor to ideokinesis, a field of bodywork and personal development that first came to prominence in the 1930s among dancers and health professionals. Todd's ideas involved using creative visual imagery and consciously relaxed movement to create refined neuromuscular coordination. Her work built on and overlapped similar work done by Heinrich Kosnick and Lulu Sweigard, who originally coined the term *ideokinesis*. Todd's work was originally published in her book *The Thinking Body* (1937), which is now considered by modern dance schools to be a classic study of physiology and the psychology of movement. Her work influenced many somatic awareness professionals of her day and is often cited along with the Feldenkrais method for its focus on the subtle influence of unconscious intention and attention on movement.

In ideokinesis, the person first has an idea or image of what she wants to have happen, and then visualizes the nervous system sending messages through the nerves to the muscles, which then contract in response to the visualized movement. For example, if someone is learning to do wall squats (deep knee bends performed by placing the back against the wall, sliding down into a sitting position, sliding back up, and repeating), she may be able to perform them better when imagining herself as a horse on a merry-go-round, rather than thinking about bending at the hips, knees, and ankles. She has an image of what her body should be doing, and her nervous system picks the most efficient way to coordinate her movements.

Ideokinesis works best when the directions from the brain are clearly stated. With daily practice of ideokinesis, the communication between the brain and the body's action becomes much clearer. Working with the body and creating changes in its health is often straightforward, and most people can see, sense, and feel the changes in their bodies as they shift their thoughts. This helps to disconnect perhaps a powerful belief some people may have that "my body is a vehicle for my brain, nothing more."

The following are several ideokinesis exercises to try:

Exercise 1

- You can begin using ideokinesis and imagery to change the level of overall tension in your body. Sit easily with your pelvis against the back of the chair and your feet resting firmly on the ground in front of you.
- Imagine your spine like the trunk of a pine tree and your ribs like the hanging branches. As you inhale, the branches will lift slightly in all directions, front, back, and to the sides. As you exhale, the branches of the pine tree fall easily and heavily down toward your waist while your spine stays long, tall, and supple. Take a few more easy breaths, slowing down your exhale, allowing the shoulders to rest on top of your ribs and your ribs to hang off your spine.
- As you continue to breathe easily, do a quick check of your body. Are there any areas that feel tight or sore? How would you describe that area? Does it feel sharp, or does it feel hard like a block of cement? Is there a color to the area?
- Imagine fresh spring water being poured into your body through the top of your head. Notice how clear and pure it is. As this water is slowly flowing into all the cells and corners and crevices of your body, it is dissolving your stress and tension. Allow the tension to drain through your feet and into the ground where it can be safely recycled.
- Your thoughts can carry tension, too, so let the water wash through your thoughts, flushing out any fear or self-criticism, anger, frustration, or doubt. Keep the flow of water filtering through your body until you feel cleansed, calm, and quiet.
- You can create different images to release the tension. You could melt the tension like butter; or send your breath slowly into the area, spreading golden light of healing energy; or imagine a beautiful color gently washing the tension away.

- There is not one right way to work with ideokinesis. With practice, you'll discover which images are more effective for you. You might get a more effective response to your visualization by first seeing yourself on a beach lying in the sun or walking through your favorite mountain meadow.

Exercise 2

- Turn your head to the left as far as you can easily and stop. Mark how far you turned your head by imagining a line stretching in front of your nose, and notice what you are looking at. Now come back to center and again close your eyes.
- Imagine yourself as a cartoon character who can twist itself around and around like a coiled spring. In your mind's eye, begin to slowly and easily turn your face toward your left shoulder. You are not actually doing this; you're just imagining doing the movement.
- As you turn your face and body toward the left in your mind's eye, you find that you can go farther, and now you are looking behind yourself and continue to twist, looking over your right shoulder, then back to the front. You've made a complete rotation with your head.
- Open your eyes and turn your head to the left. Draw an imaginary line from your nose forward and note where you are facing. Did you go farther?
- Come back to facing forward and close your eyes once more. This time you are going to imagine just your eyes rotating like slowly spinning tops turning to the left, coming all the way around. Each eye softly rests deep within your head space as you visualize them rotating without strain. Imagining the eyes moving in this way sends a message of release to the muscles at the top of the neck where so many of us store tension.
- Now open your eyes and once again rotate your head to the left and mark how far you rotated.
- You have increased your range of motion at the neck, not by doing stretches or exercises, but through ideokinesis, or giving your brain a clear direction and then getting out of the way.
- As discussed in Chapters 7 and 8, doing stretches and strengthening exercises are an important part of maintaining health in the body. If you hold tension and stress in your body, stretching is very important, and you will receive more benefit from any stretching you do if you involve the brain in visualization—focus on what you want, not what you do not want.

Exercise 3

- After finishing a treatment session, take a few minutes and imagine whatever it is that you learned or did. Can you see yourself doing it perfectly? Note the places where you cannot remember the movement easily and focus on them the next time.
- If you are injured or unable to perform any of the techniques for any reason, do a virtual workout in your mind's eye, always seeing yourself easily and effortlessly moving through space. Research shows that you can maintain some muscle engagement and patterning even when training only in your mind's eye.

Weight-Bearing Exercise

While any form of movement can help with overall well-being and achieving mindful movement, weight-bearing exercise also ensures health, vitality, and career longevity. Weight-bearing exercise helps with balance, lowers the risk of atherosclerosis, back pain, cancer, chronic lung disease, coronary heart disease, diabetes, obesity, hypertension, and osteoporosis, and it can increase energy levels.

The mind benefits as much as the body does from exercise. Research in the area of psychology and physical activity supports a relationship between physical fitness, mental alertness, and emotional stability. For example, improved endurance makes the person less susceptible to fatigue and consequently less likely to commit errors, mental or physical. Regular exercise also decreases anxiety levels. Performance on the job is enhanced, fewer breaks are needed, and the risk of injury decreases. This is certainly true of the bodywork profession. People who are physically fit usually have a better outlook, more self-confidence, and often do well in whatever their talents and ambitions prompt them to try.

More detailed information about weight-bearing exercise is covered in Chapter 8.

Wellness Profile Check-In

Looking at the Wellness Profile you completed at the end of Chapter 1, are there any challenge areas you could remedy by developing body awareness and mindful movement? If so, what are they? How would you like to improve these areas? What body awareness and mindful movement methods will you use to

Case Profile

Paul has been a bodywork practitioner for a little over 3 years, and he works at a local day spa. For most of that time, Paul typically worked 5 days a week, doing six to seven treatments per day. For the past 6 months, however, Paul has noticed that he seldom gets repeat clients and that he has been doing only two or three treatments a day, and some days he has not had any treatments scheduled at all.

Paul works in a small treatment room that also doubles as a filing room, and he often finds himself bumping into the cabinets as he performs his treatments. His table is stationary, which means that the height is not adjustable. When greeting clients, he usually rushes up to escort them back to the room as quickly as possible. He has even been known to run into the door frame of the treatment room as he practically pushes the client into the room.

When he receives treatments, Paul prefers deep pressure and vigorous techniques, which he thinks is the best way to address chronic muscle tension. He carries this into the treatments he does, and if a client requests lighter pressure, Paul states that he received an excellent bodywork education and this is how treatments are supposed to be performed.

Paul spends his Saturdays caring for his elderly mother, and Sunday is a total rest day, which he prefers to spend on the couch watching sports. If he finds the time, he will receive bodywork, but treatments are usually few and far between.

Over the last year, he has begun to feel chronic pain in his low back. His energy is low, his body is aching, he is frustrated that he is not building a clientele, and lately he has been thinking of finding another line of work.

- *What is your initial impression about Paul's overall body awareness?*

- *What are the issues Paul is facing?*

- *How do you think Paul's behavior will impact his career longevity?*

- *What advice would you give to Paul?*

improve these areas? Write down a plan for improvement that includes the methods you will use, a timeline for implementing these methods, and ways you will assess your improvement along the way.

SUMMARY

Body awareness is a person's ability to be aware of what his body is doing and feeling. Having body awareness enhances the person's sense of integrity and wholeness, and it helps promote good mental and emotional health. The level of body awareness bodywork practitioners have influences how they learn to perform techniques, how fluid their treatments are, whether they will be prone to injuries, and how much they enjoy doing bodywork. Body awareness is crucial to the development of mindful movement, which is focused and deliberate movement in the most efficient and healthy way possible. All these factors play significant roles in your career longevity.

The development of mindful movement depends on understanding three main factors: the mechanics of movement, stillness, and how to cultivate body awareness. The mechanics of movement depends on the interaction of the nervous, muscular, and skeletal systems. Nerve impulses stimulate muscles to contract, which pulls on bones, creating movement in joints. Without nerve impulses, muscles will relax. Muscles can change in length, and they can increase in tension. Developing proprioception involves enhancing a person's awareness of her body and the positions of various joints relative to each other. The three main types of proprioceptors are (1) muscle spindles, which monitor the stretch of a muscle; (2) tendon organs, which monitor the tension placed on tendons from muscular contractions; and (3) joint kinesthetic receptors, which measure the pressure placed on a joint and how fast the joint is moving.

Before practitioners can understand what mindful movement is, they need to understand what stillness is. It is a state of being in which the body is relaxed, thoughts are let go, and the focus is on being receptive to what the body is experiencing. Being still and quiet allows for the development of internal awareness. Stillness can be achieved through practicing meditation, as well as centering and grounding exercises.

Body awareness means listening to your body and paying attention to the signals it sends about feelings, sensations, and actions. You can start by concentrating on what your body is feeling during various times of the day, including all your ADL. The next step is to take the awareness of how your body feels while lying, sitting, and standing and bring it into other movements, both those for performing bodywork and ADL.

The ultimate goal of mindful movement is to learn what it feels like to be in efficient postures, where the joints are aligned, the muscles are in their strongest positions, and there is the least amount of stress on muscles, nerves, blood vessels, and connective tissues. Once you have a good sense of what an efficient posture feels like, you can practice mindful movement patterns that keep your joints within comfortable ranges of motion and allows you to use your strongest muscle groups to perform the tasks of daily living and the tasks involved in doing bodywork. You can develop mindful movement through practicing tai chi, qigong, yoga, and ideokinesis.

Review Questions

MULTIPLE CHOICE

1. The term for how a person is moving, what he is feeling, and where his body is in relation to other people and nearby objects is
   a. body awareness.
   b. thermogenesis.
   c. stillness.
   d. meditation.

2. People can walk, type, dress themselves, and perform bodywork without using their eyes because of which of the following?
   a. Thermogenesis
   b. Proprioception
   c. Reflexes
   d. Muscle tone

3. A quick, automatic, involuntary sequence of actions that occurs in response to a particular stimulus is called
   a. muscle tone.
   b. grounding.
   c. a fixator.
   d. a reflex.

4. The proprioceptors that cause muscle relaxation in response to excessive tension are
   a. muscle spindles.
   b. Ruffini corpuscles.
   c. tendon organs.
   d. lamellated corpuscles.

5. Which of the following is a way to get beyond everyday thoughts and into a deeper state of awareness?
   a. Meditation
   b. Tai chi
   c. Yoga
   d. All of the above

6. Which of the following is an ancient art that originated in India?
   a. Yoga
   b. Tai chi
   c. Qigong
   d. Ideokinesis

7. The type of yoga that is slow-paced, gentle, and provides a good introduction to the basic yoga poses is
   a. Iyengar.
   b. hatha.
   c. Kundalini.
   d. Bikram.

FILL-IN-THE-BLANK

1. Focused and deliberate movement in the most efficient and healthy way possible is known as _____ movement.

2. The _____ Method is a type of bodywork in which the practitioner communicates new sensory movement patterns to a client through performing passive movements.

3. The development of mindful movement depends on understanding the mechanics of movement, _____, and body awareness.

4. An aspect of proprioception is _____, the perception of body movements.

5. Specialized nervous tissue that responds to certain stimuli by creating nerve impulses is called a _____.

6. Using imagery to change neuromuscular pathways is the term for _____.

7. The ultimate goal of mindful movement is to learn what it feels like to be in _____ _____, where the joints are aligned and the muscles are in their strongest positions.

SHORT ANSWER

1. Explain why mindful movement is important in the performance of bodywork.

2. Describe what stillness means, three ways to achieve stillness, and the connection of stillness to body awareness.

3. Explain three ways body awareness can be enhanced.

4. Explain the three aspects of tai chi.

5. Briefly describe the health benefits of qigong.

6. Write a description of a brief ideokinesis exercise.

7. Explain how you think your performance of bodywork can be enhanced by having greater body awareness.

Activities

1. Go to a mall, park, or other recreational area and observe how the people there move. Can you identify those who seem to have body awareness and are centered and grounded? Choose five people and imitate their movements (without them seeing what you are doing). Journal what it feels like to perform these movements.

2. If you are not doing so already, practice one of the mindful movements covered in this chapter—tai chi, qigong, yoga, ideokinesis—for at least 4 weeks. Journal how you feel physically, mentally, and emotionally throughout the 4-week period by answering the following questions:
   - Before you start practicing one of the mindful movements, how much body awareness do you think you have, and how comfortable are you in your body?

   - How is your body awareness changing over the 4-week period?
   - Do you think you are moving more mindfully over the 4-week period? Why or why not?
   - After 4 weeks, how much body awareness do you think you have, and how comfortable are you in your body?

3. Choose one of the following activities. Break it down into all the individual motions needed to perform the movement. Do each motion slowly and mindfully to really feel how each movement occurs. Also, doing the movements as indicated stimulates your brain. The left side of your brain controls the right side of your body, and the right side of your brain controls the left side of your body. By

changing the way you normally do things, each side of your brain is stimulated to increase communication with the other side. You may notice that, while you are not necessarily good at first when performing the actions as indicated, you improve with practice. This means that both sides of your brain are communicating better.

- Brush your teeth with your nondominant hand
- Walk up a hill backward
- Take clothes out of a washing machine with your nondominant hand
- Start a treatment of a client from the opposite side of where you would normally begin

- Lift and carry a bag of groceries with your nondominant hand

4. Perform 10 bodywork treatments while bringing your awareness to how you move your body to perform the techniques, move around the client, and apply pressure. Journal what you discover about your movements during each of the treatments—what feels comfortable for you, what feels uncomfortable, what you find challenging, what you find successful, and so forth. Review your journals to see what awareness you are developing from each treatment, how your movements have changed, and what you still need to work on.

REFERENCES

Douillard, Dr. John. *The Encyclopedia of Ayurvedic Massage.* Berkeley, CA: North Atlantic Books, 2004.

Friedman, Suzanne. *Heal Yourself with Qigong.* Oakland, CA: New Harbinger Publications, 2009.

Kit, Wong Kiew. *The Complete Book of Tai Chi Chuan: A Comprehensive Guide to the Principles and Practice.* Boston, MA: Tuttle Publishing, 2002.

Mayo Clinic staff. Tai chi: Discover the Many Possible Health Benefits. Retrieved October 2010 from www.mayoclinic.com/health/tai-chi/SA00087.

Menehan, Karen. Trends in massage therapy research: An interview with massage therapy foundation president Diana L. Thompson. In *Massage Magazine* (Trends & Opportunities 2009 issue). Retrieved October 2010 from www.massagemag.com/News/massage-news.php?id=7039&catid=250&title=trends-in-massage-therapy-research-an-interview-with-massage-therapy-foundation-president-diana-l-thompson

Ninivaggi, Frank John. *Ayurveda: A Comprehensive Guide to Traditional Medicine for the West.* Westport, CT: Praeger, 2008.

Pizer, Ann. Yoga Style Guide, Your Guide to Popular Yoga Styles (2010). Retrieved October 2010 from http://yoga.about.com/od/typesofyoga/a/yogatypes.htm.

Tortora, Gerard J., and Bryan Derrickson. *Principles of Anatomy and Physiology*, 12th ed. Hoboken, NJ: John Wiley & Sons, 2009.

UPMC. Healthy Lifestyle Program. Retrieved May 2011 from www.upmc.com/Services/healthy-lifestyle-program/Pages/default.aspx

Posture and Its Impact on the Body

Key Terms

Alignment
Base of support
Center of gravity (center of weight)
Head-to-tail connection
Hinging
Hypertonic
Hypotonic
Ischemia
Kyphosis
Line of gravity
Lordosis
Optimal axis of rotation
Pain-spasm-pain cycle
Phasic muscles
Postural muscles
Posture
Scoliosis
Stacking the joints
Tensile stress
Tensegrity

Learning Objectives

After studying this chapter, the reader will have the information to:

1. Define balanced posture and explain its connection to career longevity.
2. Describe the components of balanced posture.
3. Explain the difference between postural and phasic muscles.
4. Explain how posture develops, including postural habits and their impact on the body.
5. Explain disorders and conditions associated with postural imbalances.
6. Evaluate what his or her balanced posture is.
7. Describe common postural imbalances.
8. Perform methods for improving personal postural balance and list additional healthful recommendations.
9. Integrate postural balance into performance of bodywork and activities of daily living.

"*A good stance and posture reflect a proper state of mind.*"
—Morihei Ueshiba

THE IMPORTANCE OF BALANCED POSTURE

Posture describes how people usually hold themselves while lying, sitting, standing, or moving. It also refers to how people hold their bodies when performing certain tasks. In the case of bodywork, this includes, of course, performing treatments. Therefore, posture involves the combination of the positions of all the joints and movements of all the muscles of the body at any given moment.

Bodywork practitioners often have many clients who present with pain from postural issues caused by muscular imbalances. In the case of bodywork that focuses on clients' energy fields, pain or other conditions result from energetic imbalances. However, since the body is viewed as having a physical component and an energetic component, the energetic imbalances can manifest as muscular pain and tension, and muscular pain and tension can contribute to energetic imbalances. In other words, the physical and energetic components of the body are intertwined. Therefore, no matter what type of bodywork the practitioner performs, he or she must have an understanding and an awareness of how clients move their bodies and how they carry themselves physically.

The same is true for all bodywork practitioners themselves. The nature of bodywork is physical, and many repetitive movements are involved. As such, the risk of injury is increased unless practitioners are aware of current and potential issues they may have with their own bodies. Therefore, an essential component of efficient body mechanics is proper postural alignment.

Overuse, misuse, and underuse of muscles can contribute to postural imbalances. Usually the body is forgiving and compensates fairly well with no symptoms. However, when postural imbalances start to cause pain, limitations, and restrictions, it is time for practitioners to pay attention and seek help. Optimally, if you have body awareness, are in tune with how your body feels, and have a balanced lifestyle, you never have to reach this point. Creating awareness of any imbalances and understanding the causes are the first essential steps to creating change for more efficient, pain-free movement. The starting point for all efficient movements is balanced posture.

DEFINING BALANCED POSTURE

When standing, balanced posture includes aligning the joints and having other parts of the body in the appropriate positions. **Alignment** means that the bones forming the joints are lined up in their proper, most efficient positions. The skeleton, specifically its joints, can easily maintain the body's balance and strength when it is in proper alignment.

Balanced posture includes the following (Fig. 3-1A, B, and C):

- Head centered over the trunk, with the chin level and the ears in line with the tips of the shoulders.
- Shoulders are not rotated forward, backward, nor elevated; they should be loose, with the scapulae flat.
- Arms hanging relaxed, with the palms of the hands facing the sides of the body.
- Chest held high but not exaggerated.
- Back maintains its natural curves; it is neither too flat nor too curved.
- Abdomen flat but not overly contracted.
- Hips tucked between extreme anterior and posterior tilt of the pelvis and in line with the knees.

- Knees straight and relaxed, neither flexed nor hyperextended, and in line with the ankles.
- Feet parallel, slightly apart, with the weight balanced evenly on the heels and the balls of the feet (bases of metatarsals I and V), like tripods.

BALANCED POSTURE AND CAREER LONGEVITY

Perhaps one of the most obvious reasons for having balanced posture is that it makes the person look better. This contributes significantly to the first impression clients will have about practitioners. Another reason is that it makes the practitioner feel better. The skeleton bears most of the body weight, taking stress off muscles and tendons. Muscles are then in their most efficient positions, joints are ready to move freely, and the body feels relaxed and stable overall.

Balanced posture contributes to career longevity because it enables you to work more proficiently. Joints, ligaments, and muscles are not strained by the positions of your body, and you have greater range of movement. Your trunk is open, allowing you to have sufficient air intake. Balanced posture also helps maintain good health. Imbalanced posture such as an exaggerated low back curve, makes practitioners more susceptible to conditions like backaches and, sometimes for female practitioners, painful menstruation. A forward head position leads to muscle tension and pain in the head, face, neck, shoulders, and arms. With a balanced posture, your upper body is in a position to receive the force generated by your lower body and then transfer it to the client's body. Having the joints in balanced positions decreases the risk of injury.

Balanced posture also encourages proper performance of techniques. The increased body awareness that balanced posture gives practitioners makes it easier for them to adjust any problems with body alignment as they work; this, in turn, allows them to perform the techniques more effectively. This can lead to greater client satisfaction with the treatments received and can increase client retention.

You should also note that by understanding your own postural imbalances, you will be better able to recognize postural imbalances in clients. Understanding the muscular and energetic changes that occur in the various postural imbalances gives you information on how to design client-centered treatments that address clients' specific needs. This, too, can lead to greater client satisfaction and increase client retention.

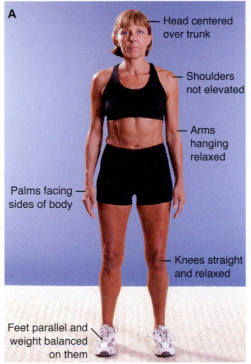

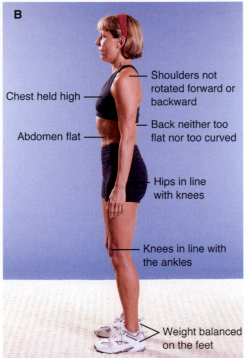

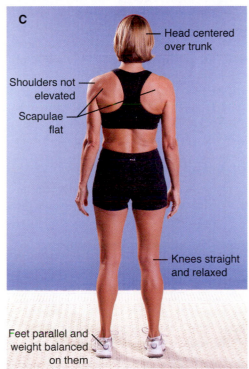

FIGURE 3-1 Balanced posture. **(A)** Anterior view. **(B)** Lateral view. **(C)** Posterior view.

BALANCED POSTURE

In order to determine their own balanced postures, practitioners need to understand the factors that affect posture. These include gravity, the body's center of gravity, the joint axes, the base of support, and a balance of strength and length of muscles. By understanding these concepts, you can strive for maximal physiological and biomechanical efficiency so you can minimize stress and strain on your body.

COMPONENTS OF BALANCED POSTURE

As mentioned, the components of balanced posture include center of gravity, base of support, and skeletal alignment and muscular support. Each of these is discussed in detail in the following sections.

Center of Gravity

Balanced posture involves the alignment and position of the body in relation to gravity. *Gravity* is defined as the force exerted by the Earth on objects in its vicinity. Because it is part of everyday life, some may not think of gravity as a force; they may just take it for granted. However, your musculoskeletal system must work hard against the pull of gravity to allow you to stand, sit, and move. Take the example of standing up from a sitting position versus sitting down from a standing position. Standing up is harder to do because you are fighting gravity; sitting is easier to do because you are simply allowing gravity to pull you down, although you are using a certain amount of muscular contraction to control how fast and how far down you sit.

Every living being has a **center of gravity (center of weight),** which is the point in the body where the

weight is concentrated. Ideally, when you are standing still, your weight is concentrated in your pelvic region, or lowermost part of your trunk. When your body's weight is appropriately centered in the pelvic region, your body is at its most stable. This stability allows your strength to come up from your legs, through your trunk, out through your shoulders, down your arms, and out through your hands as you perform techniques. This is shown in Figure 3-2A for practitioners who work on clients lying on a massage table, in Figure 3-2B for those who work on clients sitting in massage chairs, and in Figure 3-2C for those who work on clients lying on a futon.

Without this stability, the practitioner must use strength mostly from her shoulder and upper back muscles, risking injury to them and their associated joints. The **line of gravity** is one that can be visualized passing vertically through the body, from the head to the center of gravity in the lower trunk or pelvic region, down through the feet. Ideally, the line of gravity travels through the ear, tip of the shoulder, lateral hip, lateral knee, and lateral ankle for treatments performed on a massage table (Fig. 3-3A). For treatments performed on a futon, the line of gravity travels through the ear, tip of the shoulder, lateral hip, and lateral knee (Fig. 3-3B).

Base of Support

Base of support refers to the areas of contact between a person and the ground. When you are standing upright, you have two points of contact—your feet. The structure of the ankle and foot make them ideal for supporting your body's weight (Fig. 3-4). There are seven tarsal bones, five metatarsals, and fourteen phalanges. Metatarsal I is thicker than the other metatarsals because it bears more weight. In fact, the ball of the foot is the base of metatarsal I.

The foot has two arches that are held in place by ligaments and tendons: the *longitudinal arch*, which consists of a medial portion along the medial side of the sole of the foot and a lateral portion along the lateral side of the sole, and a *transverse arch*, which curves across the sole between the medial and lateral aspects. The arches enable the foot to support the body's weight, provide an optimal distribution of body weight over the tissues of the foot, and provide leverage while walking. The arches are not rigid. Instead, they give as weight is applied and spring back when the weight is lifting, which makes the arches function as shock absorbers.

During locomotion, in addition to being a shock absorber, the foot acts as a lever, lifting and pushing the body away from the ground for

Body Awareness

Keeping your back straight, start to sit down on the floor from a standing position but stop halfway. Place your hands on top of your thighs so you do not reach for the floor to balance yourself. How long can you stay in this position? Do you feel yourself getting heavier and heavier as your muscles strive to keep you upright? Can you feel how your core, hip, and thigh muscles are contracting against the force of gravity?

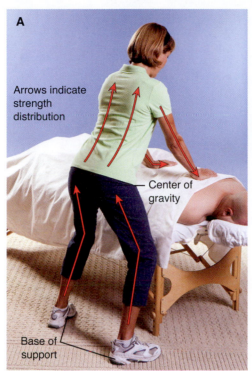

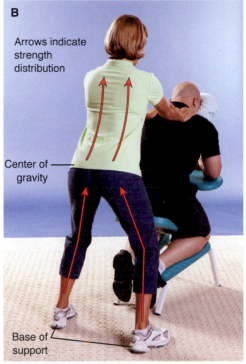

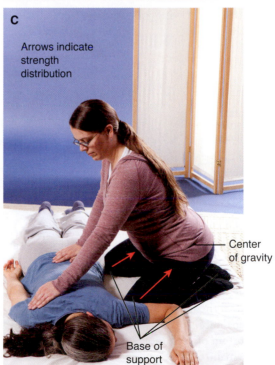

FIGURE 3-2 Practitioner's strength distribution with a stable center of gravity **(A)** working on a massage table, **(B)** working on a massage chair, **(C)** working on a futon.

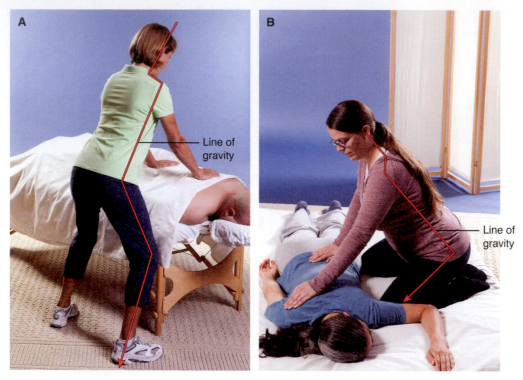

FIGURE 3-3 Line of gravity through a practitioner **(A)** working on a massage table, **(B)** working on a futon.

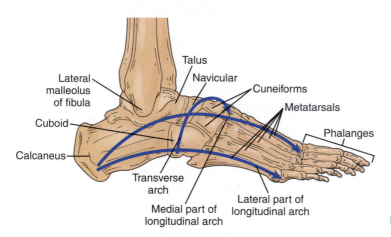

FIGURE 3-4 Bones and arches of the foot.

movement. When you are standing still, your foot helps control the movements of your lower body to maintain balance.

The bottom of each foot is actually a tripod, with the three main contact points being the calcaneus and the heads of metatarsals I and V (Fig. 3-5). Normally the heel carries about 60% of the body, with the ball of the foot (head of metatarsal I) carrying the majority and metatarsal V (and the toes) carrying the minority of the other 40% (Tortora and Derrickson, 2009).

When standing, it is important to use the entire plantar surface of the foot. Distributing your body's weight over the entire foot improves balance and postural alignment. Foot soreness and pain usually result from supporting the body weight with only one part of the foot. For example, when a person wears high-heeled shoes, the distribution of weight changes so that the ball of the foot and the toes carry up to 80% and the heel only 20%. As a result, the fat pads at the ball of the foot are damaged, joint pain develops, and structural changes in bones may occur (Tortora and Derrickson, 2009).

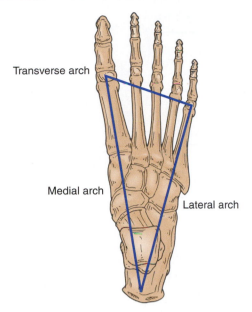

FIGURE 3-5 Tripod on the bottom of the foot.

Additionally, when a person wears high heels, the joints and muscles of the foot and lower leg are forced to not only bear the full weight of the body but to also keep it in balance. The center of gravity is off balance, increasing the stress on these joints and muscles and thus increasing the chance of injury. The pain can travel up through the rest of the body and cause knee, hip, back, and neck pain, and even headaches. This is because the muscles in these areas need to contract to compensate for the unbalanced posture (Muscolino, 2011).

Other seemingly small, insignificant imbalances can lead to major changes in the entire body. For example, if the feet are not sufficiently strong to keep the body in balance and the shins in line with the feet, the knees can change their position. This can affect the hips, which, in turn, will affect the spine, which can then affect head position. Each joint in this chain reaction will then be limited in its actions, especially when the imbalance is coupled with tight muscles on one side of the joint and weak muscles on the other.

Another example of what may seem like a minor imbalance involves a unilateral (meaning on one side of the body) pelvic tilt. This can be caused by having one arch of the foot lower than the other, greater angulation of the knee on one side, an increase or decrease in the angle on the neck of the femur, a rotation of the femoral shaft (which can make the knee point laterally or medially), and a different size and shape of one ilium as compared with the opposite one.

Having an imbalance in the body is comparable to a car with low tire pressure. The tread begins wearing unevenly, and sooner or later, the vehicle will begin to shake. As the vibration makes its way through the suspension system, the tie rods start working loose. If left unfixed, damage spreads to the motor mounts. Eventually, the engine can even sputter to a halt. Although the low tire was the root of the problem, it is tempting to blame the engine because the car no longer runs. In reality, a deflated tire started a chain of events that show up as compensations elsewhere and end up affecting the entire car.

Skeletal Alignment and Muscular Support

The individual bones and the skeleton as a whole have curves that, with the assistance of muscles, allow for balance and movement. As seen in Figure 3-6, the axial skeleton is basically a structure in which segments are stacked—the vertebrae on top of each other (with disks in between to cushion and absorb shock), the ribs on top of each other, and the skull on top of them all. The appendicular skeleton consists of structures in which the segments are lined up with each other. In the upper extremity, the humerus is lined up with the shoulder girdle; the radius and ulna are lined up with the humerus; and the carpals, metacarpals, and digits are lined up with the radius and ulna. In the lower extremity, the femur is lined up with the hip girdle; the tibia and fibula are lined up with the femur; and the tarsals, metatarsals, and digits are lined up with the tibia and fibula.

The vertebral column has four normal curves (Fig. 3-7). The cervical and lumbar curves are *convex* (bulging outward), and the thoracic and sacral curves are *concave* (cupping inward). The curves of the vertebral column increase its strength,

Body Awareness

Take your shoes off and look at the soles. Is one area more worn than the other? For example, is the lateral side of the heel or the medial surface of the shoe more worn down? If so, it is an indicator that you are not using the entire plantar surface of your foot when standing and walking.

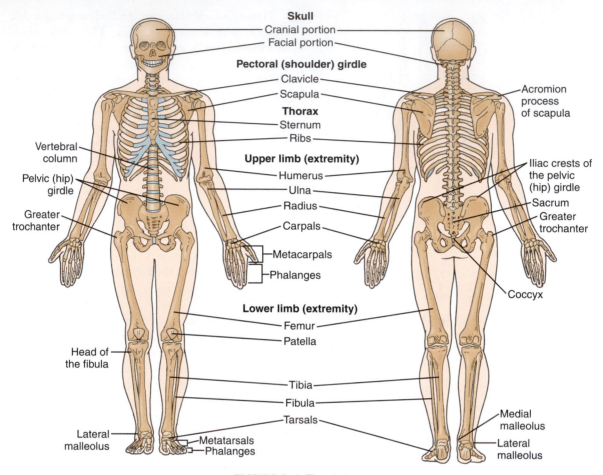

FIGURE 3-6 The skeleton.

help maintain balance in the upright position, absorb shocks while walking, and help protect the vertebrae from fracture.

During development, the fetus has only a single anteriorly concave curve. At about 3 months after birth, when the infant begins to hold his or her head up, the cervical curve develops. When the child sits up, stands, and walks, the lumbar curve develops. All the curves are fully developed by age 10, and they are the result of gravity's effect on the body. So in reality, your posture actually starts developing shortly after birth. How this posture develops can affect what happens in your body later in life. This is discussed in more detail in the "Development of Posture" section.

Muscles work most efficiently when each section of the axial skeleton is stacked vertically in proper alignment and when each joint, whether it is in the axial or appendicular skeleton, is aligned along its **optimal axis of rotation**. *Optimal axis of rotation* means the position in which the joint achieves its greatest range of motion with the most economic muscular effort.

These proper alignments evenly and symmetrically distribute the work of the postural muscles (discussed in the "Postural and Phasic Muscles" section) and reduce the amount of contraction necessary to maintain balance, freeing other muscles to move the body with ease and efficiency. This is crucial for healthy and efficient body mechanics. However, note that during prolonged standing, the average person shifts position frequently. Even when a person is standing quietly with no perceptible movements, tension in the muscles is constantly changed. This causes very slight, normal adjustments in weight distribution called *postural sway*.

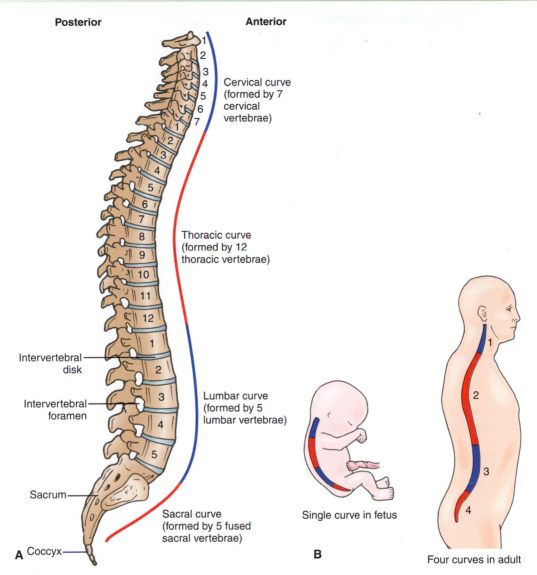

Posterior   **Anterior**

Cervical curve
(formed by 7
cervical
vertebrae)

Thoracic curve
(formed by 12
thoracic vertebrae)

Intervertebral
disk

Intervertebral
foramen

Lumbar curve
(formed by 5
lumbar vertebrae)

Sacrum

Sacral curve
(formed by 5 fused
sacral vertebrae)

A Coccyx

Single curve in fetus

B

Four curves in adult

FIGURE 3-7 Curves of the vertebral column. **(A)** Right lateral view showing four normal curves. **(B)** Fetal and adult curves.

Whenever one part of the body moves out of line, the center of gravity shifts in the direction of that section's movement, and another section must adjust in the opposite direction to bring the center of gravity back over the base. When a person is standing, postural muscles use small amounts of contraction to stabilize the body upright in gravity by continually repositioning the body's weight over the mechanical balance point. When a person stands on the heels, the center of gravity should be adjusted at the ankles, knees, and hips without disturbing the alignment of the various sections. If the backward adjustment is made at the waist, as is frequently the case, the entire alignment is affected and strain is felt in the lower back. The same principle is true in counterbalancing the added weight in the abdomen such as occurs with weight gain or pregnancy. Figure 3-8A shows how much pressure is placed on the spine from various postures. Figure 3-8B shows that for every inch the head moves forward of its normal posture, the compressive forces on the lower neck increase by 10 to 20 pounds (Kapandji, 2008; Todd, 2008).

Focus on Wellness

Dr. Lulu Sweigard researched, developed, and conceived the protocol of constructive rest position (CRP), a means of resting that creates a more efficient posture. For example, lying supine changes the orientation toward gravity by spreading the body in a horizontal alignment and having the floor support the large surface area of the body, thus helping to release tension. In CRP, it is possible to completely stop moving, so as to give up previously learned habits that you want to replace with more functional ones.

When to use CRP:

- If you feel the need to regenerate and revitalize yourself
- Before going to bed, to release tension and engage a deeper, more refreshing sleep
- In the morning, to enhance energy and coordination through the day
- Prior to, in between, or after a treatment session(s)

Try this:

- While lying supine, arms relaxed overhead, knees flexed with legs hip-width apart, feet flat on the floor, visualize the spine lengthening to send the sacrum toward your heels, the central axis growing out through the top of your head, and your trunk sinking toward the front of the spine (toward the floor).
- Check your body in its entirety, allowing yourself to be fully supported by the ground beneath you.
- You may even think of every part of your body as being fluid, like water, flowing outward and downward into the ground.
- If this doesn't work easily for you, try tensing each part of your body as hard as you can and then releasing all effort in that part completely.
- Go through each and every part of your body, beginning with your head and moving on down through your toes.

Proper alignment is also important because the body naturally wants to keep the head up and the eyes level. If postural distortions occur anywhere in the body, the entire balance is adjusted to maintain upright posture and keep the eyes horizontal. For example, if one vertebral segment between the levels of L1 and L5 becomes tipped or rotated, the segments above and below must tip or twist in the opposite direction to provide counterbalance and maintain the eye position and center of gravity. As would be expected, the next segments up and down also adjust and the eventual result is distortion from head to toe.

Tensegrity is the term for something happening in one part of the body affecting what is happening in another part of the body. *Tensegrity* is derived from the words *tension* and *integrity* and means that the integrity (stability) of these structures depends on the balance of tension within them.

All structures are supported by a balance between tension and compression, or a balance between "push" and "pull." For example, when you sit on a chair, your body is applying a compressive force on the chair's seat. In order to remain stable and not collapse, the chair's legs and seat have tension within them. This tension is distributed throughout the area of the seat and down through the legs of the chair to the ground.

Another example is thinking of the body like a balloon, which is a classic tensegrity structure. The skin is the tension part—it pulls inward to keep the inner contents of the body from spilling out. The body's internal structures are comparable to the air inside the balloon. Both the air in the balloon and the body's internal structures are the compression part—pushing out against the skin of the balloon and the skin of the body. The skin pulls in until it balances the air pushing out, and that determines the size of the balloon. The skin of the body balances the internal structures pushing out, and that determines the size of the body.

Replace the air with a group of rods, and put elastic bands in place of the balloon "skin"; the result is a classic tensegrity structure. Substitute bones for the rods and the fascial membranes (connective tissue that surrounds organs and muscles) for the balloon skin and elastic bands, and the result is structural tensegrity.

When thinking of the body in these terms—hard, inelastic bone along with soft, elastic tissues—it is easy to see that if there is a change in how the structures in one area of the body fit together, then there will be compensatory changes, occurring like a chain reaction, in another part of the body. In other words, if one area of the body starts pushing, another area of the body will start pulling; if one area of the body starts pulling, another area will start pushing. See Figure 3-9A for an illustration of balanced posture and Figure 3-9B for unbalanced, compensating posture in terms of tensegrity (Flemons, 2007; Kinesis, 2010).

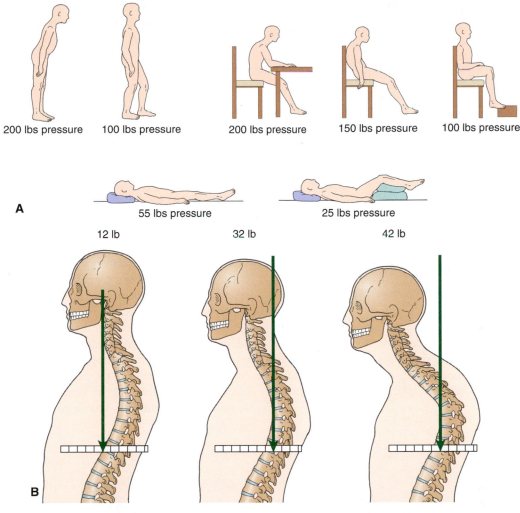

FIGURE 3-8 (A) Pressure placed on the spine from various postures. **(B)** Increased compressive forces on the lower neck by forward head posture.

Deviations in balanced posture do not lead to pain or injury if they occur once in a while. However, frequent or chronic deviations will lead to muscle tension, pain, and injury. In slumped postures, contractions in neck and back muscles increase to offset the force of gravity; the body is working against gravity instead of with it to keep the head up and the eyes level. Over time, this can lead to chronic neck and back tension, which is why this is not an efficient posture in which to stand, sit, or perform bodywork. If working in an asymmetric stance, such as with an elevated shoulder or swayed hip, the body's muscles will be working harder to maintain balance, which makes performing bodywork less efficient. Figures 3-10A, B, and C show the effect of inefficient postures while working on a massage table; Figures 3-10D, E, and F

show the effect of inefficient postures while working on a futon.

POSTURAL AND PHASIC MUSCLES

When it comes to posture and movement, there are two major categories of muscles: **postural** and **phasic muscles**. Postural muscles are used to maintain

What Do You Think?

Were you aware that you have a center of gravity? If so, how do you think of it? If not, how do you think of it now?

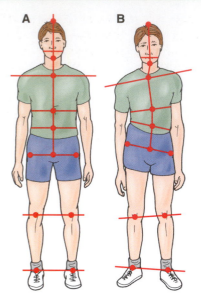

FIGURE 3-9 (A) Balanced posture. **(B)** Unbalanced, compensating posture.

the body's posture. Phasic muscles are used to move the body. Sometimes the same muscles can actually perform both functions. The main postural and phasic muscles of the body are shown in Figure 3-11.

Postural muscles are used for stamina and endurance. They tend to be smaller in structure than phasic muscles but are also physiologically different. They have a higher concentration of slow twitch, also known as *type 1 muscle fibers*. In these fibers, cellular metabolism is geared toward long periods of contraction before fatiguing. Thus they can hold the body up against gravity for long periods of time. If stimulated to respond quickly, they do not produce bursts of strength and they may end up cramping. They are the deliberate, slow, steady muscles that require more time to respond than do phasic muscles.

If posture is not balanced, postural muscles must increase their contractions to ensure stability. Postural muscles tend to shorten and have increased motor tone when under strain. This is referred to as being *locked short*. However, some postural muscles that are under low levels of constant strain, such as the cervical erector spinae, increase in muscle tone while remaining elongated. This is referred to as *locked long*. When either of these situations happens, trigger points and additional connective tissue can develop in the muscle in an effort to stabilize the body in gravity. The connective tissue freezes the body in dysfunctional positions, because connective tissue cannot actively contract and lengthen like muscle tissue.

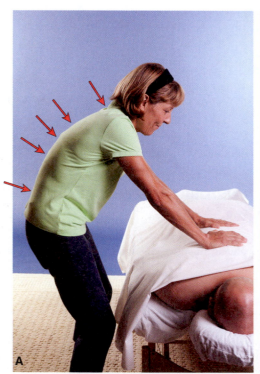

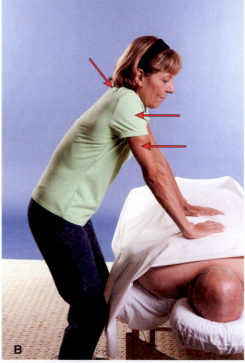

FIGURE 3-10 (A) Slumped posture. **(B)** Elevated shoulder.

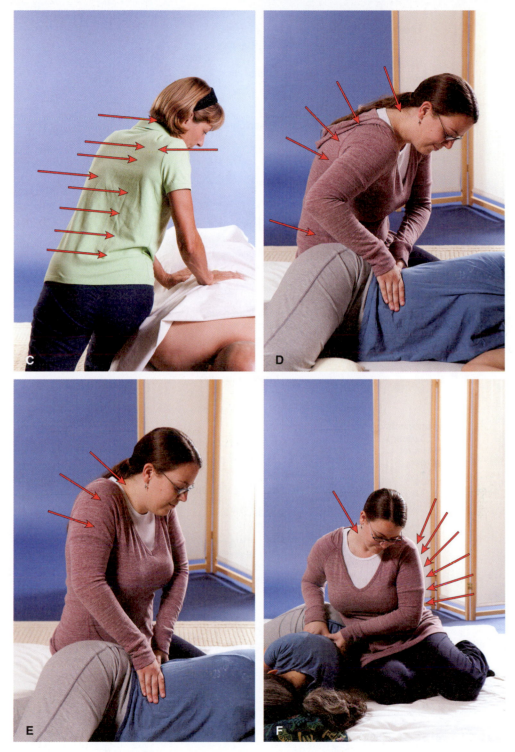

FIGURE 3-10 cont'd **(C)** Swayed hip. **(D)** Slumped posture. **(E)** Elevated shoulder. **(F)** Swayed hip.

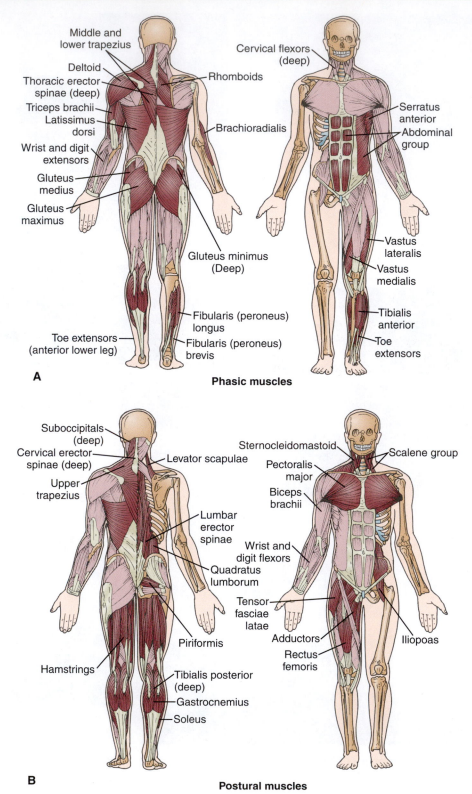

A **Phasic muscles**

B **Postural muscles**

FIGURE 3-11 Main postural and phasic muscles of the body.

Additionally, when postural muscles become fatigued because of increased contractions, they are more susceptible to becoming **hypertonic,** which means excessively tight and shortened. This can be seen when a person is really tired. His head falls forward due to neck muscle fatigue. However, the posterior neck muscles will become hypertonic and contract to pull his head back into an aligned position. This muscle interplay is responsible for the bouncing head seen in people who are falling asleep while standing or sitting. Eventually, if fatigued muscles are not allowed to rest and recover, this can lead to a heightened level of activity in the muscle, and **ischemia** (decreased blood flow into tissues), spasm, and weakness result. This can be the beginning of something called the **pain-spasm-pain cycle**. In this situation, muscles react to pain by contracting, causing them to spasm, which creates more pain. The muscles respond by contracting even more, causing more spasms and creating more pain. This catch-22 situation rarely stops on its own and usually requires intervention such as bodywork or medication to halt it.

Phasic muscles are designed to generate larger amounts of force in brief spurts and are usually under conscious control. They contract quickly but tire quickly. They have a higher concentration of fast twitch muscle fibers, known as *type 2 muscle fibers*, for rapid contraction of the muscle. In these fibers, cellular metabolism is geared toward short, concentrated bursts of contraction before fatiguing. The muscles are larger in diameter than postural muscles. Fatigue in these muscles leads them to becoming **hypotonic**, which means they have a deficient amount of muscle contraction, leading to weakness. They also tend to lengthen and become locked long.

Phasic muscles are usually inhibited or become weaker when postural muscles are locked short. However, sometimes phasic muscles can become chronically shortened in response to repetitive motions or to a sudden postural change that causes the muscles to assist the postural muscles in maintaining balance such as a fall or near fall, an automobile accident, or some other trauma. In this case, these muscles end up being locked short.

Musculotendinous junction problems are more common in phasic muscles. *Musculotendinous* refers to the connection of a muscle and its tendon. The four most common problems are the following:

- Microtearing of the muscle fibers at the musculotendinous junction

- Tendon disorders (see the box "Body Awareness")
- Adherence of muscles and tendons to underlying or surrounding tissue
- Bursitis

In order to have optimal posture and efficient muscular contraction and movements, it is important to ensure that muscle groups are in balance. The abdominal muscle group should have equal strength with the erector spinae group; the hip flexors should be equal in strength to the hip extensors; the quadriceps group should be equal in strength to the hamstrings. If one group is weaker than its antagonist group, then imbalanced posture, muscle and tendon issues, and injuries are likely to develop.

Myth: By the time people become adults, their postural and movement patterns are set.

FACT: It is never too late to change habits and patterns. As human beings, we have the most flexible nervous system of any species. We have the power to change seemingly fixed patterns of the body and the mind. Even an elderly person who has never exercised or developed body awareness can still develop his body; learn to release tension; and increase strength, endurance, and coordination.

Body Awareness

Tendinitis is an injury to a tendon that involves an inflammatory response. However, the **tensile stress** (ability to withstand tension along its length) of a tendon can be more than twice that of its associated muscle, so they are rarely torn. Ruptures usually occur at the musculotendinous junction or in the muscle fibers. Tendinosis, on the other hand, is an injury to a tendon that does not involve an inflammatory response and is generally related to collagen degeneration. Tendon overuse dysfunctions show that most overuse tendon pathologies lack inflammatory cells and instead involve a breakdown in the collagen matrix, so the term *tendinosis* is usually more applicable. (Practitioners should note that the term *tendinosis* does not specify the pathological process, only that the tendon is dysfunctional.)

Continued

> Overuse tendon disorders can take a long time to heal due to the slow rebuilding of collagen. If tendon fiber tearing (tendinitis) is the primary problem, the tissue would heal rather quickly as it moves through the various stages of inflammation and tissue-repair process. Collagen rebuilding is slow, and tendinosis can become chronic or recurring (Lowe, 2009).

DEVELOPMENT OF POSTURE

Posture is not something determined overnight. In fact, it starts in infancy. A newborn baby has minimal patterned movements. As the baby grows and develops, movement tones and strengthens her body cumulatively and forms patterns that progressively become deep-rooted over time. Infants gradually navigate more and more of their inner and outer worlds with creative and often spontaneous movements as they explore. Movement shapes their muscular and postural patterns until they become their characteristic way of holding and moving themselves.

Children learn their habitual styles of posturing and movement from their parents, mostly unconsciously. Similar postural patterns within families are so common that many may think posture is inherited, but it is, in fact, acquired. When looking at photos taken throughout people's lives, sometimes the same posture can be seen in all family members. Sometimes the same posture can be seen, for example, in the same man at the age of 60 and at the age of 20.

Congenital musculoskeletal conditions can affect posture. A person can be born with certain physical or structural conditions that cause his posture to develop in a certain way. For example, osteogenesis imperfecta (OI) is a disorder in which the bones are particularly fragile due to abnormal collagen formation. Because of this, the person may not grow to his full height, or his skeleton may twist and turn as he grows. Everyone has one leg that is slightly shorter than the other; usually this is not an issue in postural development. However, if one leg is significantly shorter than the other, then the person's posture will be considerably different from those whose leg lengths are almost the same.

Other physical conditions that can affect posture can develop throughout life. Various conditions may exaggerate the normal curves of the vertebral column. **Kyphosis** (Fig. 3-12A) is an increase in the thoracic curve. In the elderly, degeneration of the intervertebral disks leads to kyphosis. It can also be caused by poor posture and osteoporosis. **Lordosis** (Fig. 3-12B) is an increase in the lumbar curve. It may result from increased weight of the abdomen as occurs in pregnancy, extreme obesity, and osteoporosis or poor posture. **Scoliosis** (Fig. 3-12C), the most common of the abnormal curves, is a lateral curvature of the vertebral column. It may result from congenitally malformed vertebrae, chronic sciatica, paralysis of muscles on one side of the vertebral column, one leg being shorter than the other, or poor posture.

Emotions can also play a role in the development of posture. If children are in a happy home where self-expression is encouraged, they tend to develop tall and open postures. If, however, they are in a home in which emotions and thoughts are oppressed, or they are being abused in other ways, then their posture may be more shrunken inward with rounded shoulders and upper backs. People with a poor self-image carry themselves vastly different from those with a good self-image (Chaitow, 2000).

Body Awareness

This exercise is designed to explore family patterns and how they have influenced your postural tendencies. Write down your answers to the following questions. Another option is to ask your parents and grandparents (if possible) to answer the questions, and then compare your answers. After finishing this book, come back and look at your answers again to see if you would still answer the questions the same way.

- What skills do you have that your parents and grandparents also have? Are your skills mental, physical, intuitive, artistic, and so forth? How do you use your body with these skills?
- What skills do you have that your parents and grandparents do not have?
- What skills did your parents and grandparents have that you do not have?
- What was the level of physical activity for your parents and grandparents? Is your level of physical activity greater or lesser? How do your activities differ from theirs?

- How is your lifestyle more or less physically challenging than your parents' and grandparents'? More or less mentally challenging? More or less emotionally challenging?
- What were the postures of your parents and grandparents like? How is yours similar or different?
- Are you now able to see family patterns? If so, which patterns do you think are healthy and which patterns are not? How do you think your family patterns affect your posture and your level of physical activity?
- What other factors do you think affect or could affect your posture? Some of these could include self-esteem, self-image, injuries, interests, and so forth.

Children who are physically active may develop postures that are different from those who are not. Athletics and other activities that require movement such as bicycling, hiking, and playing outdoor games encourage the development of stronger muscles and more balanced posture. These can be carried into and through adulthood if the person remains active.

POSTURAL HABITS AND THE IMPACT ON THE BODY

Postural habits are patterns of movement that people repeat over and over again, often without being aware that they are using them. These include the way they move when walking, postures they hold when standing, and gestures made when talking. Bodywork practitioners are likely to transfer many of their everyday postural habits into their working environment. For example, when interviewing a new client, they probably sit the same way that they sit when watching television, or they probably adjust the height of a massage table in the same posture they use to take clothes out of the dryer. Becoming aware of postural habits is an essential step toward understanding how to improve postural balance when performing bodywork.

Some of the factors that contribute to postural habits are age, weight, self-consciousness (e.g., people who are tall may try to disguise their height by slumping), occupational conditions (e.g., a mail carrier who carries a heavy mail sack), and habitual movement patterns. These include patterns developed in response to environmental factors, such as having to bend over a low sink while washing dishes

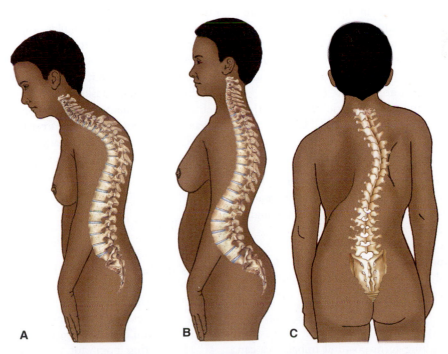

FIGURE 3-12 (A) Kyphosis. **(B)** Lordosis. **(C)** Scoliosis. *Used with permission from Gylys, B. A., Wedding, M.E. Medical Terminology Systems: A Body Systems Approach. Philadelphia: FA Davis, 2009.*

(optimal working surfaces should be at elbow height) or talking on the phone by cradling it between the head and one shoulder instead of using a headset. Sometimes postural habits develop out of a simple lack of body awareness, such as always watching television or studying while sitting in a slumped posture.

The body makes numerous changes in postures to compensate for the movements necessary to perform tasks each day. For example, the shoulders of a cyclist are medially rotated (rounded). Someone who carries her infant on one hip hikes that hip up high. This is normal, and if other pathological conditions are not present, the compensation is unlikely to be a problem. However, if there is an injury, or a certain position is maintained for a prolonged period or a body area is overused, the body may not be able to efficiently return to a balanced posture.

DISORDERS AND CONDITIONS ASSOCIATED WITH POSTURAL IMBALANCES

Disorders and conditions associated with postural imbalances may arise because of a person's lifestyle. For example, people who sit for long hours on the job are susceptible to a number of misalignments, especially when they sit in imbalanced postures. They may have tight hip flexor muscles and hamstrings and a tight pectoralis major, along with weak back and abdominal muscles. Extra weight in the abdominal area from obesity or pregnancy puts additional strain on the lumbar spine.

Postural imbalances can pull joints out of their normal, healthy positions, placing additional stress on surrounding structures and tissues. These can manifest as the following:

- Stress on vertebrae and spinal ligaments
- Intervertebral disk compression and herniation (outward bulging of the disk, possibly impinging on spinal nerves)
- Irritation or injury to spinal nerves
- Stress fractures
- Vertebral subluxation (partial dislocation)
- Muscular cramps, spasms, chronic aches and pains
- Scoliosis

Additionally, long-term postural imbalances can cause a change in proprioception, throwing off a person's sense of where his center is. This can affect balance and fluidity of movement, which are detrimental to the performance of bodywork.

DETERMINING BALANCED POSTURE

Balanced posture involves aligning the body between postural extremes, where the body is at its strongest position. The purpose of determining your balanced posture is to ensure your most optimal stability and poise so that your muscles can function the most efficiently.

As discussed previously, any deviation from this position usually reflects lifestyle, habits, injuries, and so forth. However, these deviations may also constitute postural imbalance, which can lead to various conditions such as problems with the muscular, skeletal, and nervous systems; fatigue; overuse syndromes and injury; to name a few. All of these factor into your career longevity. Remember, these issues do not happen overnight. They may actually start from birth, then be made worse by environmental factors, injury, disease, trauma, and from unhealthy choices in taking care of your body.

Another consideration is that not everyone is built the same. Some people have naturally large bodies with big bones, slower metabolisms, and higher body fat percentages than others. Some are naturally very thin, have low body fat percentages, high metabolisms, and longer, leaner builds. Yet others are naturally muscular with athletic builds, low body fat percentages, and metabolisms that are higher or lower than others. However, no matter what a person's build, it is musculoskeletal balance that enables efficient movement, protects supporting structures against injury, and enhances career longevity.

No one is absolutely balanced. The objective is to come as close to it as is comfortable. The goal is for you to get a feel for what balanced posture looks and feels like in your body. Before you begin to do anything, including sleeping or especially working, it is important for you to get into your starting balanced posture. As you work, most of your movements should be within a comfortable range. It forms the basis of your body mechanics, and you should return to it as often as possible for rest and recovery during your treatment sessions. By having body awareness, you can immediately correct your position if you deviate from your balanced posture.

The starting point for you is to do an honest evaluation of your posture. This can be done with the Postural Evaluation Form, shown in Figure 3-13. Either using a mirror or, better yet, having someone take a photo of your posture and attaching the photo to the form in the area labeled "Before Photo," you can use the checklist and ratings on the form to assess your posture before you work to improve it. Another option is to have another person make an assessment of your posture; this can be a more objective process. Ways to improve posture are discussed next and in the section "Ways to Improve Postural Balance." Once these improvements are made, you can take another photo and attach it to the form in the area labeled "After Photo," which is discussed later.

You can also secure a heavy string to the ceiling and hang a weight at the end of it. This is called a *plumb line*, which is used to determine how straight something is vertically. Stand so your nose is lined up with the string; then look in the mirror or have an anterior-view picture taken. Note if your shoulders are leaning to one side or if more of your body is on one side of the plumb line. If your body is symmetrical on both sides of the plumb line, then your posture is balanced.

You can also turn to a lateral view and line up the middle of your shoulder down to your feet with the plumb line. This gives a graphic representation of how your body weight is distributed in front and

---

POSTURAL IMBALANCES

Name: _____

Before date: _____   After date: _____

Before photo:	After photo:

Before comments:		After comments:
_____	Forward head	_____
_____	Kyphosis	_____
_____	Med rot shoulders	_____
_____	Sunken chest	_____
_____	Lordosis	_____
_____	Flat back	_____
_____	Abdominal ptosis	_____
_____	Hyperextended knees	_____
_____	Winged scapulae	_____
_____	Scoliosis	_____

Key: 0, no imbalance   X, slight imbalance

XX, needs attention   XXX, severe

FIGURE 3-13 Postural evaluation form.

behind. It will also show you if you have any major deviations in spinal curvature or positioning of your hips. Examples of balanced postures are shown in Figure 3-14A and B.

It is best to always evaluate posture from at least two different angles. For example, posture may present as balanced posteriorly or anteriorly but not from the lateral view. Figure 3-15 shows this.

Once you determine what your posture looks and feels like, you can learn to feel what balanced posture is by trying the following suggested activities. If you must strain to achieve any of the positions, then that can signal postural imbalances that need to be worked on.

- One of the best ways is to experiment with various postural extremes. For example, while standing or lying supine, tilt your pelvis posteriorly and anteriorly before stopping in the middle at the "happy medium," or balanced position.
- Visualize the pelvis as a bucket filled to the brim with water. Arching the back too much (creating an anterior tilt) will spill the water from the front of the bucket. Flattening the low back into a posterior tilt will cause the water to run out the back

(as described by Deborah Ellison, PT, in her book *Biomechanics and Applied Kinesiology*).

- Sit in a high-backed chair so that you feel your shoulders and the back of your head against the seat. Do not flatten your lumbar spine into the seat. You can choose to stand against a wall instead, with your gluteals, scapulae, and back of your head touching the wall. Slide your hand between your lumbar region and the wall to feel the natural curvature of the spine. Stand up if you are sitting down and walk away holding that posture. If you are against a wall, just walk away while holding that posture.
- While standing normally, moving from your feet up or from your head down, do the following checklist:
  - Keep your head level, with your forehead and chin perpendicular to the floor.
  - Retract your chin.
  - Keep your chest up and open.
  - Breathe naturally.
  - Relax your shoulders down and roll them back, and make sure your clavicles are parallel to the floor.

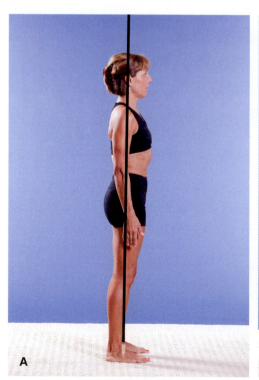
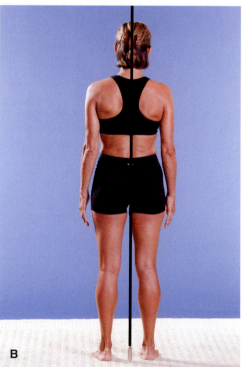

FIGURE 3-14 Balanced posture. **(A)** Lateral. **(B)** Posterior.

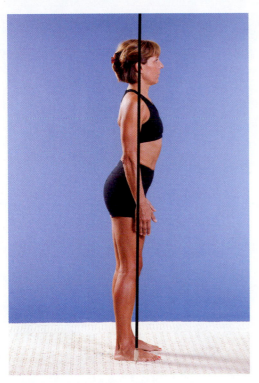

FIGURE 3-15 Posture not balanced from lateral view.

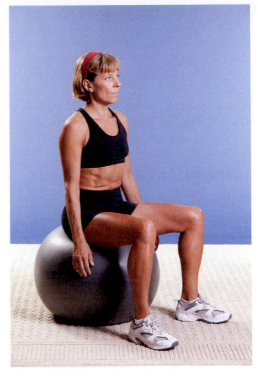

FIGURE 3-16 Finding balanced posture while sitting on a stability ball.

- Retract and depress your scapulae.
- Set your pelvis between anterior and posterior tilt.
- Comfortably contract your abdominal muscles.
- Review the natural curvatures of your spine; make sure they are not flattened or exaggerated.
- Your upper arms should hang down at your sides with your elbows slightly flexed, wrists straight, and forearms comfortably close to halfway between supination and pronation.
- Perform knee bends and end with soft knees.
- Visualize your feet as tripods centering your body and connecting to the floor.
- Check that your ears, shoulders, ribs, hips, knees, and ankles are aligned and that your feet are parallel to each other.
- While sitting on an exercise ball, also known as a *stability, balance,* or *physio ball* (see Fig. 3-16), moving from your feet up or from your head down, do the following checklist:
  - Keep your head level, with your forehead and chin perpendicular to the floor.
  - Retract your chin.
  - Keep your chest up and open.
  - Breathe naturally.

- Relax your shoulders down and roll them back, and make sure your clavicles are parallel to the floor.
- Retract and depress your scapulae.
- Set your pelvis between anterior and posterior tilt.
- Comfortably contract your abdominal muscles.
- Review the natural curvatures of your spine; make sure they are not flattened or exaggerated.
- Your upper arms should hang down at your sides with your elbows slightly flexed, wrists straight, and forearms comfortably close to halfway between supination and pronation.
- Visualize your feet as tripods centering your body and connecting to the floor.
- Check that your ears, shoulders, ribs, and hips are aligned.
- Check that your knees and ankles are aligned and that your feet are parallel to each other.

What Do You Think?

Which of the preceding methods to find your balanced posture appeal to you? Why do they appeal to you and not the other ones?

POSTURAL IMBALANCES

According to Dr. Leon Chaitow, certain muscles of the body tend to shorten in response to stress whereas others tend to elongate and become weak. As a result, the body tends to mold itself more easily into certain postures than others. Generally, a chain reaction evolves in which certain muscle groups shorten and others weaken.

COMMON POSTURAL IMBALANCES

The following are the most common postural imbalances that practitioners and clients are likely to have. In each case, the muscles that will be locked short (tight in a shortened position) and the muscles that will be locked long (tight in an elongated position) are identified. The muscles listed are not necessarily all-inclusive; more muscles may be affected depending on severity of the condition. The goal is to identify the shortened structures and release them, and follow this with reeducation in the use of the body. These are covered in the "Ways to Improve Postural Balance" section.

Sometimes more than one imbalanced posture can be present, so take into account the muscles associated with those other postures. Also, postural imbalances ultimately affect the body as a whole, since everything in the body is connected. Here are the most common postural imbalances:

- Round (medially rotated) shoulders (Fig. 3-17). The acromion processes of the shoulders are held forward and the scapulae may be protruding. This is usually accompanied by a forward head, sunken chest, and a slumped posture (kyphosis).
  - Muscles locked short: extensors of the head and neck, pectoralis major, anterior deltoid, subscapularis, latissimus dorsi, teres major, serratus anterior, abdominals
  - Muscles locked long: flexors of the head and neck, middle trapezius, posterior deltoid, rhomboids, infraspinatus, teres minor, thoracic/lumbar erector spinae group
- Slumped posture (kyphosis; Fig. 3-18). This position is often associated with other postural imbalances, such as forward head and rounded shoulders (sunken chest). Muscles involved may be the same as for round shoulders.
  - Muscles locked short: extensors of the head and neck, pectoralis major, anterior deltoid, subscapularis, latissimus dorsi, teres major, serratus anterior, abdominals

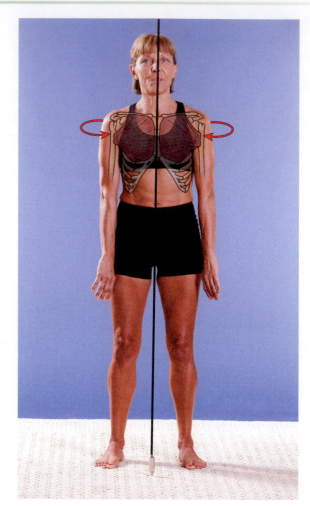

FIGURE 3-17 Round (medially rotated) shoulders.

  - Muscles locked long: flexors of the head and neck, middle trapezius, posterior deltoid, rhomboids, infraspinatus, teres minor, thoracic/lumbar erector spinae group
- Anterior tilt of the pelvis (lordosis; Fig. 3-19). This position is often accompanied by a protruding abdomen and is associated with knee hyperextension.
  - Muscles locked short: lumbar erector spinae group, quadratus lumborum, tensor fascia latae, quadriceps group, adductors, gastrocnemius
  - Muscles locked long: abdominals, iliopsoas, gluteus maximus, hamstrings group, tibialis anterior
- Posterior tilt of the pelvis (sway back; Fig. 3-20). This position is often associated with forward head, rounded shoulders (sunken chest), slumped posture (kyphosis).

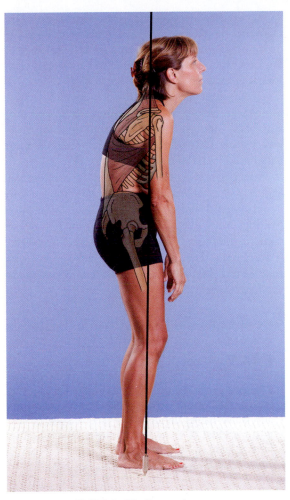

FIGURE 3-18 Slumped posture.

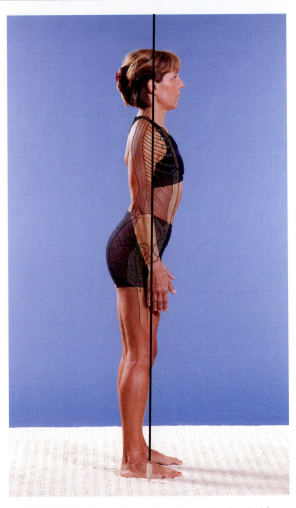

FIGURE 3-19 Anterior tilt of the pelvis (lordosis).

- Muscles locked short: abdominals, iliopsoas, gluteus maximus, hamstrings group, tibialis anterior
- Muscles locked long: thoracic/lumbar erector spinae group, quadratus lumborum, tensor fascia latae, quadriceps group, adductors, gastrocnemius

WAYS TO IMPROVE POSTURAL BALANCE

Many factors contribute to good health and improved posture. A sufficient amount of sleep and exercise is necessary, along with eating a balanced diet. Equally important is having a good understanding of what constitutes balanced posture, having kinesthetic awareness, and having the desire to possess balanced posture. However, good posture is sometimes challenging to maintain, even when you feel your best. You can stay motivated by remembering that maintaining the best health possible and the most balanced posture possible are the greatest ways to enhance career longevity.

Maintaining proper posture depends upon sufficient muscular endurance—a muscle's ability to perform work for a sustained period as happens in bodywork. Muscles that fatigue easily will be unable to maintain correct body alignment.

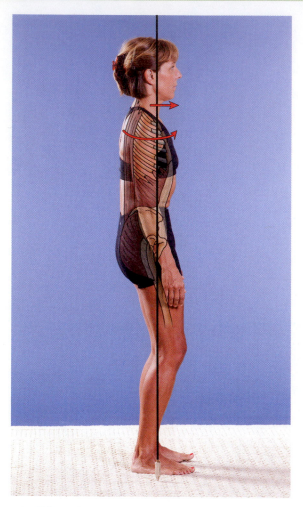

FIGURE 3-20 Posterior tilt of the pelvis (sway back).

As discussed in Chapter 2, muscles work in antagonistic pairs, and both pairs must be exercised in order to prevent or alleviate postural imbalances. For example, exercising the chest muscles (pectorals) could cause medially rotated shoulders and a sunken chest unless the upper and middle back muscles are also developed. In general, weak muscles need strengthening, and the tight or short muscles need stretching. This is covered in more detail in Chapters 7 and 8.

After performing the exercises and stretches for at least 3 weeks, you can check to see how your posture has changed. Using your Postural Evaluation Form (see Fig. 3-13), check your posture using a mirror or taking a photo and placing it in the section labeled "After Photo." By comparing your "after photo" with your "before photo," you can see what improvements you have made.

Myth: Posture cannot be changed because it is inherited.

FACT: Although genetic factors determine the shape and physiology of our tissues, posture is largely a learned pattern; therefore, it can be unlearned. Our thoughts, emotions, attitudes, developmental history, and family habits underlie the unique style of each posture. Most of these are elements over which we have at least some control.

Focus on Wellness

Based on the Postural Evaluation Form (see Fig. 3-13) you filled out, the following are exercises you can do to improve your postural balance. Exercises in the lying position should be done on the floor or a table, using a pad or mat for comfort if needed. All exercises should be done *slowly*. It is best to stretch muscles after they have been warmed such as through exercise or a hot shower (more information can be found about this in Chapter 7). Hold the stretch for 10 seconds or more.

Be sure to breathe in the following manner for every exercise or stretch: Inhale on the easiest part of the movement, and exhale on the most difficult part of the movement. Usually, the inhale is done during the lengthening of the muscle and the exhale is done on the shortening of the muscle.

Before beginning any exercise program, check with your physician to see if there are any contraindications for you for any of the exercises.

Protruding Abdomen (these are also good for lordosis)

- Abdominal setting (stretch and strengthen abdominals): While on your hands and knees, drop your abdomen and arch your back downward (Fig. 3-21A). Then flatten your abdomen by pulling it in, and arch your back upward. It should look

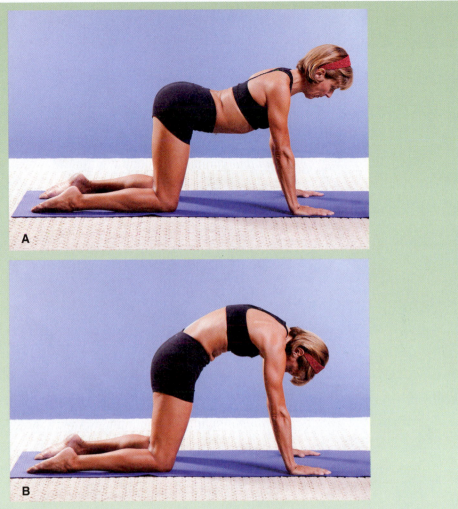

FIGURE 3-21 **(A)** Drop your abdomen and arch your back downward. **(B)** Flatten your abdomen by pulling it in, and arch your back upward.

like you are rounding your back (Fig. 3-21B). Hold for 4 seconds, and then relax for 5 seconds. Repeat three or four times.

- Pelvic tilt (strengthens abdominals): This is an isometric exercise done in a supine position, with your arms at your sides or behind your head, knees flexed and slightly apart, and feet flat on the floor (Fig. 3-22A). Press your spine down to the floor and hold it while tightening (contracting) your abdominal and gluteal muscles (Fig. 3-22B). Hold for 4 seconds, then relax. Repeat five times.
  - Challenging modification: Start the exercise the same, except place your hands behind your head and, as you contract your abdominal and gluteal muscles, *slowly* extend and lower one leg (Fig. 3-22C) until it is fully extended (Fig. 3-22D).

Hold for 4 seconds, and raise and return your leg to the flexed position (Fig. 3-22E). Repeat with your other leg.

Lordosis

- Wall exercise (strengthens abdominals and stretches lower back): Stand with your back to the wall, with your heels about an inch away from the wall (Fig. 3-23A). Flatten your lower back against the wall (Fig. 3-23B), then walk away while maintaining the flattened back (Fig. 3-23C). Return to the wall and check to see if you have kept that position.
  - Challenging modification: Sit on a stool, then place your back against the wall while keeping your upper back straight (Fig. 3-23D). Lift your arms

Continued

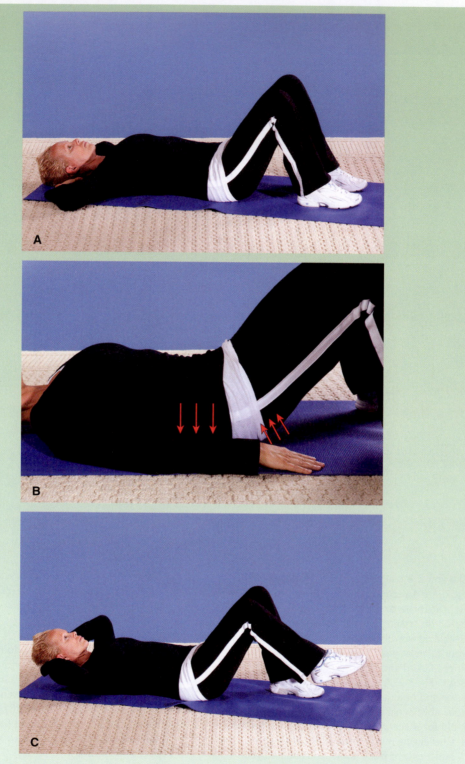

FIGURE 3-22 **(A)** Lie in a supine position, with your arms at your sides, or behind your head knees flexed and slightly apart, and feet flat on the floor. **(B)** Press your spine down to the floor and hold it while tightening (contracting) your abdominal and gluteal muscles. **(C)** Place your hands behind your head, and as you contract your abdominal and gluteal muscles, slowly lower one leg at a time.

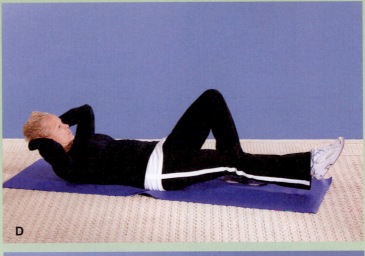

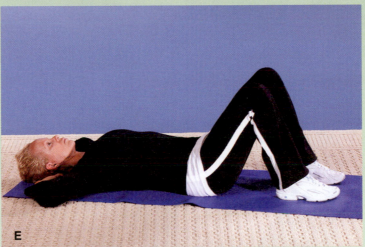

FIGURE 3-22 cont'd (D) until leg is fully extended. **(E)** Raise and return your leg to the flexed position.

overhead against the wall, then retract your chin and flatten your lower back (Fig. 3-23E). Hold for 4 seconds, and then relax. Repeat five times.

- Knee raise (stretches lower back and deep lateral rotators of the hip): Stand against the wall in a neutral position, feet hip-width apart and your arms down to the side (Fig. 3-24A). Raise one knee as high as possible, grasping it with both your hands and pulling it to your body while maintaining a straight back (Fig. 3-24B). Hold for 4 seconds, then relax and lower the leg. Repeat with your other leg. Alternate right and left legs, repeating four times with each leg.
  - Challenging Modification: This can also be done on the floor, one leg at a time (Fig. 3-24C) or both legs simultaneously (Fig. 3-24D).

Medially Rotated Shoulders, Sunken Chest, Kyphosis, and Winged Scapulae

- Doorway exercise (stretches pectorals): Stand in a doorway with arms bent at the elbows and parallel with the floor (Fig. 3-25A). Slowly lean into the doorway. Hold for 4 seconds then relax.
  - Modifications: Try varying the position of your arms, as this will stretch the different pectoral fibers (Fig. 3-25B, C, and D).
- Arm circles (strengthens upper back and shoulders, stretches the pectorals, and can help alleviate forward head posture): Keeping your chin retracted, abduct your arms to shoulder height (Fig. 3-26A) and move them in a large circle backward five times (Fig. 3-26B and C). Also while keeping your chin retracted, abduct arms to

Continued

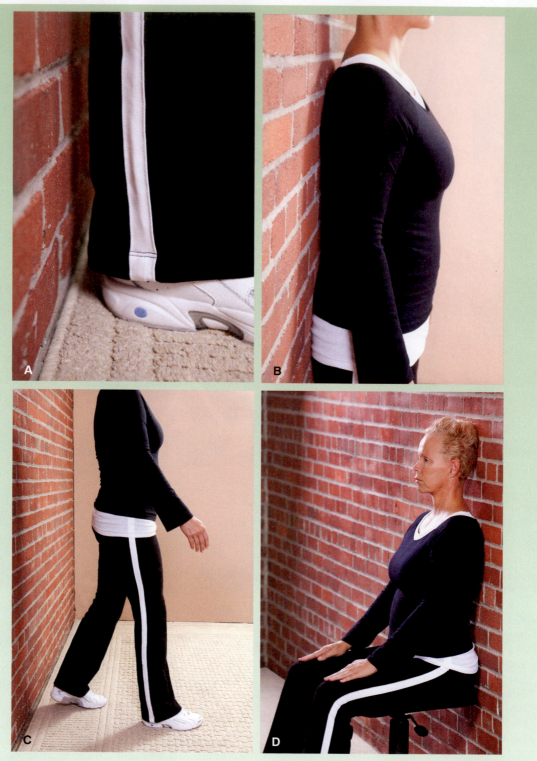

FIGURE 3-23 (A) Stand with your back to the wall, with your heels about an inch away from the wall. **(B)** Flatten your lower back against the wall. **(C)** Walk away while maintaining the flattened back. **(D)** Sit on a stool, then place your back against the wall while keeping your upper back straight.

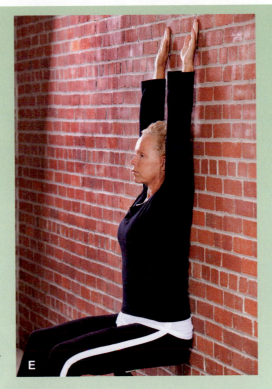

FIGURE 3-23 cont'd (E) Lift your arms overhead against the wall, then retract your chin and flatten your lower back.

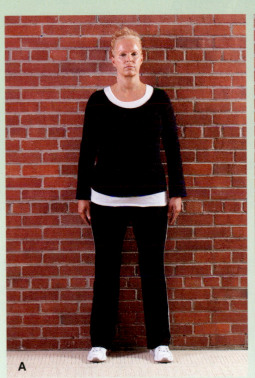

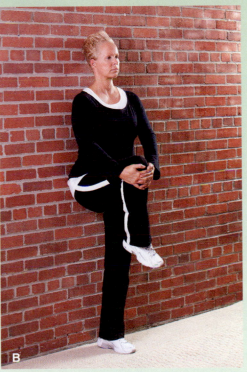

FIGURE 3-24 (A) Stand against the wall in a neutral position, feet hip-width apart and your arms down to the side. **(B)** Raise one knee as high as possible, grasping it with both your hands and pulling it to your body while maintaining a straight back. This can also be done on the floor,

Continued

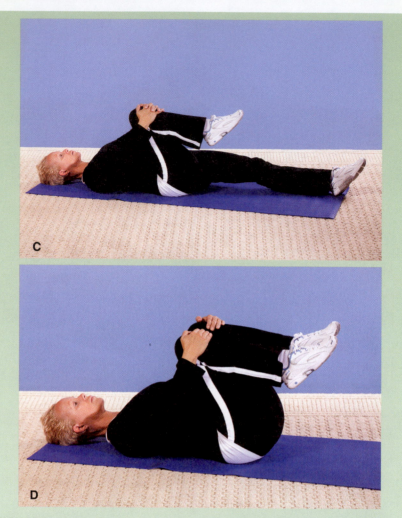

FIGURE 3-24 cont'd (C) one leg at a time, **(D)** or with both legs simultaneously.

shoulder height, flex at your elbows (Fig. 3-26D), and retract your scapulae (Fig. 3-26E). Hold for 4 seconds, and then relax. Repeat five times.

- Supine arm raise (strengthens back and shoulders): Lie in a supine position on the floor, knees flexed and feet flat on the floor (Fig. 3-27A). Stretch both arms straight up toward the ceiling (Fig. 3-27B), then bring them down. Stretch one arm straight up toward the ceiling (Fig. 3-27C), bring it back down, and then raise the other arm. Repeat the movements five times.
- Backstroke (strengthens back and shoulders; great for increasing shoulder range of motion): Place the back of your right hand on the right side of your face, then press your elbow straight back (Fig. 3-28A). Keeping your elbow back, reach backward with your right arm (Fig. 3-28B), then

relax that arm. Repeat with your left hand and arm. Alternate left and right arms, repeating four times on each arm, as in swimming the backstroke.

Forward Head

- Wall press (strengthens neck muscles): Stand with your back to the wall with your heels 2 or 3 inches from the wall (Fig. 3-29A). Press the back of your head against the wall, keeping your chin neutral and not increasing your lumbar curve (Fig. 3-29B). Hold for 4 seconds, and then relax for 5 seconds. Repeat three or four times.
- Head lift (strengthens neck muscles): Lie in a prone position, with your hands clasped behind your head (Fig. 3-30A). Apply slight resistance with your hands while raising your head from the floor (Fig. 3-30B). Hold for 4 seconds and then relax. Repeat five times.

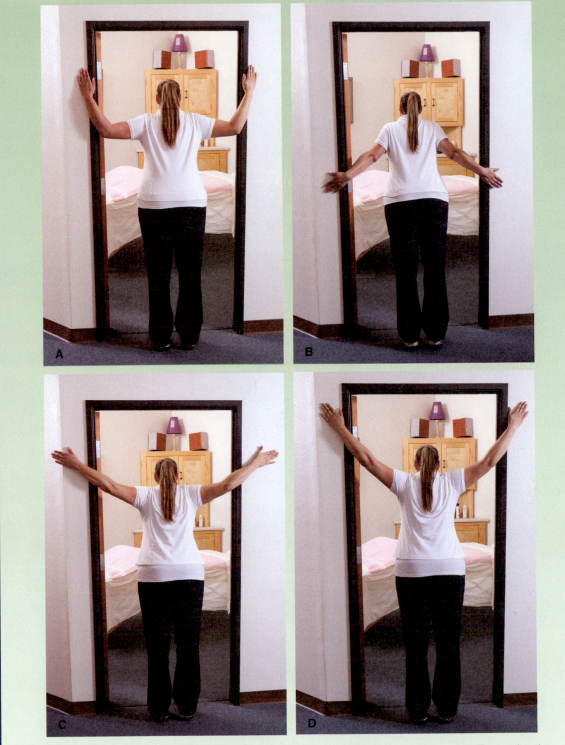

FIGURE 3-25 (A) Stand in a doorway with arms bent at the elbows and parallel with the floor. Try varying the position of your arms **(B, C,** and **D)**, as this will stretch the different pectoral fibers.

Continued

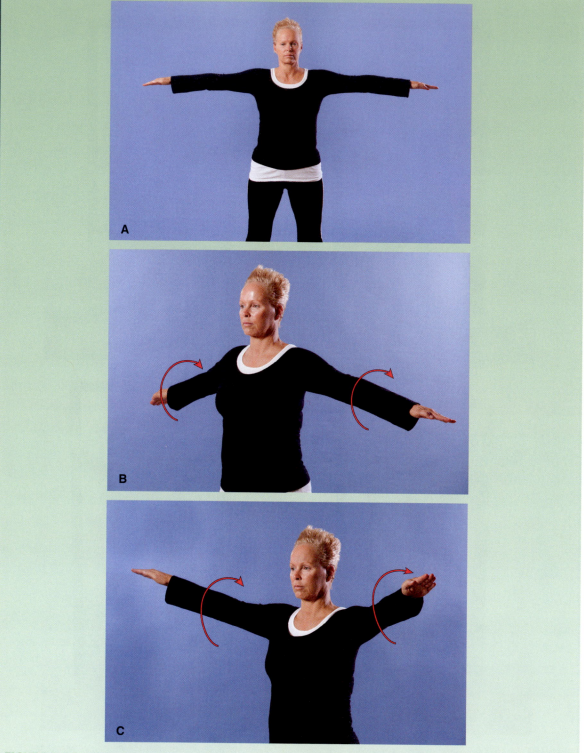

FIGURE 3-26 (A) Keeping your chin retracted, abduct your arms to shoulder height. **(B, C)** Move them in a large circle backward five times.

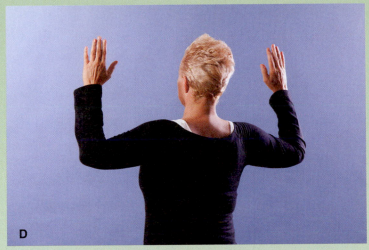

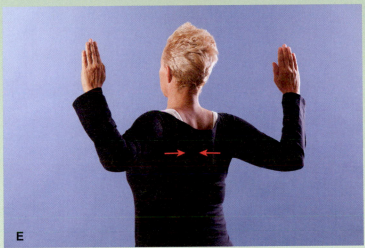

FIGURE 3-26 cont'd (D) Flex your elbows. **(E)** Retract your scapulae.

Scoliosis

- S-curve with left dorsal and right lumbar curves. If curves are the opposite of this, reverse the exercise position.
  - Chair hang (stretching): With the seat of the chair facing away from you, stand far enough away from the chair to place your hands on the back of the chair and bend over comfortably with your arms outstretched. Keep your back flat and your vertebral column aligned while stretching (Fig. 3-31A). Hold for 4 seconds, and then relax. Repeat five times. Ideally, you will work your way up to stretching for 30 to 60 seconds at a time. This stretch can also be done using a bar.

  Hang from a bar by your hands with your arms fully extended.
  - Standing stretch: While standing, stretch your right arm over your head. At the same time, stretch your left arm down and across your back, keeping the arm extended but with a soft elbow (Fig. 3-31B). Hold for 4 seconds and then relax. Repeat five times. Ideally, you will work your way up to stretching for 30 to 60 seconds at a time.
  - Supine stretch: Lie supine. Draw your knees to your chest and clasp your hands around your knees (Fig. 3-31C). Hold this position for 4 seconds and then relax. Repeat five times. Ideally, you will work your way up to stretching for 30 to 60 seconds at a time.

Continued

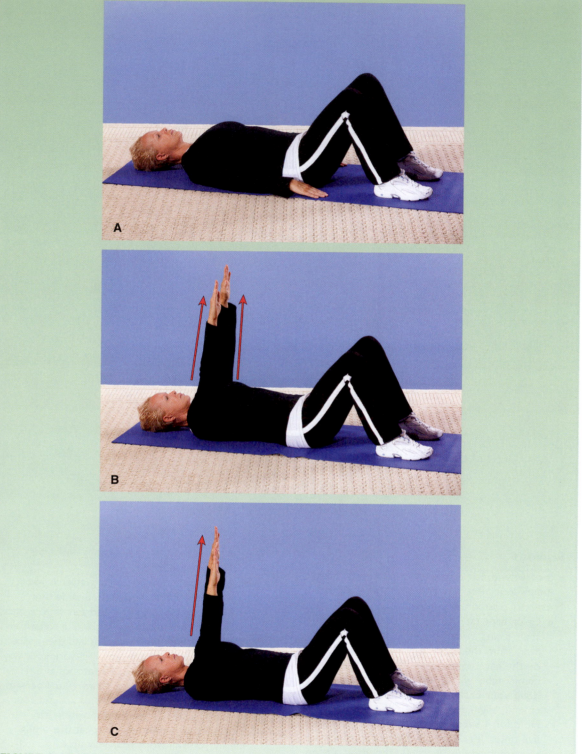

FIGURE 3-27 **(A)** Lie in a prone position on the floor, knees flexed and feet flat on the floor. **(B)** Stretch both arms straight up toward the ceiling. **(C)** Stretch one arm straight up toward the ceiling.

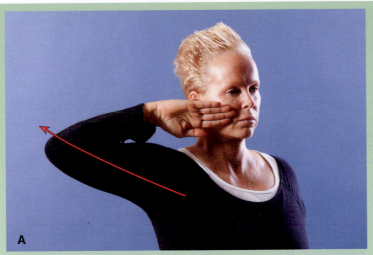

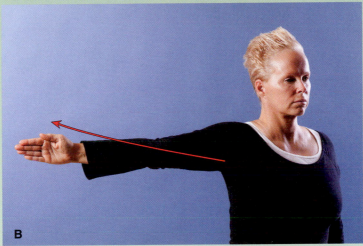

FIGURE 3-28 **(A)** Place the back of your right hand on the right side of your face and then press your elbow straight back. **(B)** Keeping your elbow back, reach backward with your right arm.

- C-curve to the left. If the curve is to the right, reverse the exercises.
  - Chair hang: Perform it the same as for the S-curve.
  - Stretch down: Stand with your hands by your sides (Fig. 3-32A). Stretch your left arm down at your side, pushing down firmly while raising your right arm over your head (Fig. 3-32B), then relax. Do not bend your body toward the left side. Repeat five or six times. Stretch your right arm up overhead while pressing your left hand against your rib cage at a point that comfortably forces your spine into a straighter position (Fig. 3-32C), then relax. Repeat five or six times.

Flat Back

- Shoulder lift (strengthens muscles in lower back): Lie supine; place a pillow under your knees for support if needed (Fig. 3-33A). Place your hands behind your neck, and then raise your shoulders off the floor, slightly arching your back while keeping your hips in contact with the floor (Fig. 3-33B). Hold for 4 seconds and then relax. Repeat five times.
- Lumbar arch (strengthens muscles in lower back): Stand and interlock your fingers behind your back in the lumbar region (Fig. 3-33C). Have your elbows flexed and out laterally (Fig. 3-33D). Press your elbows down and back; try to bring your elbows together while slightly arching your back in the lumbar area (Fig. 3-33E). Hold for 4 seconds and then relax. Repeat five times.

Continued

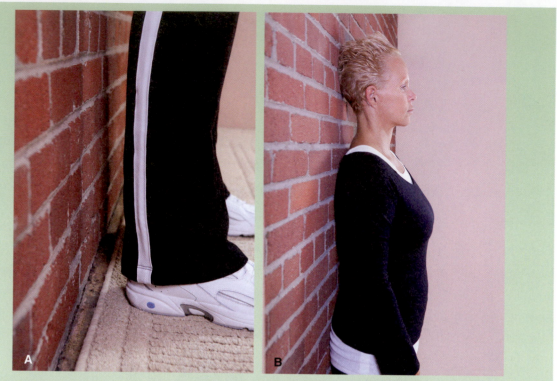

FIGURE 3-29 (A) Stand with your back to the wall with your heels 2 or 3 inches from the wall. **(B)** Press the back of your head against the wall, keeping your chin down and not increasing your lumbar curve.

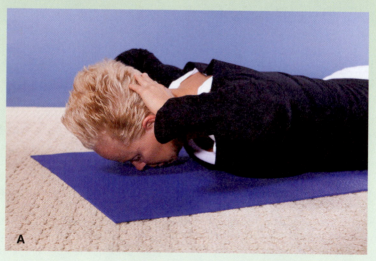

FIGURE 3-30 (A) Lie in a prone position, with your hands clasped behind your head.

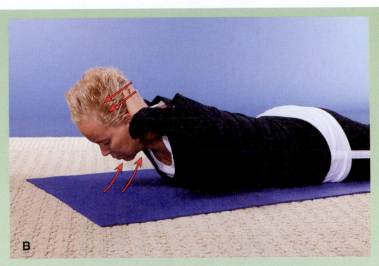

FIGURE 3-30 cont'd **(B)** Apply slight resistance with your hands while raising your head from the floor.

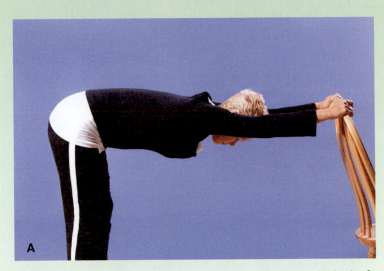

FIGURE 3-31 **(A)** With a straight, flat back, stretch while holding on to the back of a chair.

Continued

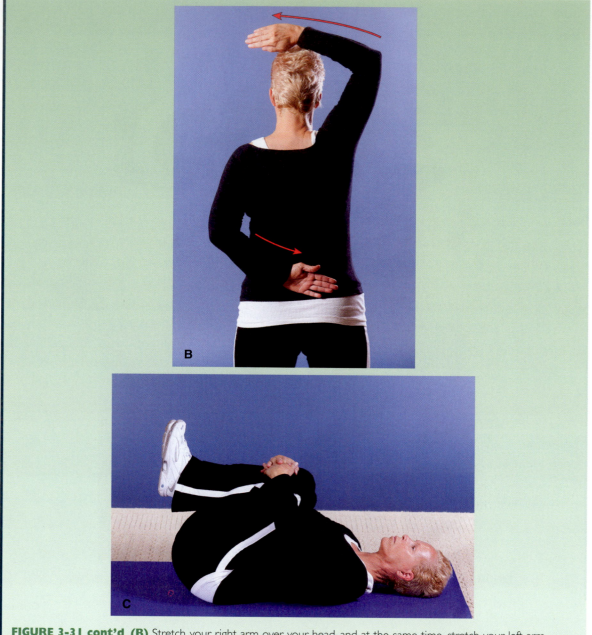

FIGURE 3-31 cont'd (B) Stretch your right arm over your head, and at the same time, stretch your left arm downward and across your back. **(C)** Draw your knees to your chest and clasp your hands around your knees.

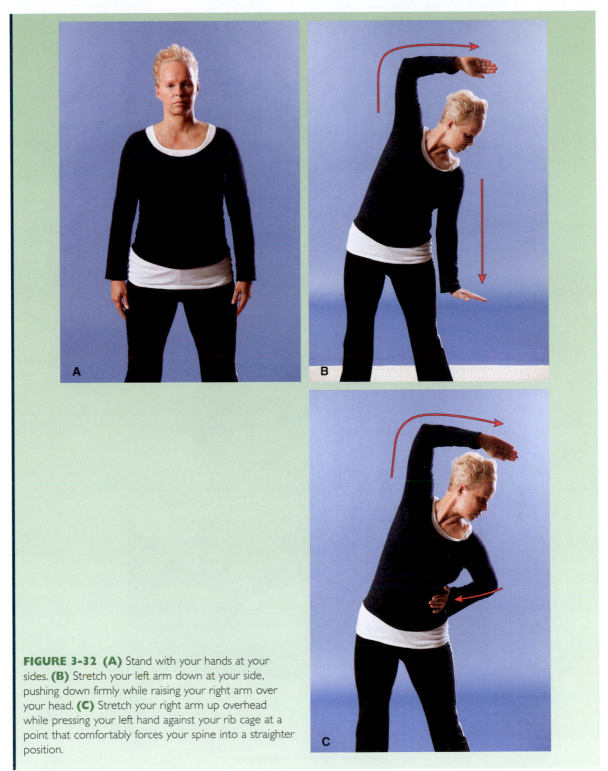

FIGURE 3-32 **(A)** Stand with your hands at your sides. **(B)** Stretch your left arm down at your side, pushing down firmly while raising your right arm over your head. **(C)** Stretch your right arm up overhead while pressing your left hand against your rib cage at a point that comfortably forces your spine into a straighter position.

Continued

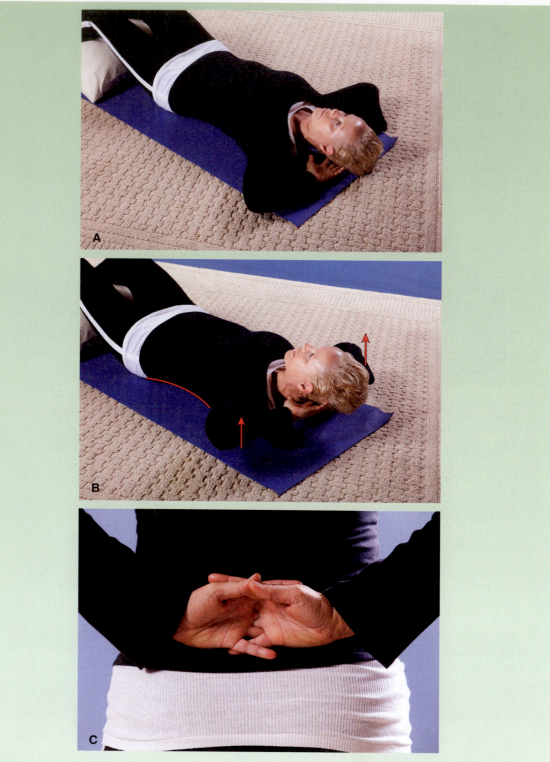

FIGURE 3-33 **(A)** Lie supine and place your hands behind your neck, then **(B)** raise your shoulders off the floor, slightly arching your back while keeping your hips in contact with the floor. **(C)** Stand and interlock your fingers behind your back in the lumbar region.

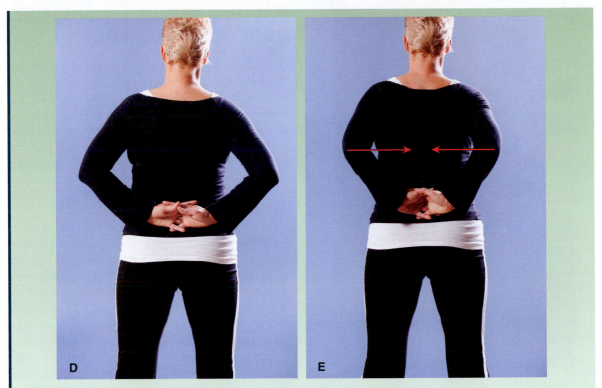

FIGURE 3-33 cont'd (D) Have your elbows flexed and out laterally. **(E)** Press your elbows down and back, and try to bring your elbows together while slightly arching your back in the lumbar area.

Additional Recommendations

The following are additional recommendations for improving health and fitness while performing bodywork and activities of daily living. These are also discussed in more detail throughout the rest of this book.

- Keep your body in as balanced a posture as possible as often as possible. Your joints will be naturally aligned and muscles relaxed.
- Avoid fatigue by:
  - changing position often to increase circulation to muscles.
  - stretching whenever possible.
  - taking deep, efficient breaths.
  - keeping objects close to your center of gravity.
  - staying hydrated by drinking plenty of water throughout the day. Each day, you can drink 6 to 8 glasses of water, ½ ounce of water for every pound of body weight, or divide your body weight in half and drink that number of ounces of water. However, if you increase your

levels of activity, make sure to also increase your water intake.

- Find a good, adjustable chair with proper support specific for any activities you do while sitting, including performing bodywork.
- Keep your feet flat on the floor when seated or use a footrest. Make sure your ankles are aligned with your knees, and your knees are aligned with your hips.
- Keep frequently used items close at hand to avoid twisting or reaching movements.
- Wear the proper shoes based on the activity you do while wearing them.
- Avoid repetitive lifting or reaching overhead; use a stepstool or ladder.
- When picking things up, lift with your legs by flexing your knees so you do not bend over at the waist to lift. You could also kneel down or squat to pick something up, while maintaining a balanced posture. For example, Figure 3-34 shows the proper way to lift a massage table.
- Seek pain relief when necessary.

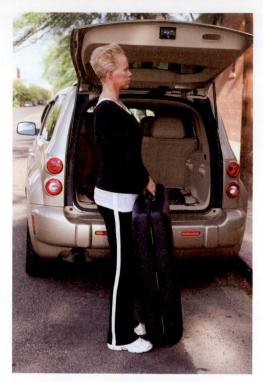

FIGURE 3-34 Lifting a massage table using proper posture.

- Always be aware of the correct joint alignment of your body to reduce wear and tear.
- Participate in strength training with emphasis on the muscles that are weak and stretched (Chapter 8 has more information about this).
- Participate in stretching with emphasis on the muscles that are tight and shortened (Chapter 7 has more information about this).

Body Awareness

Many practitioners need reminders to aid in achieving and maintaining balanced posture. These key words might be helpful:

- Stand tall
- Sit tall
- Walk tall
- Think tall

POSTURE WHILE PERFORMING BODYWORK AND ADL

Generally, the lower a person's center of gravity and the wider the base of support, the more stable the person's body is. For example, when lying down, the body is completely stable because the base of support is the posterior body, and weight is extended throughout, as opposed to being centered in one area of the body. The standing position is much less stable because the base of support is much smaller, and the center of gravity is higher and concentrated in a smaller area of the body.

When the line of gravity passes through the center of the base of support, as happens in balanced posture, less muscular strength and energy is required to maintain balance. For example, standing with the feet close together makes the body sway in an attempt to maintain balance and not fall over. But if the feet are moved apart to shoulder-width or wider, there is an immediate increase in stability.

These principles certainly carry into the performance of bodywork. When standing while working on clients lying on a massage table or sitting in a massage chair, the practitioner is less stable when the feet are closer together (Fig. 3-35A). To increase the base of support and lower the center of gravity, the practitioner can widen the stance and flex the knees to drop the trunk. The practitioner should also maintain a **head-to-tail connection** so that the line of gravity is as straight as possible. Head-to-tail connection means being aware that the skull is connected to the vertebral column, that the vertebral column is a line down the back, and that the vertebral column ends in the coccyx (Fig. 3-35B). This means practitioners must pay attention to balanced spinal posture as they work and must choose the proper stance for doing the work, whichever one allows them to move in the direction of their work.

The practitioner can use a symmetric stance (horse stance), with weight equally distributed on both feet, or an asymmetric stance (lunge), which allows the weight to be shifted back and forth between the two feet. This allows for brief muscular rest periods. The practitioner should also be **hinging** at the hips, which means flexing the thigh at the hip joint—as though going into a squat. This keeps the practitioner from bending at the waist (which will eventually cause lower back issues) and ensures

FIELD NOTES

I developed significant wrist pain while still in massage school. The problem originated with an inadequate computer workstation in my previous field (and reflected my mother's history of wrist problems) but was clearly exacerbated by giving massage. I sought input from massage teachers and books and used a combination of strategies to resolve the problem:

1. Maintaining neutral wrist alignment: Careful attention to maintaining neutral wrist alignment is key. It has proven critical for me to be rigorous about not applying firm pressure with wrists extended beyond even a very slight angle. Besides this "absolute" rule, I also avoid stressing my wrists in other ways during treatments; instead I modify some massage techniques and replace or eliminate other techniques.

2. Avoiding compounded stress: I've discovered that it is essential for me to temper other activities that could stress my wrists. For example, at drum jams, instead of packing an evening with vigorous drumming, I alternate drumming with light percussion. Doing projects at home, I avoid focusing on a single task all afternoon; for example, when doing yard work, I rotate between activities like digging, tree trimming, and raking, and so on. I've adjusted my bicycle handlebars, I avoid yoga poses that involve supporting my body weight on extended wrists, and so on.

3. Performing wrist-strengthening exercises: For several months I did various strengthening exercises. Eventually I settled down to just doing wrist extensions (with 5-pound dumbbells), since that was the most important exercise in the sense that neither massage nor other daily activities strengthened the extensors.

4. Doing hydrotherapy: When the problem started, and I was feeling wrist pain at the end of the day, hydrotherapy proved very helpful. I purchased two small plastic planter boxes, just long enough to immerse my forearms from fingertips to elbows, with those pesky wrists in a neutral position. Sometimes I just used ice water immersion, and sometimes I alternated between ice water and hot water. Now I've cultivated healthy wrist habits to the extent that I haven't needed hydrotherapy for quite some time.

Although it's possible to create long lists of ways to remain injury-free, I think the bottom line is awareness. There are two aspects or two keys to this awareness. One key is careful attention to principles of body mechanics. Follow expert advice on body mechanics, even when it seems unimportant or inconvenient. This means stick with the principles even when you think you're so young or strong it doesn't matter for you, or your client really needs this move, or you're not doing enough massages that it should matter, or whatever other excuse you have. Body mechanics is a whole field of study in itself; trust that there are experts who know more than you and whose guidance you will benefit by following.

The second key is careful attention to messages from your body. Always listen to the earliest signs that your body is stressed. So, for example, if your thumbs even once feel stiff at the end of the day, take this as a call to action! There's no need to wait until you experience real pain. Start watching your thumbs like the proverbial hawk, assess what specifically aggravates them, and take action to eliminate or change that. Ideally you are listening carefully enough that you can address a situation before it becomes a full-blown problem.

Laura Key, BA, MS, LMT, NCTMB, Owner, Lotus Massage and Wellness Center, Tucson, AZ. Massage therapist since 2006.

efficient alignment (maintaining a constant head-to-tail connection). It also allows the practitioner to maintain a proper stance. The lunge stance and hinging at the hips are shown in Figure 3-35C.

When performing bodywork on a futon on the floor, practitioners naturally have a more stable stance because their points of contact include the knees and feet, and sometimes the shins. Even when kneeling, with their knees close together, they have quite a bit of stability (Fig. 3-36A). They can also place their knees farther apart to widen their stance more. In this way, their bodies can form a tripod if they keep their feet together (Fig. 3-36B) or a four-point stance if they keep their feet apart (Fig. 3-36C). Practitioners also need to make sure they drop their center of gravity down into their abdomen and pelvic floor. This area of the body is the source of the practitioner's strength, as kneeling postures mean the practitioner needs to rely on their core and leg muscles for balance, movement, and application of pressure.

Body mechanics are covered in more detail in Chapter 5, but it is never too soon to focus on posture. Therefore, the following are some postural guidelines to keep in mind while performing bodywork. These principles apply to the performance of all types of bodywork, whether the treatments are on massage tables, massage chairs, or futons.

Since it usually takes approximately 21 days to make or break a habit, it is recommended that you focus on one area of your posture you find challenging. You can then choose the guideline that addresses it and

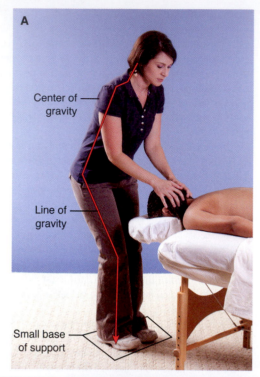

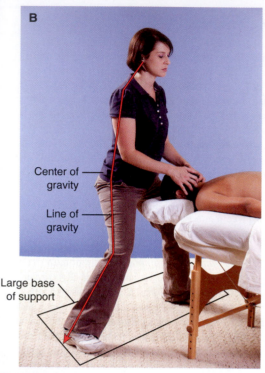

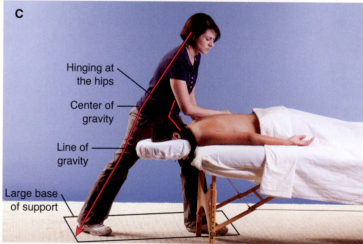

FIGURE 3-35 (A) Stance with feet too close together for optimal stability. **(B)** Stance with feet apart for greater stability. **(C)** Lunge stance.

practice it for 3 weeks. During this time, monitor your progress and body awareness. After 3 weeks, if you have other postural challenges to address, try a different focus area for 3 weeks, monitoring your progress. Keep doing this until you have a balanced posture.

- Make sure you choose the proper stances for your work throughout your treatments. They are the ones that allow you to go in the direction of your work and allow you to hinge at your hip joints. You should keep in mind that different stances

can be used as needed to ensure you are working as efficiently as possible.

- It is important to keep moving while performing treatments. Static positions lead to static treatments, and contracted muscles use more energy than relaxed muscles.
- Deep, efficient breathing is the root of all muscular activity. Remind yourself to keep breathing, even as you remind your clients to breathe.
- Maintain a head-to-tail connection.

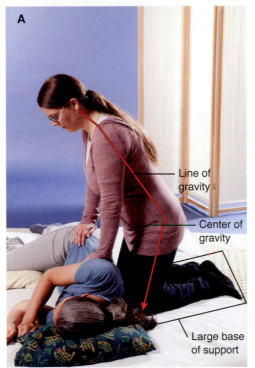

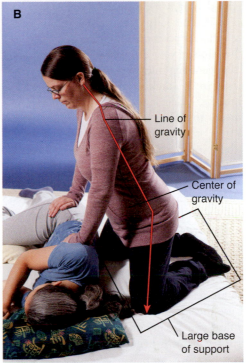

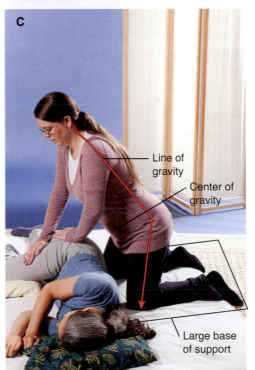

FIGURE 3-36 (A) Kneeling practitioner. **(B)** In a tripod stance. **(C)** In a four-point stance.

- Stay behind your work instead of rising up over the top of it. This keeps your joints and muscles in more efficient positions.
- Keep the joints in your fingers, wrists, elbows, and knees aligned along their axes of movements. This is referred to as **stacking the joints** and is the most healthy, efficient way to work. The alignment means the joints are in their strongest position so their associated muscles work less at stabilizing the joint and more at generating force. It also reduces your chance of injury.
- Keep your body moving in the direction of your work. This eliminates unhealthy rotation and twisting of your body as you perform treatments. It also allows you to apply more pressure, using your body weight, during the treatment while decreasing your risk of injury.
- Keep your arms close to your midline. If it feels like you are reaching, you are. Reaching postures do not use the strength in your core and leg muscles. Unless you are intentionally incorporating a stretch for your own benefit into the treatment, applying pressure while in reaching postures greatly increases your chance of injury.

Remember, if you *feel* like you are working hard, and you *look* like you are working hard, chances are you *are* working too hard.

Voice of Experience

As a massage therapy instructor and a full-time massage therapist, I have witnessed many students and practitioners dealing with pain due to imbalanced postures or misalignments. The nature of our work is very physical and repetitive, and the risk of injury is increased unless we address the problem. Even using correct body mechanics will not eliminate the risk of injury if we don't have balanced postures.

A few key points for our clients and ourselves:
- Seek pain relief
- Have awareness of correct joint alignments
- Perform strength training with emphasis on the muscles that are weak and elongated
- Perform stretching with emphasis on the muscles that are tight and shortened
- Practice correct joint alignment to reduce wear and tear
- Establish a maintenance program

Christiane Testa-Rekemeier, NCTMB, licensed massage therapist since 1998, massage therapy instructor since 2001.

POSTURE DURING ACTIVITIES OF DAILY LIVING

The same principles of postural balance for performing bodywork can be applied to activities of daily living. Once practitioners have awareness of where their balanced posture is and are working on improving their posture, they can carry these into the movements and tasks they do on a daily basis, thus increasing their body awareness. These habits then become natural.

For example, while sitting at a computer or driving, be mindful of how your neck and back are feeling and reposition yourself as needed to keep your joints in alignment (Fig. 3-37). Instead of bending over to take groceries out of the car (Fig. 3-38A), keep your vertebral column aligned, flex your knees, and sink down, using your leg strength (Fig. 3-38B). Instead of twisting to replace a lightbulb in an overhead light fixture (Fig. 3-39A), stand so your joints are aligned while performing the task (Fig. 3-39B).

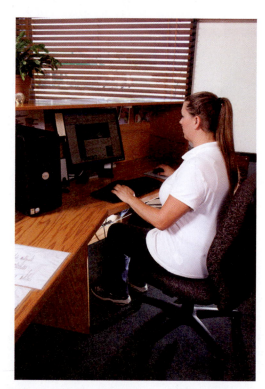

FIGURE 3-37 While sitting at a computer, practitioners can be mindful of how their necks and back are feeling and reposition themselves as needed.

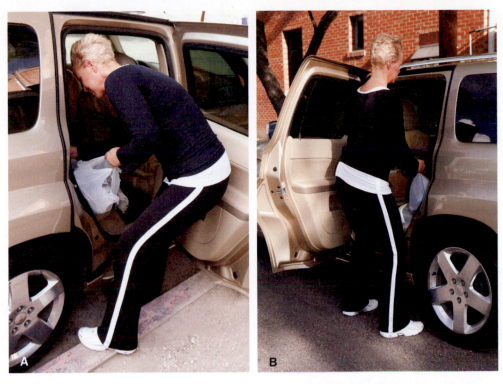

FIGURE 3-38 (A) Instead of bending over to take groceries out of the car, **(B)** they can stand so their joints are aligned while performing the task.

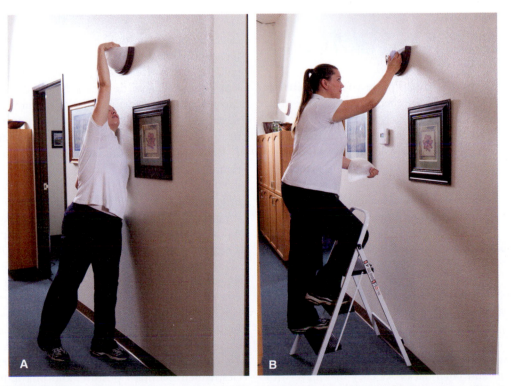

FIGURE 3-39 (A) Instead of twisting to replace a lightbulb in an overhead light fixture, **(B)** they can stand so their joints are aligned while performing the task.

Case Profile

Rebeccah is 26 years old and has been a bodyworker for 6 months. She works at a wellness center where she typically sees four or five clients a day, 5 days a week. Prior to going to bodywork school, she worked as a nanny for triplets who kept her on the run. When she was in bodywork school, she was a very ambitious student. She practiced what she was learning quite a bit outside of class and got favorable feedback from the clients she worked on in the student clinic. She had a reputation for being able to apply deep, specific pressure; for being willing to try all new techniques right away; and for saying that she planned to work hard enough to own her own bodywork business 2 years after graduating. No one else in her class worked as hard as she did.

However, during class, she would listen impatiently as the instructor talked about and demonstrated the importance of balanced posture and aligning the joints while working. Rebeccah thought this took valuable time away from learning how to do techniques. She thought, "I'm young and healthy. That stuff is for old people. I won't have to worry about that for years."

Lately Rebeccah has been noticing pain in both of her wrists, upper back, neck, and shoulders. Periodically she has some discomfort in her low back. Her friends have recommended that she see her physician, but she is afraid to since she thinks he may say she has carpel tunnel syndrome or thoracic outlet syndrome, which would severely hamper her professional plans. She is not sure what to do and is upset because nothing has ever stopped her from doing anything before.

■ *Even though she is active, why do you think Rebeccah is experiencing pain and discomfort as a bodyworker?*

■ *Based on her symptoms, what specific postural imbalances could Rebeccah have?*

■ *How do you think the way Rebeccah is currently working will impact her career longevity?*

■ *What suggestions would you give Rebeccah to help her alleviate the symptoms she is experiencing?*

Wellness Profile Check-In

Looking at the Wellness Profile you completed at the end of Chapter 1, are there any challenge areas in which you could improve your postural balance? If so, what are they? How would you like these areas improved? What methods will you use to improve postural imbalances? Write down a plan for improvement that includes the methods you will use, a timeline for implementing these methods, and ways you will assess your improvement along the way.

SUMMARY

Posture involves the combination of the positions of all the joints and movements of all the muscles at any given moment. Since bodywork is physical and many repetitive movements are involved, the risk of injury is increased unless bodywork practitioners are aware of current and potential issues they may have with their bodies. Overuse, misuse, and underuse of muscles can contribute to postural imbalances. Balanced posture contributes to career longevity because it enables practitioners to work more proficiently, makes them look better to clients, decreases the risk of injury, and encourages proper performance of techniques. All of these can lead to greater client satisfaction with the treatments received and can increase client retention.

Balanced posture involves aligning and positioning the body in relation to gravity. Factors involved in balanced posture include a low center of gravity and a wide base of support. The foot is the primary base of support for the body, and its unique structure makes it ideal for this purpose. These factors contribute to the practitioner's stability while performing treatments. Additionally, the structure and functions of the bones and muscles allow balance and movement. These include curves in the bones and vertebral column, as well as finding the optimal axis of joint rotation and the balanced strength of antagonistic pairs of muscles. Two broad categories of muscles are postural muscles, which maintain posture, and phasic muscles, which move the body.

There are many influences on postural development such as genetics, family life, congenital disorders, levels of physical activity, environment factors, trauma, and lack of body and postural awareness. Postural habits are patterns of movement that people repeat over and over again, often without being aware that they are actually using them. The body makes numerous changes in postures to compensate for the movements necessary to perform tasks each day, but unhealthy postures can lead to more serious conditions if they are not addressed.

There are many different imbalanced postures that practitioners are likely to encounter in clients and that they themselves might have. Some examples include rounded shoulders, slumped posture, and anterior pelvic tilts. Practitioners should be able to recognize these postures and understand what muscles are involved and what the quality of contraction those muscles have. These can provide a focus for the client's bodywork treatment and can give practitioners crucial information about their own postures.

Becoming aware of postural habits is an essential step toward understanding how to improve postural balance when performing bodywork. You should determine what your balanced posture is and what your current posture is, then decide what exercises and stretches you would like to do and what lifestyle changes you would like to make to improve your postural patterns. Several of these are offered in this chapter.

Review Questions

MULTIPLE CHOICE

1. The area in the body where weight is concentrated is called
   a. base of support.
   b. alignment.
   c. center of gravity.
   d. joint axes.

2. The areas of contact between a person and the ground is called
   a. line of gravity.
   b. base of support.
   c. plumb line.
   d. head-to-tail connection.

3. What parts of the foot provide optimal distribution of body weight over the tissues of the foot?
   a. Arches
   b. Phalanges
   c. Tendons
   d. Tarsals

4. Normally, the heel carries what percentage of body weight?
   a. 20
   b. 40
   c. 60
   d. 80

5. The muscle that is locked short in round shoulders is
   a. middle trapezius.
   b. rhomboid.
   c. infraspinatus.
   d. pectoralis major.

6. Which of the following is a way postural imbalances can manifest in the body?
   a. Muscular spasm
   b. Stress fracture
   c. Intervertebral disk compression
   d. All of the above

7. Which of the following contributes to improved posture?
   a. Sufficient sleep
   b. Kinesthetic awareness
   c. Muscular endurance
   d. All of the above

FILL-IN-THE-BLANK

1. How a person usually holds himself or herself while lying, sitting, standing, or moving is called _____.

2. The _____ can be visualized passing vertically through the body, from the

head to the center of gravity in the lower trunk or pelvic region, down through the feet.

3. The four normal curves of the vertebral column are the _____, _____, _____ and _____.

4. In order to have optimal posture and efficient muscular contraction and movements, it is important to ensure that muscle groups are in _____.

5. A lateral curvature of the vertebral column is called _____.

6. Being aware that the skull is connected to the vertebral column, that the vertebral column is a line down the back, and that the vertebral column ends in the coccyx describes _____.

7. In a proper bodywork stance, flexing the thigh at the hip joint means that the practitioner is _____ at the hips.

SHORT ANSWER

1. Describe what balanced posture looks like.

2. Explain how balanced posture can enhance career longevity.

3. Briefly explain the characteristics of postural muscles and the characteristics of phasic muscles.

4. Describe at least four factors that contribute to postural development.

5. Describe three activities practitioners can do to feel what balanced posture is.

6. Describe at least five exercises or stretches practitioners can do to improve their postural balance.

7. Explain at least five ways postural balance can be used during activities of daily living.

Activities

1. Look at members of your family. What kind of postures do they have? List at least three different ways your posture is similar and three ways it is different.

2. Go to a mall, park, or other recreational area and observe how the people there move. What specific postures can you observe? What muscles might be affected because of this posture? How might they be affected (e.g., which ones are locked short and which ones are locked long)? In which areas of their bodies might people with these postures be having tension or pain? What activities do you think might help improve postural imbalances?

3. Try each of the following for at least 3 weeks. Keep a journal of how you feel before you start, and what you feel at the end of each week.
   - Maintain wrist alignment while brushing your teeth.
   - Try vacuuming while keeping your arms close to your body's midline.
   - While cooking, maintain your head in a balanced posture, using only your eyes to look down at what you are doing.
   - When lifting bags of groceries or anything else heavy, maintain a head-to-tail connection, keep your knees soft, and lift with your legs.

4. After trying some of the suggestions in this chapter, revisit your wellness wheel. Are there any shifts in any of the areas? If so, what are they? Color in a blank wellness wheel to reflect the changes that have occurred for you.

REFERENCES

Chaitow, Leon. *Palpation Skills, Assessment and Diagnosis Through Touch.* London, England: Churchill Livingstone, 2000.

Flemons, T. E. The Geometry of Anatomy and the Bones of Tensegrity (2007). Retrieved October 2010 from www.intensiondesigns.com/geometry_of_anatomy.html.

Kapandji, I. A. *The Physiology of the Joints,* volume 3. St. Louis, MO: Churchill Livingstone, 2008.

Kinesis. Tensegrity (2010). Retrieved October 2010 from www.anatomytrains.com/explore/tensegrity/explained.

Lowe, Whitney. *Orthopedic Massage,* 2nd ed. St. Louis, MO: Elsevier Mosby, 2009.

Muscolino, Joseph E. *Kinesiology, the Skeletal System and Muscle Function*, 2nd ed. St. Louis, MO: Elsevier Mosby, 2011.

Todd, Mabel Elsworth. *The Thinking Body*. Gouldsboro, ME: Gestalt Journal Press, 2008.

Tortora, Gerard J., and Bryan Derrickson. *Principles of Anatomy and Physiology,* 12th ed. Hoboken, NJ: John Wiley & Sons, 2009.

Breathing for Best Practice, Health, and Wellness

Key Terms

Alveoli
Bronchioles
Chest (shoulder or
shallow) breathing
Diaphragm
Diaphragmatic
(abdominal) breathing
Eupnea
Metabolism
Pulmonary
Pulmonary ventilation
Respiratory center
Respiratory membrane
Respiratory pump

Learning Objectives

After studying this chapter, the reader will have the information to:

1. Explain the importance of breathing efficiently.
2. Describe the components of the respiratory system, and explain their functions.
3. Explain the mechanics of breathing.
4. Describe different ways of breathing.
5. Perform breathing methods, activities, and exercises to improve respiratory function, increase endurance and stamina, and clear and center the mind.
6. Integrate efficient breathing into his or her performance of bodywork.
7. Encourage clients to breathe effectively while receiving bodywork to help them during the treatment and in their everyday lives.

> "Breath is a connecting force. It creates a bodily equilibrium and balance and helps us to make inner and outer impressions interchangeable. It connects the human being with the outside world and the outside world with his inner world."
> —Ilse Middendorf, founder of the Institute for Breath Therapy in Berlin, Germany

THE IMPORTANCE OF BREATH

Breathing is one of those functions that most people do not always think about and perhaps even take for granted. This could be because breathing happens automatically; it started with the first breath of life when coming into this world. Babies have to learn to do many things, such as how to contract their muscles to maintain posture and to create movement such as for walking or reaching for things, how to talk, how to develop reasoning skills so they can understand their environments and interactive skills so they can understand how to relate and communicate with other people. But one thing babies do not have to learn is how to breathe.

Because conscious effort is not required in order to breathe, many people may not be aware of how essential proper breathing is to maintaining health. When breathing efficiently, blood and lymph flow are enhanced, muscles relax, and mental clarity and feelings of calm increase. Oxygen is constantly needed by your body, whether you are resting, moving, relaxing quietly, feeling angry, exercising strenuously, or sleeping. Whatever you are doing, your breathing needs to adequately support you. Efficient breath is needed to perform tasks without becoming worn out, to withstand stress, and to recuperate from strain.

This is true for everyone, no matter their circumstances. It is most certainly true for bodywork practitioners. Because bodywork is such a physical profession, practitioners need to have effective breathing methods to ensure efficient oxygen intake and carbon dioxide release. The breath and the way it fills the body serves as a support to internal musculature as they stand and move. Expansion of the thorax balances the skeletal muscles that move the shoulders, arms, and hands. All of these factors give you the stamina and strength needed to perform treatments of varying lengths. It also gives you the ability to have a long career in the bodywork profession.

In addition to performing treatments on clients, bodywork practitioners are also educators. In this role, you should be modeling healthy behavior for your clients. This includes dressing appropriately for the work you do, having a balanced posture, being physically fit, and breathing properly. You should not be out of breath with the slightest exertion, nor should you breathe so shallowly it is difficult for you to talk or it seems you are hyperventilating, or breathe so deeply it is distracting to the client. Some practitioners may also choose to educate their clients more directly on how they can focus on their breath as a means of relaxation and calming. Ways to do this are covered in the "Encouraging Clients to Breathe" section.

FACTORS THAT AFFECT BREATHING

While breath is vital to sustaining life and is completely automatic, it can be altered in a wide variety of ways. Your breathing is affected by everything that happens to you—physical or emotional strain, injury, frustration, and even great success. Anything that goes on in and around you will affect your breathing. The free flow of air can be hampered, exhalation may be inhibited, and inhalation may become insufficient.

Breathing rhythm and rate not only reflect the body's physical and emotional conditions, but also help create them. Breathing is an excellent indicator of emotional and mental states. When people are worried or excited, their respiration rate increases and may become more irregular, and their breaths become shallower. When people are more calm and centered, their breathing rate slows down and becomes more regular, and their breaths become fuller.

Feelings, whether momentary or constant, manifest in the body in characteristic postures and actions, and in characteristic respiratory rhythms. For example, consider the posture and breathing patterns of someone who is sobbing inconsolably. They are quite different from someone who is laughing joyfully. They are both different from someone who is meditating peacefully, and all are different from someone who is exercising strenuously.

Proper breathing is important, yet many people do not breathe efficiently. For some, the stress of busy lives may make them in too big a hurry to breathe efficiently. Excessive heat, high humidity, and air pollution are environmental factors that can interfere with breathing easily. Smoking and breathing in secondhand smoke severely compromise efficient breathing. Illness can strongly influence breathing patterns, including respiratory illnesses that can interfere with the ability to take in or let out air. Sudden, severe pain can cause the person to hold his breath, but prolonged somatic pain, such as in the muscles, joints, and connective tissues, can increase the rate of breathing (Tortora and Derrickson, 2009).

Many people have suffered physical, mental, or emotional traumas that can affect how they breathe. Breathing is a self-regulating function, and it has the capacity to recover from strain and stress as soon as the situation that causes the trauma is over. However, unconsciously and unintentionally, many people maintain the changed ways of breathing even after the events that brought on the trauma have passed (Chaitow, 2009; Fritz, 2009).

However, people can consciously change their patterns of breathing. By bringing their awareness to their breath, they can choose to breathe more efficiently. Their breath will always be affected by what happens in their lives. By focusing on establishing good breathing habits, they create a great therapeutic tool that allows them to connect their bodies and minds. This will help them develop healthier and more responsive bodies that are better able to weather the ups and downs of life.

Bodywork practitioners need to create an environment within their bodies that allows for a sufficient oxygen supply to muscles and other organs and for carbon dioxide to be removed efficiently. The more this occurs, the more vital and healthy practitioners are likely to be. In order to do this, there needs to be an understanding of what happens within the body during breathing. This information is foundational to understanding how to perform various breathing exercises and learning the benefits of doing them.

Body Awareness

Take a moment now and, without changing it, just notice your breath. Where does it feel like you are breathing in your body? Your chest? Your abdomen? Or into your throat? Is this your normal pattern of breathing? How do you think your energy levels and muscular strength are affected by your normal pattern of breathing?

THE MECHANICS OF BREATHING

Cells continually use oxygen for the metabolic reactions that release energy from nutrient molecules. **Metabolism** refers to all the chemical reactions that occur in the body. The released energy is used throughout the entire body for processes such as protein synthesis, nerve impulse conduction, and muscle contraction. A by-product of oxygen use in metabolism is carbon dioxide. An excessive amount of carbon dioxide produces acids that can be toxic to cells. Therefore, excess carbon dioxide must be eliminated quickly and efficiently.

The two body systems that work together to supply oxygen and eliminate carbon dioxide are the cardiovascular and respiratory systems. The respiratory system is responsible for gas exchange—intake of oxygen and elimination of carbon dioxide. The cardiovascular system transports the blood containing the gases between the lungs and the body cells. Failure of either system has the same effect on the body, namely disruption of homeostasis and rapid cell death from oxygen deprivation and buildup of wastes.

Besides the function of gas exchange, the respiratory system also does the following:

- Helps regulate blood pH (by eliminating carbon dioxide and thus decreasing acidity)
- Contains olfactory receptors (for sense of smell)
- Filters incoming air
- Produces sounds
- Eliminates some water and heat in exhaled air

Air movement in and out of the body and gas exchange are performed by the anatomical structures of the respiratory system. These include the nose and nasal cavity, pharynx (throat), larynx (voice box), trachea (windpipe), bronchial tree, and lungs.

Inhaled air is first affected in the nasal cavity. The entire respiratory tract is lined with mucous membrane. In the nasal cavity, the sticky mucus traps particles, and the air is moistened and warmed. The air continues down through the pharynx and larynx and into the trachea. At about the level of the fifth thoracic vertebra, the trachea divides into right and left primary bronchi, which enter each lung (Fig. 4-1).

The lungs are in the thoracic cavity and rest on the diaphragm. Each lung is a separate organ. If one collapsed, the other would continue to function. The right lung has three lobes and is thicker and broader than the left lung because the liver, a large organ, is underneath the diaphragm on the right side. The left lung has two lobes and an indentation called the *cardiac notch*. The heart, whose inferior portion tilts to the left, fits into this notch.

Inside each lung, the primary bronchi branch into smaller airways, which, in turn, branch into even smaller airways called **bronchioles**. This extensive branching of airways resembles an inverted tree and is referred to as the *bronchial tree*. The bronchioles are composed mainly of smooth muscle and elastic connective tissue. This allows them to stretch to accommodate incoming air. Eventually the bronchioles branch into **alveoli** (*alveolus* is singular). Alveoli are the air sacs in the lungs. They have very thin walls that contain a lot of elastic tissue, and they stretch as they fill with air, like little balloons.

The **pulmonary** (from Latin *pulmonarius*, meaning "lung") capillary network surrounds the alveoli and is fused to the outer wall of the alveoli. The pulmonary capillaries are derived from pulmonary arteries, which transport deoxygenated blood from the heart to the lungs. Between the wall of the pulmonary capillaries and the walls of the alveoli is the **respiratory membrane**. The respiratory membrane is the site of gas exchange. Oxygen diffuses from the air in the alveoli across the respiratory membrane into blood in the pulmonary capillaries. Carbon dioxide diffuses from the blood in the pulmonary capillaries to the air in the alveoli.

After the blood in the pulmonary capillaries becomes oxygenated, it flows into pulmonary veins that carry it back to the heart so that it can be pumped to all the tissues of the body. At the tissue level, the oxygen diffuses from the blood into the cells, and carbon dioxide from the cells diffuses into the blood. The deoxygenated blood then travels back to the heart so that it can be pumped to the lungs to become oxygenated again (Tortora and Derrickson, 2009).

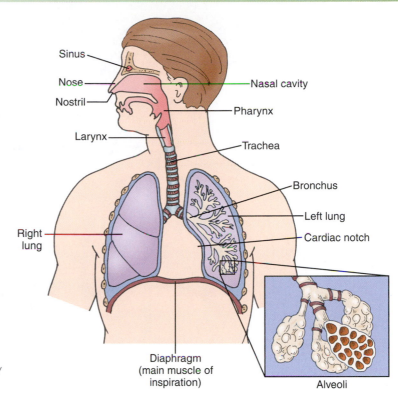

FIGURE 4-1 Overview of the respiratory system.

Focus on Wellness

There are several reasons why someone who smokes may become easily winded during even moderate exertion (Fig. 4-2). These include the following:

- The constriction of small air passageways; this decreases airflow into and out of the lungs.
- Carbon monoxide, a toxin in cigarette smoke, binds to hemoglobin, the oxygen-carrying part of red blood cells. This reduces the amount of oxygen that red blood cells can transport to cells.
- Irritants in smoke cause increased mucus secretion and cause the linings of the respiratory tract and bronchial tree to swell, impeding airflow into and out of the lungs.
- Irritants in smoke inhibit the movement of cilia, which are microscopic, hairlike appendages of cells that move mucus and what is trapped in the mucus up and out of the lungs and respiratory tract. Over time, the irritants in cigarette smoke can even destroy the cilia. Thus, excess mucus and foreign debris are not easily removed, which further adds to breathing difficulty.
- With time, smoking destroys elastic fibers in the lungs and is the prime cause of emphysema, a disease in which the alveoli can no longer push air out. This causes less efficient gas exchange.

The following are websites that offer information about how to quit smoking:

The American Cancer Society:
www.cancer.org/docroot/PED/content/PED_10_13X_Guide_for_Quitting_Smoking.asp

The American Heart Association:
www.heart.org/HEARTORG/GettingHealthy/QuitSmoking/Quit-Smoking_UCM_001085_SubHomePage.jsp

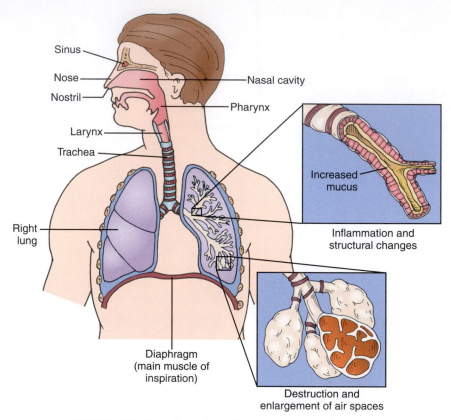

FIGURE 4-2 The effects of smoking on the respiratory system.

PULMONARY VENTILATION

The trunk of the body is divided into two main sections: the thoracic cavity and the abdominopelvic cavity. The thoracic cavity includes everything contained in the rib cage, which extends from the base of the neck to a few inches above the navel. In effect, it is a sealed-off container for the lungs, with the heart resting in between. The abdominal cavity is the part of the trunk that begins at the inferior border of the rib cage and fills the space down into the pelvis. This cavity contains the digestive organs, the urinary system, and the reproductive organs. The two cavities are separated by a strong muscle called the *diaphragm*. It attaches all around the inferior border of the rib cage and down to the lumbar spine. It looks like an open parachute that curves up into the thoracic cavity, forming both the top of the abdominal cavity and the bottom of the thoracic cavity (Fig. 4-3).

Air movement into and out of the lungs is called **pulmonary ventilation**, and it consists of inhalation

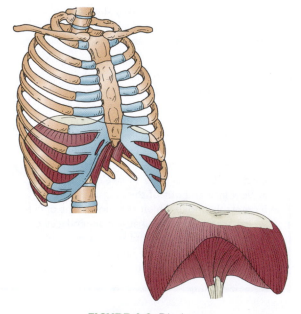

FIGURE 4-3 Diaphragm.

(inspiration) and exhalation (expiration). Pulmonary ventilation is a mechanical process because it involves muscular contraction, muscular relaxation, and elastic recoil of the alveoli. Air moves from high pressure to low pressure. Just before each inhalation, atmospheric pressure equals air pressure in the lungs. To move air into the lungs, the air pressure in the lungs needs to become lower than atmospheric pressure. This is accomplished by enlarging the thoracic cavity.

The **diaphragm** is the main muscle of inhalation; it is responsible for about 75% of air that enters the lungs during quiet breathing. When it contracts, it descends and enlarges the thoracic cavity. The external intercostal muscles also assist in inhalation by lifting the ribs and the sternum; they are responsible for about 25% of the air that enters the lungs during normal, quiet breathing. Air pressure in the lungs drops, air is drawn in, and normal, quiet inhalation occurs. This is an active process. The alveoli fill up with air. Normal, quiet inhalation draws in approximately 500 milliliters (1/2 liter) of air.

Normal, quiet exhalation occurs when the diaphragm relaxes and descends, and elastic recoil of the alveoli pushes air out. This is a passive process. Approximately 500 milliliters of air is moved out.

The added benefits of the diaphragm's movement are that it assists in venous blood return to the heart from the lower extremities and in the flow of lymph in the lymphatic vessels of the lower extremities. This is referred to as the **respiratory pump**. During inhalation, as the diaphragm moves downward, the decrease in pressure in the thoracic cavity and the increase in pressure in the abdominal cavity compresses the abdominal veins and lymphatic vessels. As a result, a greater volume of blood and lymph moves from the compressed abdominal veins and lymphatic vessels into the decompressed thoracic veins and lymphatic vessels. The respiratory pump is one of the ways the body combats gravity to move blood and lymph upward.

During deep, forceful inhalation, the secondary muscles of respiration are used. These include the scalenes, which lift ribs 1 and 2; sternocleidomastoid, which lifts the sternum and clavicle; pectoralis minor, which lifts ribs 3, 4, and 5; and serratus posterior superior, which lifts ribs 5, 6, and 7 (Fig. 4-4). All of these contract to greatly increase the size of the thoracic cavity and to assist in drawing in air. Deep, forceful inhalation can result in approximately 3,600 milliliters (3.6 liters) of air per breath for the

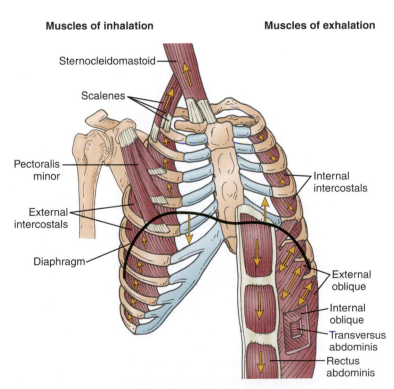

Muscles of inhalation   **Muscles of exhalation**

Sternocleidomastoid

Scalenes

Pectoralis minor

External intercostals

Diaphragm

Internal intercostals

External oblique

Internal oblique

Transversus abdominis

Rectus abdominis

Anterior view

FIGURE 4-4 Accessory muscles of respiration. The arrows indicate the direction in which the muscles contract to either elevate or compress the thoracic cavity.

average man and approximately 2,400 milliliters (2.4 liters) of air per breath for the average woman. This difference is because, in general, men have a larger body size than women.

During deep, forceful exhalation, secondary muscles of respiration will also be used. These include the abdominal muscles, which assist in pushing the diaphragm upward; the internal intercostals, which depress the ribs; and serratus posterior inferior, which depresses ribs 9, 10, 11, and 12 (see Fig. 4-4). All of these muscles contract to greatly decrease the size of the thoracic cavity and assist in pushing out air (Tortora and Derrickson, 2009).

CONTROL OF RESPIRATION

At rest, about 200 milliliters of oxygen are used each minute by body cells. During strenuous exercise, this rate increases 15 to 20 times as much in normal healthy adults and up to 30 times as much in endurance-trained athletes. Performing bodywork falls under the category of exercise and, depending on the type of bodywork being performed, can sometimes be strenuous exercise. The body has several mechanisms that help increase respiration to match metabolic demands.

A **respiratory center** is located in the brainstem. It has sections that control the basic rhythm of breathing and ensure smooth transitions between inhalation and exhalation. During quiet breathing, the respiratory center sends nerve impulses to the diaphragm and external intercostal muscles, causing them to contract, and inhalation occurs for about 2 seconds. At the end of 2 seconds, the impulses stop, the diaphragm and external intercostal muscles relax, and elastic recoil of the alveoli push air out. Exhalation occurs for about 3 seconds. During forceful inhalation and exhalation, nerve impulses are sent to accessory muscles of respiration, causing them to contract.

Normal breathing consists of a shorter inhale and a longer exhale. Adults actually take between 12 and 16 breaths per minute. Men breathe slightly slower, about 12 to 14 times a minute, while the rate for women is typically 14 to 16 breaths per minute. With an average respiratory rate of 14 breaths per minute, a person breathes 840 times an hour, or 20,160 times a day, throughout her life.

The basic rhythm of respiration can be modified in response to input from other parts of the brain, receptors in the peripheral nervous system, and other factors. Because the cerebrum has connections with the respiratory center, people can voluntarily alter their patterns of breathing. For example, they can hold their breath. However, this is limited by the buildup of carbon dioxide and acidity in the bloodstream. When they reach a certain level, the respiratory area is strongly stimulated. Nerve impulses are sent to inspiratory muscles and breathing resumes.

Proprioceptors play a role in stimulating respiration. As a person starts increasing her levels of activity, her rate and depth of breathing increase, even before changes in blood levels of carbon dioxide, acidity, and oxygen occur. Proprioceptors that monitor movement of joints and muscles respond quickly to send nerve impulses into the respiratory center to ensure there is no lag time between starting to exercise and increasing air intake. This is so respiration will instantly match metabolic demands.

Anticipation of activity, such as thinking about hiking or cycling or performing bodywork, or emotional anxiety may stimulate the limbic system, which then sends excitatory input to the respiratory area, increasing the rate and depth of ventilation. This is another way the body prepares to meet the demands of metabolic needs of increased movement (Tortora and Derrickson, 2009).

TYPES OF BREATHING

The term for the normal pattern of quiet breathing is **eupnea** (from Latin *eupnous* meaning "breathing freely"). Eupnea can consist of shallow, deep, or a combination of shallow and deep breathing. There are several other ways breathing can be characterized as well.

Chest, Shoulder, or Shallow Breathing

Chest, shoulder, or **shallow breathing** is a common way of breathing that involves minimal movement of the rib cage or diaphragm. This leaves the rest of the thorax compressed and contracted (Fig. 4-5). This breathing pattern can so significantly restrict the

What Do You Think?

What do you think of the statement, "Breathing has its own inherent movement and rhythm." Do you agree or disagree? Why did you answer the way you did?

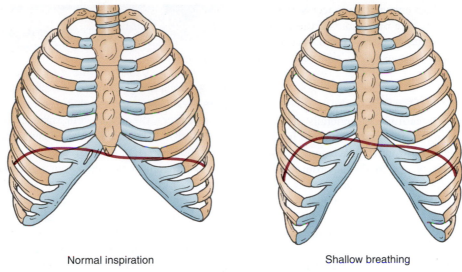

Normal inspiration   Shallow breathing

FIGURE 4-5 Changes in size of the thoracic cavity during inhalation and exhalation.

movement of the diaphragm that the work of respiration is largely taken over by the accessory respiratory muscles. The shoulders rise toward the ears during inhalation and then fall back down during exhalation; therefore, this is sometimes called *shoulder breathing*. It is usually accompanied by muscular tightness in the shoulders and upper back.

During chest breathing, a person is moving less than 500 milliliters of air into and out of the lungs. As a result, there is minimal exchange of oxygen and elimination of carbon dioxide. Continuous chest breathing results in fatigue, which can cause injury and susceptibility to illness, since there is always a large residual volume of air in the lungs with each breath. This large residual volume of air contains waste products, such as carbon dioxide, moisture, and particles of substances. Additionally, since the air is relatively static, mucus cannot be removed from the lungs and the upper respiratory tract. This increases vulnerability to respiratory infections, such as colds, flu, and pneumonia.

Diaphragmatic or Abdominal Breathing

During **diaphragmatic** or **abdominal breathing**, the person focuses quite directly on engaging the diaphragm as fully as possible in the movements of breathing. The rib cage is greatly expanded and muscles of the abdomen assist the diaphragm in fully descending and ascending during the breathing cycle. The abdomen balloons during inhalation and

flattens during exhalation (see Fig. 4-5). This is why diaphragmatic breathing is also commonly referred to as *abdominal breathing*. This is the most effortless way to breathe because it decreases the work of the accessory muscles of respiration, with the exception of the abdominal muscles, which are larger and stronger than the rest of the accessory muscles.

This is a much deeper form of breathing, with up to an average of 3,600 milliliters of air for men and 2,400 milliliters of air for women being moved with each breath. Diaphragmatic breathing allows the body to eliminate large amounts of carbon dioxide and other wastes with each breath. It also decreases heart rate, stress, muscle tension and fatigue, and the perception of pain (Rosen, 2010).

Many methods of relaxation—including meditation, yoga, visualization, and exercise—use this form of breathing. This is because by consciously engaging in diaphragmatic breathing, the focus is on the breath. This allows the mind to calm and the body to relax.

To develop a supportive breathing pattern, become mindful of when your breathing is interrupted because of stress or pain, and then consciously return to diaphragmatic breathing. When breathing is impaired, your entire body becomes restricted and strained, and injuries can occur. A healthy and supportive breathing pattern allows your body to have more fluid movements, giving you more freedom to be dynamic in your body mechanics. When your diaphragm is not fully engaged, your accessory respiratory muscles must take over more of the work of breathing. This results in excessive muscular effort, and in turn leads to tension in the neck, chest, abdomen, and back.

Nose or Nostril Breathing

Nose or nostril breathing is generally a slower process of bringing air into the lungs, and it allows the air to gently move from the environment to the lungs and then back out to the environment. Air brought into the body through the nose is filtered through the nasal hairs, and many impurities are removed as they stick to the nasal cavity mucus. Additionally, the air is warmed and moistened before it enters the lungs.

This method is also frequently used in meditation, relaxation, yoga, and many breath-work methods. Nose breathing can affect the higher reasoning centers of the brain, as well as certain regulatory areas such as the hypothalamus and the pituitary gland. The endocrine and immune systems can be affected as well. The optimal overall effects are increased mental awareness, levels of consciousness, meditative states, and internal states of awareness (Rosen, 2010).

Body Awareness

This is an exercise in nose or nostril breathing. Sitting upright and comfortable, breathe in and out slowly and evenly three times. Inhale once more, then close your right nostril with your right thumb, and exhale fully through the left nostril. When the exhalation is complete, close the left nostril with your right index finger, release your right nostril, and inhale through your right nostril. It is important that the inhalation and exhalation are of equal length and depth. Repeat this cycle of exhaling through your left nostril and inhaling through your right nostril two more times. Switch to repeat the process by exhaling through the right nostril and inhaling through the left nostril. Repeat this three times to complete another cycle.

Try practicing this exercise twice a day. Your focus is to increase the length of your inspiration and expiration and to keep each of them equal. See if it helps you relax and allows for a greater focus on the task at hand.

Body Awareness

This is an exercise in diaphragmatic breathing. Gently place your hands on your abdomen. Exhale slowly through your mouth until you feel as if all the air has slowly and gently left your body. Now slowly breathe in, first filling the lungs so that your hands over your abdomen begin to move up. Once this area is filled, continue to breathe until your rib cage is fully expanded. At this point, you have used your diaphragm to fully fill your lungs with air. After a few seconds, exhale fully, contracting your abdominal muscles. Repeat this process for several breaths. Make sure you do not inhale and exhale so quickly you start hyperventilating. How do you feel? Do you feel lighter and more energized? If not, what do you think happened?

Mouth Breathing

Expiration of air through the mouth or pursed lips is frequently used in breathing exercises. Exhaling in this way forces more air out of the lungs to make space for more air to come in during inspiration. This promotes better exchange of oxygen and carbon dioxide. Mouth breathing tends to be more rapid and is usually associated with activity that is stressful on the body, such as exercise or emotional issues. The advantage of mouth breathing is that air can be brought into the lungs more quickly, but the quality is less conditioned. When a person breathes in through the mouth, the air is not cleaned by the nasal hair and nasal passages, nor is it warmed and moistened. In this way, the focus is on quantity of air rather than quality.

Practitioners should note that rapid mouth breathing can result in hyperventilation. This rapid, uncontrolled breathing occurs when blood levels of oxygen become too high and carbon dioxide levels become too low. Recall from the "Control of Respiration" section that high blood levels of carbon dioxide stimulate the respiratory center to cause inhalation. The best method to alleviate hyperventilation is to have the person breathe into his hands or into a paper bag, thus inhaling carbon dioxide he just exhaled. Within a few minutes, his blood levels of carbon dioxide should increase, and his breathing will become slower and deeper.

FOCUS ON BREATHING

The physical structure of the body suffers from inefficient breathing patterns. One way to think of this is that, with over 20,000 breaths per day, the muscles associated with breathing will be used incorrectly over 20,000 times per day. During efficient breathing, all the primary and secondary muscles of respiration function in a balanced way. On the other hand, incorrect breathing can mean chronic muscle dysfunction, muscle pain, and syndromes like chronic headache and backache.

Voice of Experience

The most important aspect of breathing that will most benefit your clients and your stamina as a bodyworker is to learn how to breathe through your nose all the time. Here are some reasons and helpful tips.

With nose breathing, the air circulates throughout the entire chest cavity or through all five lobes of the lungs. It distributes air more evenly, helping the body to relax and receive a more sustainable amount of air over the long run. This method can help us stay more relaxed during the day and make breathing easier.

Mouth breathing results in chest breathing, which is useful in emergencies when you need a lot of air in a hurry, like when you are in "fight or flight." Using our mouths to breathe can dry out our airway, bring polluted air into our lungs, and force our lungs to adjust to air that may be the wrong temperature. The nasal passage helps to moisturize the air; balance the air for the correct temperature to enter the lungs, which is body temperature; and filter 95% to 98% of the pollutants in the air before it enters your lungs.

Do yourself a favor during the day that will help you recover from breathing challenges—pace yourself in your daily activities so that you can breathe through your nose all the time.

Robert Litman, certified Buteyko Institute Method of Breathing Retraining Educator since 2003; authorized Continuum Movement Teacher since 1999 and a member of the Continuum Movement faculty in Los Angeles since 2000; certified in the Duggan/French Approach to Somatic Pattern Recognition in 1988 and advanced certification in 1992.

Regardless of age or fitness level, people can focus on their breathing and take steps to improve it. Unconscious and conscious breathing patterns can be altered to truly affect long-term health and well-being. Once efficient breathing patterns are established and integrated so that they become an unconscious process, resistance to stress and disease increases, metabolic functions improve, and chronic pain patterns may be alleviated. However, the way to focus and enhance breathing is not by just doing a few deep-breathing exercises once in a while or whenever the thought strikes. They must be done daily to reset the respiratory center in the brainstem.

RESPIRATORY POSTURE

Because pulmonary ventilation involves coordinating the contraction and relaxation of many different muscles, you can start by honestly evaluating your posture, as discussed in Chapter 3. You can do this by standing in front of a mirror; having someone take your photo; honestly assessing your posture; and being receptive to what trusted mentors, colleagues, and friends say about how you hold yourself.

Classic signs of poor breathing include:

- Mouth breathing
- Forward head posture
- Rounded shoulders
- Thoracic kyphosis
- Sunken chest
- Rigidity in the body

Check to see if you are able to take a normal, deep, diaphragmatic breath. Ask yourself the following questions:

- Does my abdomen distend and my lower ribs move up and widen?
- Does my abdomen stay flat and my shoulders rise toward my ears?
- Do my shoulders and upper chest stay relatively still?
- Can I take a deep, satisfying breath?
- Does my breath feel shallow and constricted?

Another step is to have an experienced bodywork practitioner, such as a massage therapist, assess your primary and secondary muscles of respiration through palpation. Does the margin of the diaphragm along your ribs feel tight? Does your rib cage feel constricted with tightness in the intercostal muscles? How do your abdominals and serratus posterior inferior feel upon palpation? Are the scalenes, sternocleidomastoid, and serratus posterior superior exhibiting a great deal of tension and tightness?

Postural muscles—such as upper trapezius and the medial scapular group, including levator scapula—will also tend to be tight. Additionally, quadratus lumborum and psoas may be chronically shortened. Shortening in quadratus lumborum or shoulder pain is often not identified as resulting from inefficient breathing patterns when that may indeed be the root cause.

> **Myth:** Slouching feels more comfortable, so that must be more efficient for the body.
>
> **FACT:** Slouching compresses the thoracic cavity, impairing the function of the primary and secondary muscles of respiration. As a result, insufficient oxygen is inhaled, and insufficient amounts of carbon dioxide are exhaled. The body cells do not have the oxygen they need for metabolism, which means the body operates less efficiently.

MUSCLE MOVEMENT

During inhalation, the thoracic cavity must be enlarged so that air can rush into the lungs. This cavity increases in size when the diaphragm descends, and the external intercostal muscles contract to expand the rib cage up and out. In the case of an extremely deep inhalation, accessory muscles elevate the rib cage even more. Each rib articulates with a vertebra so that during inhalation, each rib can move up and out from the vertebral column. This means that while the rib cage tends to move as a whole, individual segments can also be moved. It also means that when the rib cage expands, there is movement around the entire trunk, posteriorly and anteriorly.

During exhalation, the thoracic cavity reduces in size through a reversal of the inhalation process. The muscles between the ribs and in the upper chest lengthen, allowing the rib cage to compress downward due to the pull of gravity on the ribs. The diaphragm elevates. Because of this, breathing fairly deeply, with

Body Awareness

While sitting in a chair, slouch down (into an imbalanced posture) and focus your attention on your breathing. Notice how your body feels during inhalation. In particular, feel how the weight of your head and upper trunk compress the anterior rib cage and then must be pushed upward as part of the intake of air. Come back into balanced posture and check your breathing again. What changes do you feel in your breathing while in balanced posture as opposed to breathing while in an imbalanced posture?

The purpose of bringing your attention to breathing is to sharpen your sensory awareness so that you can feel corrective feedback more readily. This is part of your body awareness. Over time, you will need to give less conscious attention toward correcting your inefficient breathing patterns.

Focus on Wellness

The following are suggestions to improve respiratory posture:

- Receive regular massage therapy or other types of bodywork that specifically address the primary and secondary muscles of respiration.
- Participate regularly in activities that focus on movement and breath such as yoga, dancing, or martial arts.
- Do a pectoral stretch. This helps open the chest. Lie supine on a massage table or bench. Take a deep breath and exhale as you horizontally abduct your arm off the massage table or bench and stretch your pectorals (Fig. 4-6).
- Do arm movements. The advantage of this exercise is that it quickly increases oxygen in the lungs. Begin by standing with your knees slightly bent and feet shoulder-width apart. Move your arms so they are straight ahead at shoulder height. Breathe out in three short exhalations through pursed lips, making the final expiration a long one, as if blowing a feather across a room. As you are exhaling, bring your arms down to your sides. Then do a slow inspiration, moving your arms up to their starting position. Repeat three or four times.

For another exercise, try focusing on a full expiration of breath through pursed lips, followed by three rapid inspirations.

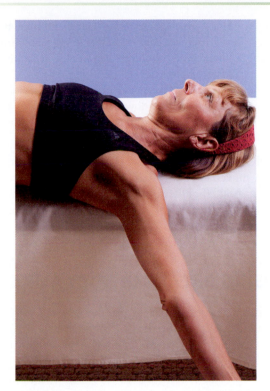

FIGURE 4-6 Pectoral stretch on a massage table.

specific attention paid to the exhalation, is a way to help ease tension and pain in the neck, shoulder, and back regions.

BREATHING ACTIVITIES

When changing your breathing patterns so they become more efficient, the challenge is to become aware of breathing without controlling it—to focus attention on unconscious and spontaneous actions without converting them into formal, directed activities. There are, of course, many occasions when breathing needs to be controlled for various reasons such as during athletics, while singing, performing certain yoga exercises, and meditation. However, the purpose of the breathing activities in this section is to become aware of breathing without controlling it. It is not necessarily an easy thing to do, but it is well worth learning.

As with support of the body's core (which is discussed in more detail in Chapters 5 and 8), the goal is to let go of voluntary nervous system control of breathing. Do not expect to achieve a perfect release of control, especially at the beginning. Just keep in mind that the intention is to focus on breathing in order to perceive, not manage, your breathing. The only factors you should be aware of are where you are directing your attention, how you are adjusting your balance, and the muscle tension you feel releasing, especially in your trunk and neck. You may find that when you quiet and focus your attention on your breath, your breathing changes, sometimes dramatically.

Breathing activities promote relaxation in the following ways:

- Achieve overall relaxation by tensing and relaxing the muscles of respiration. A deep inhalation tenses the muscles of inhalation and relaxes the muscles of exhalation; a deep exhalation relaxes the muscles of inhalation and tenses the muscles of exhalation.
- Allow for more oxygen to be absorbed into the bloodstream. This will improve body functions by assisting the body's response, repair, and recovery from stress.
- Slow the heart rate by increasing the amount of oxygen in the bloodstream. This produces a calming effect.
- Focus on breathing allows the person to pause and plan responses to a stressful situation. This can result in mental clarity and calmness during times of stress (Courtney, 2003).

Suggested Activities

Breath can be speeded up or slowed down, but it can also feel like it is being initiated in different parts of the body. Here are some exercises to try:

- Inhale through your nose so the air can be filtered. Exhale four times longer than you normally do, or until you feel that all the air has been released, and then exhale some more. The more you release through exhalation, the greater amount of air you can take in during your next breath.
  - With each inhalation, imagine life is filling inside of you, and with each exhalation, imagine you are releasing pain, discomfort, or stress.
  - Visualize breath as not just coming from your abdomen, diaphragm, or chest, but as a movement of life that affects every cell in your body.
  - Notice how you feel before, during, and after this activity.
- Stage 1 breathing. This is a basic technique for getting connected to yourself and realizing the importance of breath in everything you do.

1. Lie on your back with your legs extended out in front of you. Place your hands on your chest, one on top of the other.
2. Close your eyes and breathe gently into your nose and out of your mouth.
3. Pay attention to how it feels when you breathe into each of the following places and ask yourself, "Is there movement?"
4. As you breathe in, expand your chest by bringing the breath into it. Feel how easy or difficult this is.
5. Repeat for several breaths, and then move your hands to the area at the bottom of your sternum, just below where your ribs come together.
6. Breathe there several times. Feel how easy or difficult this is.
7. Now move your hands on top of your navel and take several breaths. Feel how easy or difficult this is.
8. Decide where the easiest and most difficult places in your body are to breathe, and place one hand in each of those areas.
9. Alternate your breath in between those two areas, enjoying the ease of one place and acknowledging the tension, discomfort, or restriction in the other.
10. Notice what changes.

- Qigong exercise. Recall from Chapter 2 that the ancient practice of qigong is performed specifically to help the practitioner focus on developing qi, breath, and awareness. This exercise is a lung and breathing revitalizer. It is designed to move your arms to maximize your chest expansion, which allows your lungs to expand more fully. This exercise involves qigong breathing, which means you should push your abdomen out when inhaling and pull it back in on the exhale. Make sure your shoulders are relaxed and down throughout all the movements.

  1. Place your arms straight in front of your body at shoulder level, as if you are about to start swimming the breaststroke. Turn your palms outward. Your arm muscles should be loose so that your arms feel as if they are resting on water (Fig. 4-7A).
  2. Inhale very slowly and horizontally abduct your arms. Squeeze your scapulae together while keeping your shoulders relaxed (Fig. 4-7B).
  3. Once you have abducted your arms as far as is comfortable for you, turn your palms up.

Exhale slowly, and move your arms back toward your starting position. Keep your arms and hands at shoulder level in front of your body (Fig. 4-7C).
4. As your hands reach your starting position, turn your palms down then outward. Inhale, and horizontally abduct your arms to repeat the exercise (Fig. 4-7D).

Repeat this exercise for 5 to 10 minutes. Your arm movements will help to release tension from your chest, shoulders, and upper back. Over time, your arm muscles will also strengthen (Friedman, 2009).

USING BREATH IN BODYWORK

When practitioners become tired or stressed, fatigue can affect their awareness of themselves and their movements, their clients and their needs, and the bodywork treatments. An important thing to keep in mind is that when the body is moving during walking, running, dancing, or even performing bodywork treatments, there is an automatic increase in mental awareness. This is because instinctively the body wants to avoid injury, and the way to do this is to be alert and mentally clear. Methods to increase this awareness, which will help you stay injury-free throughout your career, involve focusing on your breath while performing bodywork.

Breath and the way it fills your rib cage also serves to support internal musculature as you stand and move. Expansion is especially important in your thorax, as it balances the movements and contractions of the skeletal muscles that move your shoulders, arms, and hands. Observe the rhythmic contracting and relaxing of your primary breathing muscles. Your breath needs to fill your upper lungs as well as the lower portion. Also remember to breathe in a smooth and natural rhythm throughout the treatment.

What Do You Think?

If you perform a treatment with a sunken chest, what does that do to the rest of your body alignment? On the other hand, if you have an upright and open chest, how does your posture feel?

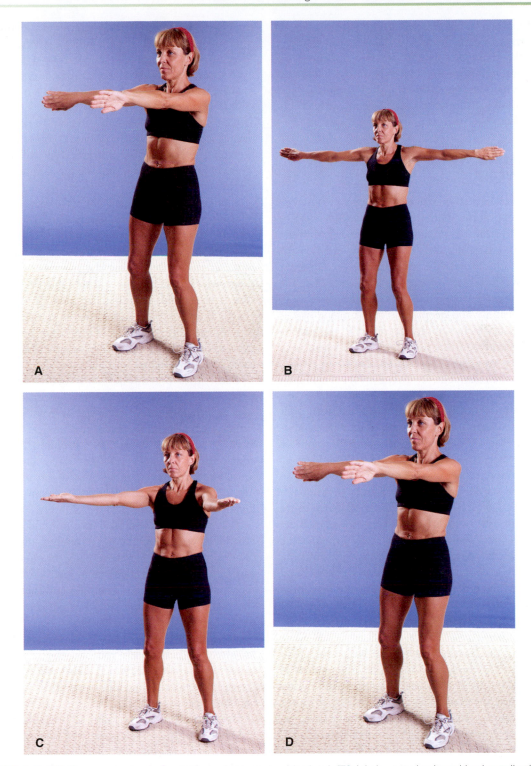

FIGURE 4-7 **(A)** Place your arms in front of your body at shoulder level. **(B)** Inhale very slowly and horizontally abduct your arms. **(C)** Bring your arms back toward the starting position with your palms up. **(D)** Turn your palms down, inhale, and horizontally abduct your arms to repeat the exercise.

Breathing in a forced manner or holding your breath can detract from focus on the client. It can also decrease the amount of oxygen necessary for the muscular contraction required to perform the bodywork movements. Carbon dioxide and other wastes can also build up, leading to muscle tension and soreness in your body.

BREATHING WHILE PERFORMING BODYWORK

Emphasis needs to be placed on the proper rhythm of breathing during bodywork, both with delivery of technique and the practitioner's internal rhythm. Breathing efficiently assists in the delivery of techniques and ensures the practitioner's endurance. Also, how the practitioner breathes can often cue the client to breathe the same way. If the practitioner breathes calmly and deeply, the client may do so as well, enhancing her ability to relax. If the practitioner breathes quickly and sharply, the client may start doing so as well and not be able to let go and ease into the treatment.

Before beginning a treatment, bring your awareness to your breath. You can do this by assessing your posture, seeing if you have any muscle tension anywhere in your body, and noticing whether you are breathing deeply or shallowly. Are your shoulders up around your ears? Do you feel out of breath? Do you feel upset or nervous? If so, chances are you are breathing shallowly. Does your abdominal area move in and out as you breathe? Do you feel relaxed yet energized? Are you focused and ready to begin the treatment? If so, chances are you are breathing deeply. By taking a moment to center yourself and breathe diaphragmatically, you can make any shifts in posture you need to, release any muscle tension your are feeling, and begin the treatment feeling calm and focused.

During the treatment, check in with yourself to see how you are breathing and make adjustments as necessary to ensure you keep breathing efficiently and diaphragmatically. You should also synchronize your breathing with the rhythm you are using to perform techniques. Breathe more slowly with techniques that are performed slowly, such as gliding strokes in massage therapy and palming techniques in shiatsu. Techniques that are performed more rapidly, such as vibration and percussion in massage therapy, should be accompanied by faster breathing to ensure you have adequate breath for the physical exertion. Other techniques involve no movement at all, such as certain holds in craniosacral therapy and Jin Shin Jyutsu. In these cases, quiet, even breathing allows the practitioners to stay focused and aware of what is going on in their clients' bodies.

With the intensity and concentration needed for deeper work into tissues, you should make sure your breathing does not become restricted and shallow. This can lead to tension and mental fatigue in your body during treatments. Also, sometimes a great deal of patience is needed to feel clients' tissues relax and release tension. Breathing consciously and mindfully through this can signal the client to do so as well, causing him to enter into more of a parasympathetic mode and possibly causing the muscles to relax on their own. This can allow you to apply deeper pressure, if warranted, and not have to work so hard to get the results needed. Generally, as you exhale, you should feel your weight fall into your hands, and then transfer this weight as a comfortable, deeper pressure to the client.

Sometimes practitioners will inadvertently restrict their breathing when they are lifting items such as a massage table or futon, or even when elevating a client's leg to perform a range-of-motion technique. During lifting, the abdominal muscles contract, which also restricts the diaphragm's movement. However, remember to breathe when lifting by inhaling before the lift, then exhaling during the lift.

Practitioners should also be mindful of their breathing when performing stretches on clients. Generally, inhale as you are moving the client's body part into position for the stretch. Just before you do the stretch, ask the client to inhale, and then both of you should exhale as the stretch is performed. Both the client and you should then breathe calmly and evenly while the stretch is held. Breathing this way for stretches helps both you and the client be in parasympathetic mode, which allows you to perform the stretch smoothly and allows the client's tissues to be more receptive to the stretch.

Breathing consciously helps to revitalize the entire body and can aid in comforting specific areas of stress or pain. If, for example, you experience discomfort in your neck, you can consciously focus your breath into your neck as you are working. By taking deep, slow breaths, you may be able to reduce your discomfort and keep your focus and attention on the client.

What Do You Think?

How do you think music choice affects the rhythm of your breath and techniques during the treatment? How do you think it affects the rhythm of the client's breath during the treatment?

ENCOURAGING CLIENTS TO BREATHE

When they notice practitioners using conscious breathing, some clients will remember to breathe deeply as well. Other clients may need a gentle reminder to breathe during the treatment. All deep muscle palpations should be done slowly, and the client should breathe with the palpation process in a slow and rhythmic manner. Ask the client to take in a moderate to deep breath; then as the client slowly exhales, slowly sink into the muscle. Next, ease off the pressure slightly and ask the client to take in another breath, then continue to slowly sink in deeper as the client slowly exhales again.

The following are guidelines you can give clients about relaxing and breathing into their treatment. These suggestions can be given to clients ahead of time so they can get the most out of their treatment:

- Encourage the client to settle onto the treatment table, massage chair, or futon by feeling the weight of his body sink in. Ask him to allow himself to be supported by the structure; then have him begin to notice his breathing.
- Ask the client to feel where his breathing is most noticeable in his body, and invite his breath to move into the parts of his body that feel less full.
- When the treatment starts, have the client notice the pressure and rhythm. While maintaining a comfortable rhythm in his breathing, suggest the client notice when you let up on pressure and breathe in. When you apply pressure, he should breathe out.
- If there is an area on the client's body that is particularly tender when you work on it, encourage the client to pay special attention to his breath. He can work with the tenderness on the exhale, imagining that he is breathing out the pain.
- As you work on different areas, ask the client to imagine his breath moving there to meet you. He can send his breath wherever you are working. Tell the client that you can work on the outside of his body while he works on the inside.
- Notice the changes as the treatment progresses. The client can notice his thought patterns and his comfort and stress levels change as he sends breath to the various areas of his body.
- When the session is complete and the client sits up, ask him to notice how his breath feels. He can also pay attention to what he notices about his body.

For clients experiencing minor physical discomfort, such as from a mild headache, backache, upset stomach, or menstrual cramps, leading them through some of the simple breathing techniques presented in this chapter may help to relieve them. Practitioners can encourage these clients to focus their breath into the area of discomfort, and then guide them through slow and deep cycles of breathing.

FIELD NOTES

I spend a great deal of time working on my body mechanics. I also make an effort to schedule at least a 30-minute break between each client so that I can take the time to rest, stretch, hydrate, and eat if need be. I am also very careful to adjust the table height for each client and for the type of work I am going to be doing on that individual. I do my best to take care of any minor issues as soon as they come up and not let them become a problem (minor aches and pains unrelated to my work).

Do all you can to take care of yourself. Preparation prior to work is all-important. Make sure that you have plenty of time between clients, hydrate properly, stretch often, and get proper nutrition. If you notice a problem developing, don't assume it will get better on its own; take care of it right away.

David Blum, LMT, Certified in Kinesio Taping. Massage therapist since 2006.

Case Profile

Tricia is 24 years old and has been a massage therapist for 3 years. Her massage therapy school offered optional movement and body awareness courses along with the required anatomy, physiology, kinesiology, pathology, and basic and advanced technique classes. However, Tricia preferred learning deep-tissue and sports-massage techniques and did not see the point in taking any of the movement and body awareness courses. During her technique classes, her instructors gave her feedback on how she would hold her breath and did not seem to work with her practice partner's breath while performing certain techniques. Tricia thought they were being too critical, especially since she was young, healthy, in shape, and did not smoke. She thought her breathing was just fine.

Tricia is currently working at her dream job. She gives treatments to elite athletes at a training center, and she is kept quite busy. One of her regular clients, Chiwetal, is a professional cyclist. He has been happy with the results of Tricia's treatments and tells her he is recommending one of his friends, Jose, to come see her.

Jose arrives the next week for a scheduled treatment. While Chiwetal did say that Jose is 30 years old, he did not mention that Jose uses a wheelchair, as he has a T8 spinal cord injury from a car accident he was in when he was 20. Jose tells Tricia that he is having shortness of breath when he manually uses his chair. Tricia feels confident in giving him a treatment to address muscular tension through his clothing while he is in his chair but does not know how to help him improve his breathing any other way.

■ *What breathing methods and activities would you recommend to Tricia to help Jose?*

■ *How would you recommend Tricia instruct Jose in the practice of these methods and activities?*

■ *What would you recommend Tricia do for herself to learn more about breathing methods and activities?*

Wellness Profile Check-In

Looking at the Wellness Profile you completed at the end of Chapter 1, are there any challenge areas you could remedy with efficient breathing patterns? If so, what are they? How would you like to improve these areas? What breathing exercises or activities will you use to improve these areas? Write down a plan for improvement that includes the methods you will use, a timeline for implementing these methods, and ways you will assess your improvement along the way.

SUMMARY

Efficient breath is needed to perform tasks without becoming worn out, to withstand stress, and to recuperate from strain. Practitioners need to have effective breathing methods in order to ensure efficient oxygen intake and carbon dioxide release. The breath and the way it fills the body serves as a support to internal musculature as they stand and move. It also gives practitioners the stamina and strength needed to perform treatments of varying lengths, which is part of having a long career in the bodywork profession.

Proper breathing is important, yet many people do not breathe efficiently. This can be due to the stress of busy lives; excessive heat; high humidity; air pollution; pain; and physical, mental, and emotional traumas. It can also be due to smoking or breathing in secondhand smoke. However, people can consciously change their patterns of breathing. By bringing their awareness to their breath, they can choose to breathe more efficiently.

The respiratory and cardiovascular systems provide a continual supply of oxygen to cells for metabolism. Besides the function of gas exchange, the respiratory system also helps regulate blood pH, detects smells, filters incoming air, produces sounds, and eliminates some water and heat. The respiratory system consists of the nose, nasal cavity, pharynx, larynx, trachea, bronchial tree, and lungs. Between the wall of the pulmonary capillaries and the walls of the alveoli is the respiratory membrane, which is the site of gas exchange.

Air movement into and out of the lungs is called *pulmonary ventilation*. The primary muscle of inhalation is the diaphragm. Accessory muscles of respiration include the external intercostals, scalenes, sternocleidomastoid, pectoralis minor, serratus posterior superior, abdominal muscles, internal intercostal muscles, and serratus posterior inferior. The respiratory center is located in the brainstem and controls the basic rhythm of breathing. The basic rhythm of respiration can be modified in response to input from the limbic system, other parts of the cerebrum, and proprioceptors. Breathing occurs automatically but can be consciously controlled as well. The four types of breathing are chest, diaphragmatic, nose, and mouth breathing. The most efficient is diaphragmatic. Many methods of relaxation, meditation, yoga, visualization, and exercise use this form of breathing.

A healthy and supportive breathing pattern allows the body to be less restricted, giving practitioners more freedom to be dynamic in their body mechanics. No matter the age or fitness level, people can focus on their breathing and take steps to improve it. These include determining what their respiratory posture is, performing activities to improve it, and becoming aware of breathing without controlling it.

You should be mindful of using your breath when performing bodywork to keep from becoming tired or stressed. You need to make sure you are breathing diaphragmatically, breathing rhythmically with the techniques you are using, allowing breathing time to work more deeply in the client's tissues, and breathing while lifting. You can also educate clients on how to breathe while receiving treatments and how to use breathing to stay calm and centered in their everyday lives.

Review Questions

MULTIPLE CHOICE

1. When someone is worried or excited, his respiration rate tends to become
   a. slower.
   b. deeper.
   c. regular.
   d. shallow.

2. The two body systems that cooperate to supply oxygen and eliminate carbon dioxide are the respiratory and
   a. cardiovascular system.
   b. endocrine system.
   c. nervous system.
   d. muscular system.

3. Which of the following is a function of the respiratory system?
   a. Help regulate blood pH
   b. Detect smells
   c. Eliminate water and heat
   d. All of the above

4. Which of the following muscles or group of muscles is primarily responsible for inhalation?
   a. Internal intercostals
   b. Diaphragm
   c. Abdominals
   d. Psoas major

5. Air movement into and out of the lungs occurs due to a process called
   a. eupnea.
   b. respiratory pump.
   c. pulmonary ventilation.
   d. qigong.

6. Which of the following is a classic sign of poor respiration?
   a. Nose breathing
   b. Backward head posture
   c. Rounded shoulders
   d. Open chest

7. Breathing activities promote relaxation by
   a. allowing less oxygen to be absorbed into the bloodstream.
   b. allowing the chance to pause and plan responses to stress.
   c. causing the heart to beat harder and faster.
   d. causing overall chronic tension in the muscles.

FILL-IN-THE-BLANK

1. Breathing rhythm and rate reflect the body's _____ and _____ conditions.

2. The term for all the chemical reactions that occur in the body is _____.

3. Between the wall of the pulmonary capillaries and the walls of the alveoli is the _____.

4. After the blood in the pulmonary capillaries becomes oxygenated, it flows into pulmonary veins that carry it back to the _____.

5. At rest, about _____ milliliters of oxygen are used each minute by body cells.

6. The challenge in becoming efficient at breathing is to become aware of breathing without _____ it.

7. The breath and the way it fills the rib cage also serve as a support to internal _____ as the practitioner stands and moves.

SHORT ANSWER

1. Explain how bodywork practitioners are educators for clients in terms of breathing efficiently.

2. Give at least four reasons why most people do not breathe efficiently.

3. Explain how cigarette smoking decreases respiratory efficiency. Give at least four specific reasons why.

4. Explain how the respiratory center controls breathing. Include how people can voluntarily control their breathing.

5. Briefly describe chest, diaphragmatic, nostril, and mouth breathing.

6. Describe how breathing efficiently is essential to performing bodywork.

7. Explain at least four ways practitioners can encourage their clients to breathe when receiving bodywork.

Activities

1. To deepen your breath while inviting the child within you to come out and play:
   - Spread your arms up and out as if they are wings and breathe deeply
   - Blow up balloons
   - Blow bubbles
2. Use the Internet to research the lung capacities of elite athletes like Lance Armstrong and Serena and Venus Williams.
3. Participate in a yoga or qigong class for at least 3 weeks. Journal how your breathing changes throughout each of the classes and how it changes over time.

4. Perform 10 bodywork treatments while bringing your awareness to how you breathe while performing the techniques. How does your breathing change as you apply pressure? Journal what you discover about your breathing during each of the treatments—what feels comfortable for you, what feels uncomfortable, what you find challenging, what you find successful, and so forth. Review your journals to see what awareness you are developing from each treatment, how your breathing has changed, and what you still need to work on.

REFERENCES

Chaitow, Leon. *Palpation and Assessment Skills: Assessment Through Touch.* London, England: Churchill Livingstone, 2009.

Courtney, Rosalba, D.O. Breathe Easy (2003). Retrieved October 2010 from www.massagetherapy.com/articles/index.php/article_id/307/Breathe-Easy.

Friedman, Suzanne B. *Heal Yourself With Qigong.* Oakland, CA: New Harbinger Publications, 2009.

Fritz, Sandy. *Fundamentals of Therapeutic Massage,* 4th ed. St. Louis, MO: Mosby Elsevier, 2009.

Rosen, Richard. Inhale, Exhale, Relax (2010). Retrieved October 2010 from www.yogajournal.com/practice/1523.

Tortora, Gerard J., and Bryan Derrickson. *Principles of Anatomy and Physiology,* 12th ed. Hoboken, NJ: John Wiley & Sons, 2009.

Body Mechanics

Key Terms

Archetypes
Circular force
Compressive force
Cumulative trauma
    disorders (CTD)
Fulcrum
Hypermobile
Kneeling stance
Lifting force
Lunge (archer, bow)
    stance
Occupational overuse
    syndromes (OOS)
Pushing force
Pulling force
Repetitive movement
    injuries (RMI)
Repetitive stress injuries
    (RSI)
Stances
Static loading
Straight (horse) stance

Learning Objectives

After studying this chapter, the reader will have the information to:

1. Explain the importance of using efficient body mechanics.
2. Describe the forces involved in the performance of bodywork.
3. Integrate the components of efficient body mechanics into treatments.
4. Evaluate his or her body positions for the performance of bodywork and make corrections as needed.
5. Demonstrate the stances for working on a massage table and a futon, and incorporate them into treatments.
6. Describe the archetypes of poor body mechanics, and give suggestions to improve them.
7. Define repetitive stress injuries (RSI), including their causes, symptoms, and risk factors.
8. Explain how environmental factors affect efficient body mechanics.

> "Movement is life. Life is a process. Improve the quality of the process and you improve the quality of life itself."
> — Moshe Feldenkrais

INTRODUCTION

Care of clients, self-care, and career longevity are enhanced when proper thought and action are given to body mechanics. Bodywork is, of course, a physical profession. Because of the physical effort involved, massage therapists who work 15 to 30 hours per week consider themselves full-time workers (Bureau of Labor Statistics, 2010). Therefore, these and practitioners of other types of bodywork need to be able to provide treatments without excessive fatigue or pain for as long as they wish to practice. When problems caused by repetitive motion and fatigue are reduced, potential earnings and career longevity are increased. Healthy lifestyles that include efficient body mechanics will also positively influence a practitioner's ability to maintain long-term career goals, including earnings.

In order to maintain a long career in bodywork, it is important to pay attention to body mechanics not only when working on clients but also when doing any other activity. For example, do you notice how you use your body when you put dishes away, run a vacuum cleaner, and lift groceries out of the car? If you like to read, how do you hold the book? How do you sit while reading? Do you keep your vertebral column in alignment, or do you slump or slouch? If you play sports, do you use your body in the most efficient way? Or do you simply relax back into habitual postural patterns and movements?

Once learned, body mechanics should be used throughout a practitioner's entire career. It takes time, effort, awareness, and a willingness to learn and use them. New practitioners need to consciously incorporate them into their bodywork treatments until they become second nature; more experienced practitioners who are in tune with their own bodies may not necessarily need to check in with themselves regularly to see how their bodies are feeling.

Improving body mechanics includes knowing your particular challenges and how to make changes to meet them. That way, when you do position your body inefficiently, you will immediately know it and can make corrections. Eventually, your body will become used to efficient body mechanics, and this will be your habitual way of standing and moving.

EFFICIENT BODY MECHANICS

Because every person's body is different, there is no one way to use the human body efficiently. The important thing is to be relaxed and comfortable and not strain when performing bodywork. If practitioners are comfortable, unstrained, and relaxed while they work, the client will benefit from rhythms that can induce relaxation and comfort. If you find yourself straining or working hard during a bodywork treatment, chances are you could improve your body mechanics.

Recall from Chapter 1 that body mechanics involve practitioners using their bodies in a careful, efficient, safe, and deliberate way to perform bodywork. This means using balanced posture, balance, leverage, and the strongest and largest muscles to perform the work. Fatigue, muscle strain, and injury result from improper use and positioning of the practitioner's body.

There are, of course, many different bodywork modalities. Each is unique, so it would be impossible to outline in this book the proper body mechanics for every individual modality. However, the same body mechanic principles apply to all modalities. Instead, the focus will be on those modalities that involve applying pressure, lifting parts of the client's body (such as lifting the leg to position it for certain techniques or to drape properly), and stretching and range-of-motion (ROM) techniques. Additionally, efficient body mechanics will be discussed for bodywork performed on a massage table and bodywork performed on a futon or mat on the floor.

Internal rhythm is important to body mechanics and treatment sessions. It keeps you moving; helps you avoid fatigue, muscle strain, and injury; conserves energy; and keeps your joints lubricated. It also keeps the treatment from becoming stagnant. A stagnant treatment is not therapeutically beneficial and can be a cause of client dissatisfaction or injury to the practitioner.

One way to think of bodywork is as a dance. Every time your hands move, your weight needs to shift as well. Also, every time the direction of your technique changes, your body should change as well. This is why it is important to use postural positions that allow for freedom of movement. As part of the dance, use a variety of techniques. This helps to avoid repetitive movements that cause stress and strain. Also, use a variety of techniques that are appropriate for your muscles, body style, and the client.

FORCES INVOLVED IN THE PERFORMANCE OF BODYWORK

In hands-on bodywork modalities, **compressive force** refers to applying pressure. *Compress* means to press or squeeze together, and *force* means strength or power exerted on an object. Therefore, compressive force is using strength or energy to apply pressure to the client's body. The pressure can be applied lightly, as when resting the hand on the client's body, or it can be applied more deeply, as with compressions

What Do You Think?

With deep, specific work, how would you minimize strain that could build in your body? How would you change your body positions? What would you do with your massage table or futon?

into muscle bellies (Fig. 5-1). It can also be applied broadly, as with the palm of the hand or the forearm, or it can be applied specifically, as with the thumb, knuckle, or fingertips. Other techniques involve **pushing** and **pulling force**. *Pushing force* means using strength or energy to move forward such as using the gliding stroke (Fig. 5-2). *Pulling force* means using strength or energy to cause motion toward the force such as applying mild traction on the client's neck (Fig. 5-3) or the pulling involved in performing stretches.

Lifting force means using strength or energy to raise an object from a lower to a higher position, such as lifting the client's leg. The client's arms, neck, head, shoulders, low back, hips, and legs can be lifted (Fig. 5-4A, B, and C). Some ROM techniques involve using **circular force**. This means using strength or energy to move a client's extremity in a circle such as for the shoulder and hip joints (Fig. 5-5A, B, and C). ROM techniques for other joints, such as the hinge joints of the elbow and knee, require pushing and pulling force.

As can be seen, every technique a bodywork practitioner performs requires the use of strength or energy. This strength or energy comes from the practitioner's body. There is a transfer of energy from the practitioner's body to the client's body, and it is how this energy is transferred that determines how effective the techniques will be. When performing bodywork properly, more of the energy is applied as force to the client's body, rather than being "lost" in the practitioner's movements.

More specifically, nerve impulses (electrical energy) travel to the practitioner's muscles. The muscles contract and pull on bones at the joints, creating movement (the electrical energy gets converted to mechanical energy). Recall from Chapter 2 that bones act as levers at the joints. The joint itself acts as a **fulcrum**, which is a support around which levers

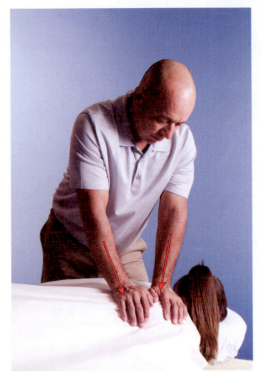

FIGURE 5-1 Application of compressive force using compressions.

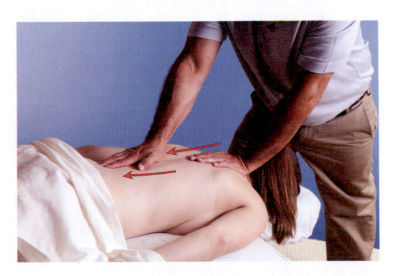

FIGURE 5-2 Application of pushing force in the gliding stoke.

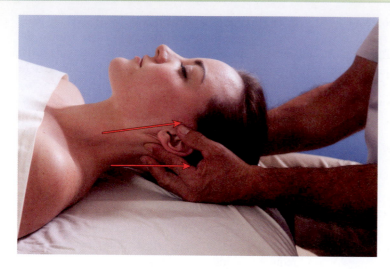

FIGURE 5-3 Application of pulling force in the neck traction.

turn. Levers and fulcrums increase mechanical force. Therefore, muscles contracting and pulling on joints actually multiply the mechanical force the practitioner's body is generating. This mechanical force is then transferred to the client's body in the form of a gliding stroke, thumbing pressure, hip ROM technique, and so forth. Therefore, to maximize the mechanical force generated, your joints need to be in their most optimal positions as you work. Otherwise, you might work harder than you need to, placing unnecessary strain on your body. Figure 5-6 shows this transfer of energy.

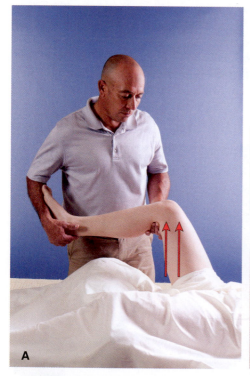

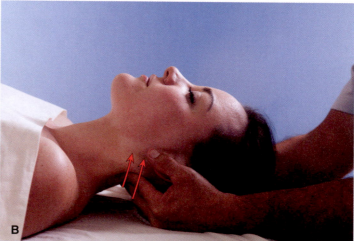

FIGURE 5-4 (A) Application of lifting force on the client's leg. **(B)** Application of lifting force on the client's head.

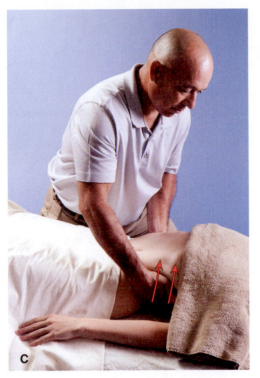

FIGURE 5-4 cont'd (C) Application of lifting force on the client's low back.

Myth: Upper body strength is most important for delivery of techniques.

FACT: Although upper body strength is important, core and leg strength serve the practitioner much better. The pelvis and lower extremities generally have larger bones and joints than the shoulder girdle, and leg muscles are larger and stronger than shoulder and arm muscles. By moving from the core and legs, the practitioner's body is in better alignment and is much more stable, and less muscle strength is needed to perform techniques. This lessens the possibility of upper body muscle strain and fatigue, thus conserving energy.

COMPONENTS OF EFFICIENT BODY MECHANICS

The human body is designed for movement and strength. However, unless practitioners use efficient body mechanics, they will not be able to apply the forces necessary to perform bodywork techniques for long periods of time without risking injury to themselves and to clients. Therefore, it is important to understand the components of efficient body mechanics. These components include stability, balance,

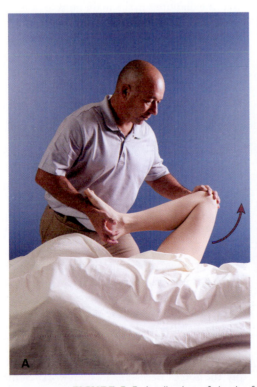

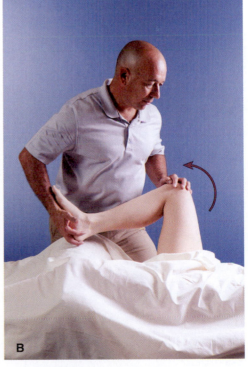

FIGURE 5-5 Application of circular force in hip range-of-motion technique.

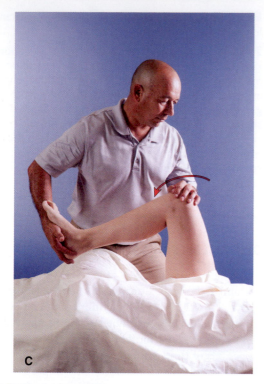

FIGURE 5-5 cont'd

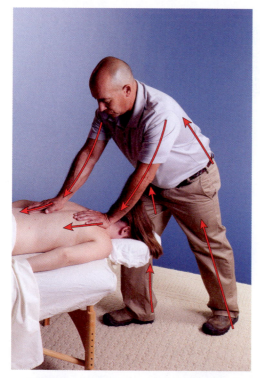

FIGURE 5-6 Transfer of energy from the practitioner's body to the client's body.

coordination, and stamina. The keys to all of these are body awareness and mindful movement (discussed in detail in Chapter 2), balanced posture (discussed in detail in Chapter 3), an understanding of center of gravity (discussed in Chapter 3), and core stability.

Recall from Chapter 1 that the core muscles are those that are in the center of the body (Fig. 5-7). The strength for performing many types of bodywork comes up through the practitioner's legs, through the torso, and then out the arms. Thus, leg strength and core strength are the foundations of body strength (in fact, some types of bodywork, such as shiatsu and Thai massage, involve techniques applied with the practitioner's knees and feet). To shift the center of gravity forward to lean and use body weight to apply force during a treatment, practitioners need core stability to keep their posture balanced and their joints stacked. Figures 5-8A and B show the shift in the practitioner's center of gravity to apply force for techniques on a massage table. Figures 5-8C and D show the shift in the practitioner's center of gravity to apply force for techniques on a futon.

Breathing is important in providing the core stability for moving and lifting. Recall from Chapter 4 that the diaphragm, the main muscle of inhalation, is located in the center of the body, separating the thoracic and abdominal cavities. When it contracts, it enlarges the thoracic cavity and compresses the contents of the abdominal cavity. When the core muscles (the abdominals) contract during exhalation, they apply compressive force on the contents of the abdominal cavity. This compression, during both inhalation and exhalation, provides support to the vertebral column and pelvic girdle during movement.

Core fitness also allows for better breathing, better posture, and better transfer of energy, especially for movements that require extra effort such as lifting. Without core stability, the lower back is not supported from inside and the smaller muscles of the back, such as the deep paraspinal group, can be injured from straining. Insufficient core stability can result in lower back pain, poor posture, and fatigue. Exercises to increase core muscle strength (and core muscle stability) are presented in Chapter 8.

If practitioners do not have core stability, they will use muscular strength instead of body weight to apply the forces necessary in bodywork. Some practitioners think if they are doing only two or three

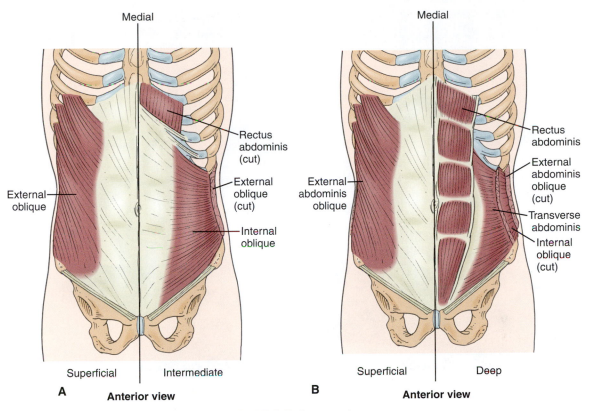

FIGURE 5-7 Core muscles.

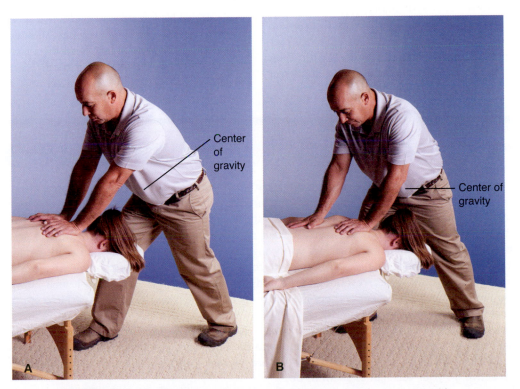

FIGURE 5-8 (A, B) Shifting center of gravity for techniques on a massage table.

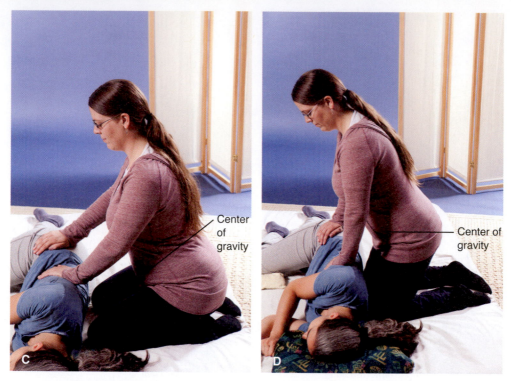

Center of gravity

Center of gravity

C

D

FIGURE 5-8 cont'd (C, D) Shifting center of gravity for techniques on a futon.

treatments a week, they can rely on muscular strength. However, risk of injury is greater than if they use proper body mechanics. Also, focusing on muscle contraction to provide the desired effect may interfere with the ability to connect with their clients, to palpate tissues effectively, or to detect changes as the techniques are applied.

PROPER BODY POSITIONS

Basic principles for efficient body mechanics involve correct positioning, movement, and awareness. Recall from Chapter 3 that head-to-tail connection means being aware that your skull is connected to and in line with the vertebral column, that your

Body Awareness

Figure 5-9A shows a practitioner using muscular strength from his arms to apply pressure on a client lying on a massage table. Figure 5-9B shows a practitioner using muscular strength from her arms to apply pressure on a client on a futon. Figure 5-10A shows a practitioner using strength coming from his legs up through his core to apply pressure on client on a massage table. Figure 5-10B shows a practitioner using strength coming from her legs up through her core to apply pressure on client on a futon.

Imitate the practitioner using muscular strength to apply pressure on a client on either a massage table or a futon (whichever corresponds to the bodywork you practice). How does it feel? How easily can you move around your client? Where in your body do you feel tension or stress? How effective do your techniques seem to be?

Now imitate the practitioner using leg and core strength to apply pressure on a client on either a massage table or a futon (whichever corresponds to the bodywork you practice). How does it feel? How easily can you move around your client? Where in your body do you feel tension or stress? How effective do your techniques seem to be?

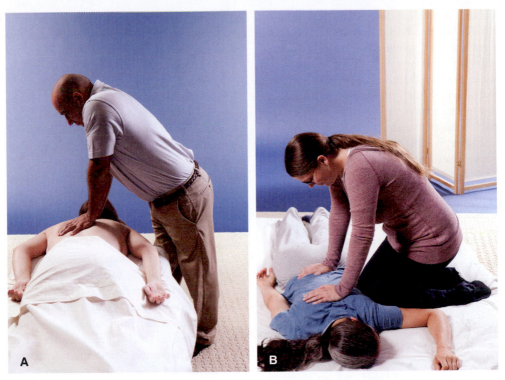

FIGURE 5-9 Practitioner using muscular strength to apply pressure **(A)** on a massage table and **(B)** on a futon.

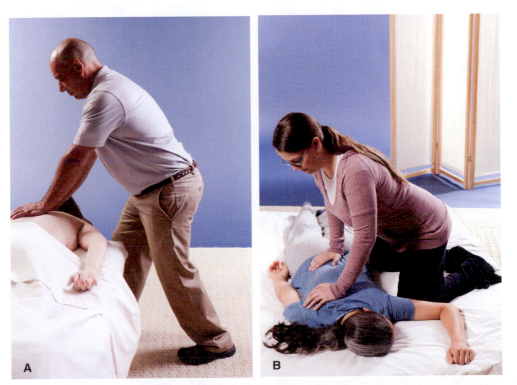

FIGURE 5-10 Practitioner using leg and core strength to apply pressure **(A)** on a massage table and **(B)** on a futon.

vertebral column is in a line down your back, and that your vertebral column ends in your coccyx. This means that you need balanced spinal posture as you work. If you maintain a proper head-to-tail connection, your head will be in a neutral position. Use your eyes to look down at your client while you are working instead of flexing your neck. Flexing your neck disrupts your head-to-tail connection and increases the strain on your neck. Figure 5-11A shows a practitioner maintaining proper head-to-tail connection and using his eyes to look at his work. Figure 5-11B shows the practitioner not maintaining a proper head-to-tail connection and straining his neck to look at his work.

Here are other body positions practitioners should have for efficient body mechanics:

- **Hinging:** To maintain a stacked vertebral column, you must hinge from the hips (discussed in Chapter 3) and remember to *not* tuck your pelvis and round your back. A good rule to remember is to keep your heart over your hands or slightly behind. This means that you are not leaning too far forward or back but are hinging the way you should.
- **Shoulders:** Keep these relaxed and not elevated. Remember to keep them moving (rhythmically)

so they are not stuck in a static position. This will decrease your neck stress and back tension.

- **Arms:** Keep these close to your midline, not medially rotated or reaching. If you feel like you are reaching, you are. The better option is to move your whole body to place yourself where your arms and hands can work easily.
- **Elbows:** Keep these soft, which means they are not locked in extension, and keep them close to your midline.
- **Wrists:** Have these in a neutral, relaxed position (less than 90 degrees) as shown in Figure 5-11A. If you find that you are hyperextending your wrists, step back and decrease the wrist angle. This will help you avoid excessive compressive forces on your wrists. These compressive forces are responsible for repetitive stress injuries (RSI) in the wrists, a common complaint among bodywork practitioners. Also, tension in your wrists can transfer to your shoulders and can result in problems there. RSI are discussed in more detail in the "Repetitive Stress Injuries" section.
- **Hands and fingers:** It is essential to brace and support your hands, fingers, and thumbs while

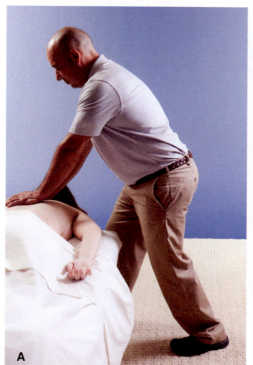
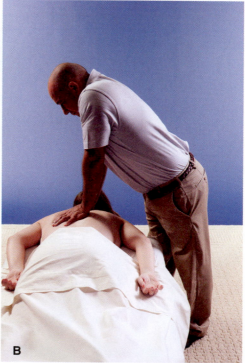

FIGURE 5-11 (A) Practitioner with proper head-to-tail connection. **(B)** Practitioner without proper head-to-tail connection.

working. This is especially important if your thumbs are easily hyperextended. The joints in the hands, fingers, and thumbs are not built for compressive forces; limit their use to prevent RSI. Keep your fingers close to the midline of your hands. This will help to keep your hands injury-free by bracing the joints of the metacarpals and phalanges, and it conserves energy. Figure 5-12A shows how to brace your hand, Figure 5-12B shows how to brace your fingers, and Figure 5-12C

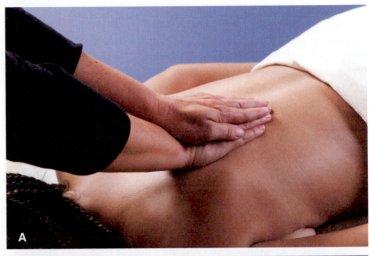

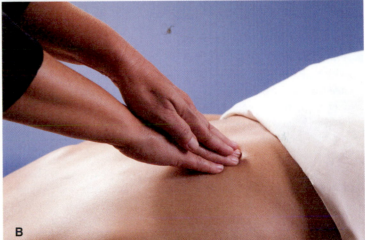

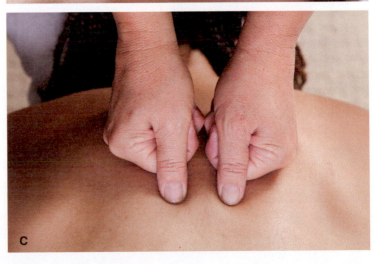

FIGURE 5-12 (A) Bracing the hand. **(B)** Bracing the fingers. **(C)** Bracing the thumbs.

shows how to brace your thumbs. Make sure you do not do repetitive ulnar and radial deviation with your hand. Ulnar deviation is a movement of the wrist where the hand moves toward the ulna. Radial deviation is a movement of the wrist where the hand moves toward the radius. Transfer your body weight into your hands to provide appropriate pressure; avoid using muscles in the hands and arms to give that pressure. You can also save your fingers and thumbs for more specific work in smaller areas of the client's body. Use your forearms to apply pressure in broader areas of the body, and use your elbows instead of your thumbs wherever you can.

- **Leg position:** Align your feet with your knees, align your knees with your pelvis, and align your pelvis with your shoulders.
- **Knee position:** Keep your knees soft, which means not locked in extension. Flex your knees as needed to achieve the correct height and angle at which you need to work. When lunging (described in the "Stances for Working on a Massage Table" section), do not allow your knee to go past your foot, because this will place undue stress on your knee.
- **Foot position:** Keep your feet at least shoulder-width apart. This gives you the most stability. If needed, you can use an even wider stance. Your feet need to be pointed in the direction of your work. Otherwise, you will be placing undue stress on your knees. Frequently shift your weight from foot to foot. This gives rhythm to your work, assists in returning blood flow back to your heart, and keeps you from locking your knees, which can cause muscular tension.
- **Sitting on the massage table:** If you sit on the massage table while performing techniques such as working on the client's feet, avoid twisting your trunk. A way to prevent this is to keep one foot on the floor while placing one knee on the table next to the client's feet. This is a good way to stay grounded and stable. It also allows you to maintain your head-to-tail connection and to hinge from your hips.

What Do You Think?

Do you listen to your client's body with your hands or your ears? How does listening to your client's body affect your body mechanics?

STANCES FOR WORKING ON A MASSAGE TABLE

There are several body positions practitioners can use when performing bodywork. These are referred to as **stances**. A stance is defined as a way of standing or, for practitioners who use futons, as ways of kneeling or sitting. It is important to choose the proper stance for the techniques you are performing—that is, whichever one allows you to move in the direction of your work.

However, before discussing stances, you need to be aware of keeping your work centered around your core. The massage table should be of a width and height that allows you to perform techniques centered at the level of your core muscles. What determines the height of the massage table? The best answer to this is the client's size and the treatment goals. Does the client need stretching? Deep, specific techniques? Is the client more than 3 months' pregnant and so needs to be in a side-lying position to have her back worked on? These are just some of the considerations to keep in mind.

Optimal table height allows you to apply techniques without bending over at the waist. You are also able to apply pressure efficiently and safely. There are two methods you can use to determine your best table height. Both involve standing perpendicular to the massage table with your legs touching it. Relax your shoulders and have your arms at your sides. With the hand closest to the massage table, do the following:

- Extend your wrist and fingers. Your optimal table height is where your fingertips slightly brush the top of the table.
- Make a fist. Your optimal table height is where the table touches your fist or knuckles.

Additionally, the table should be wide enough to accommodate your client comfortably and allow you to easily access areas of the client's body.

If the table is too low or too wide, practitioners typically end up leaning forward over the table. Their abdominal, hip, and leg muscles will contract to compensate for the force of gravity pulling down the mass of their upper bodies. For women, this is about half their body weight, and for men, it can end up being much more than half their body weight (because they generally have larger and, therefore, heavier upper bodies than women). Then the low back muscles contract to counteract that pull of gravity. This puts quite a bit of strain on the vertebral column (Fig. 5-13).

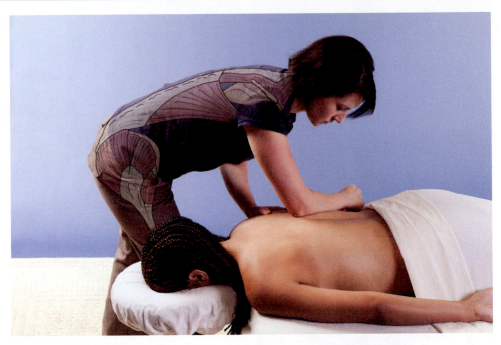

FIGURE 5-13 Practitioner leaning over the table, straining the vertebral column.

When stretching or performing ROM techniques on areas such as the legs, there is the potential of placing an additional 300 pounds of pressure on the lumbosacral area. Most low back injuries that occur from this type of loading are minor strains and sprains of muscles and ligaments. However, repeated loading of this type can cause cumulative damage to intervertebral disks, increasing the risk of herniation.

A table that is too high causes elevated shoulders, and work is not centered around the core. This can cause upper back, shoulder, and neck problems. Some practitioners may even try to reach across the table, causing upper body strain and fatigue. Figure 5-14A shows a table too low for the practitioner, Figure 5-14B shows a table too high, and Figure 5-14C shows a table at the appropriate height.

Lunge Stance

One of the primary stances used in bodywork is a **lunge stance**, also known as the **archer** or **bow stance**. In this stance, the practitioner has balanced posture, one foot is placed in front of the other, toes of both feet are parallel, and the hips face the same direction as the feet. Both feet, and the practitioner's entire body, should be in alignment with the area where pressure will be applied. The practitioner can increase the width of her stance to enlarge her base of support.

In this stance, the practitioner's center of gravity drops into the abdomen, thus allowing her sense of balance and force of energy to come from the center of her body. This focus allows her to be stable, and the strength she applies is not due to her contracted muscles (which can tire quickly) but more from using the force of gravity when leaning forward. This relationship with gravity is important because it allows the practitioner to apply pressure simply by leaning forward, allowing the body weight to do the work.

The practitioner's body weight is kept on the back leg and foot, and the client's body is in front of the practitioner. This position provides adequate leverage. If the weight is placed on the front leg and the client's body is directly under the practitioner's pressure, there is no leverage. All pressure will result from the practitioner pushing with the upper body muscles instead of using body weight. The practitioner should be able to lift his front leg off the floor and still maintain a stable balance point when contacting the client's body. This demonstrates that muscle strength is not a big factor in applying pressure, but leverage is essential.

The practitioner's strength comes from the back leg. As she pushes forward off her back foot, the front knee flexes somewhat but the majority of the weight is transferred through the arms and hands to

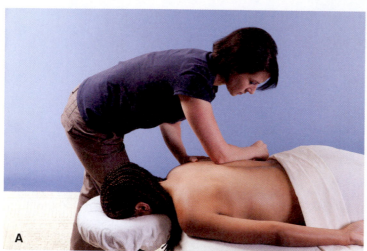

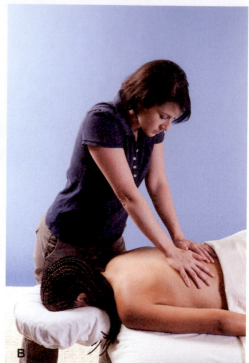

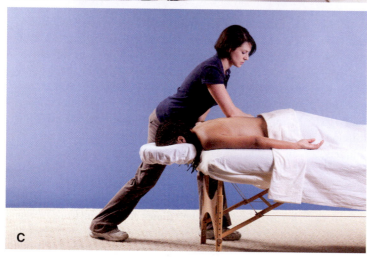

FIGURE 5-14 (A) Massage table too low for the practitioner. **(B)** Massage table too high for the practitioner. **(C)** Massage table at the appropriate height.

the client's body. The arm generating the pressure is opposite of the weight-bearing leg, which allows for proper counterbalance and prevents twisting of the body (Fig. 5-15A). The more the practitioner flexes her front knee, the more weight she transfers to the client's body. However, the practitioner's knee should not go past her toes, as this places undue stress on the knee. If this happens, the practitioner needs to widen her stance (Fig. 5-15B). Thus, the practitioner controls the amount of weight (pressure) she places on the client's body by adjusting the movements of

her legs, not by increasing muscular strength from the shoulder and arm muscles.

It is important to stay behind, not on top of, the techniques being performed. When pressure is applied, the compressive force on the shoulder and arm joints should be minimized by passing straight through the joint, not at an angle. Therefore, the arms are approximately at a 45-degree angle from the shoulder, the shoulder is lined up behind the elbow, and the elbow is lined up behind the hand (as in Fig. 5-15A). Recall from Chapter 3 that this is

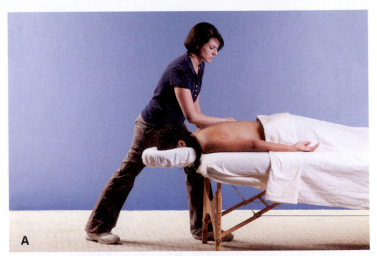

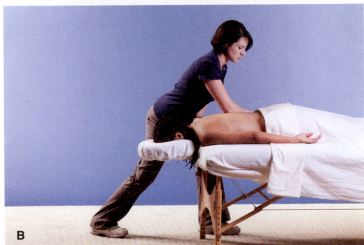

FIGURE 5-15 (A) Practitioner in lunge stance. **(B)** Practitioner shifting weight to apply more pressure.

called *stacking the joints*. If the angle of the arm at the shoulder joint is 90 degrees, then the practitioner is on top of the technique, and muscle tension in the arm will result.

Myth: Wrist positions are not that important, as long as the practitioner is able to deliver the technique and it feels good to the client.

FACT: A neutral wrist position helps avoid excessive compressive forces from the delivery of bodywork techniques. Tension in this area transfers up the practitioner's arms and could result in shoulder and neck problems, as well as compression in the carpal tunnel.

The shoulders are relaxed, the elbows are relaxed, the wrists are neutral, and the hands are placed forward onto the client. Relaxed elbows means that

they are not locked in extension. Instead, the joints are soft or slightly flexed. Neutral wrists means they are not hyperextended; they are less than 90 degrees (in reference to the posterior forearm; Fig. 5-16A). Hyperextended wrists are more than 90 degrees (in reference to the posterior forearm; Fig. 5-16B). Injuries can occur if the wrists are kept in a chronically hyperextended position throughout the treatment. (There are some strokes in which the wrists are not in a 100% neutral position; however, these strokes should be applied briefly and without undue pressure.) Relaxed wrists and hands decrease tension that can be transferred to the shoulders, possibly leading to shoulder and neck problems.

The key to this stance is the practitioner becoming adept at easily shifting her weight backward and forward, applying pressure on the forward movement and releasing pressure on the backward movement. This creates a rhythm in applying pressure and

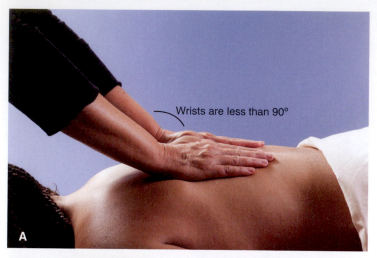

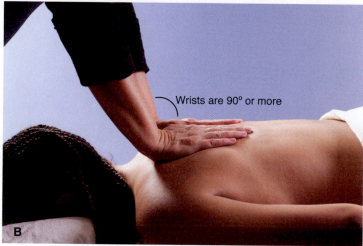

FIGURE 5-16 (A) Neutral wrists at 180 degrees. **(B)** Hyperextended wrists, more than 90 degrees.

lets body weight, not muscular strength from the arm, provide the pressure. The pressure should be applied and released evenly and steadily.

An optimal way to apply techniques is to exhale while moving forward to apply pressure and inhale while moving backward to release pressure. This ensures that the practitioner is not holding the breath while working and also helps establish rhythmic movement.

The lunge stance is efficient for body mechanics when performing stretches and ROM techniques. For example, during a shoulder stretch, the practitioner and the client inhale as the client's arm is brought into position. Sinking down into a lunge gives the practitioner more leverage to apply the stretch (Fig. 5-17). Then as the practitioner applies the stretch, both she and the client exhale.

With ROM techniques, such as for the hip muscles, the practitioner and the client exhale while lifting the leg into position. The lunge position provides a stable stance for circumduction (Fig. 5-18). As the ROM technique is applied, both practitioner and client breathe normally.

Straight Stance

Some techniques require precision but not necessarily a lot of pressure. In these instances, the practitioner can use the **straight stance** (also called the **horse stance**; Fig. 5-19). With a balanced posture, the practitioner faces the area she is working on. The feet are parallel and at least shoulder-width apart (or wider, if needed), with the weight evenly distributed. The practitioner is hinging at the hips and her knees are slightly flexed.

As the practitioner places her hands forward onto the client, her shoulders are relaxed, the elbows are relaxed (soft joints that are not locked into position), and the wrists are neutral. Pressure is applied by

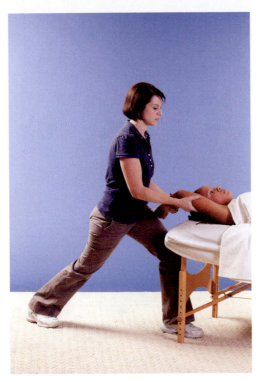

FIGURE 5-17 Practitioner lunging while stretching the client's shoulder muscles.

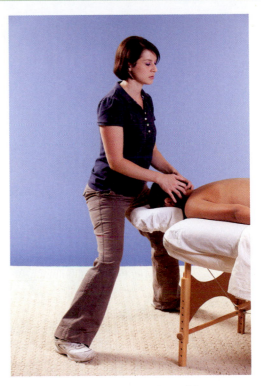

FIGURE 5-19 Practitioner in straight stance.

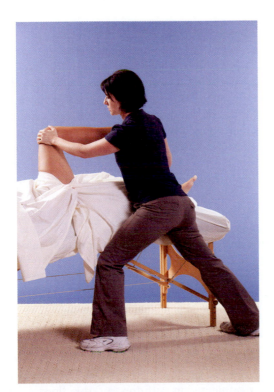

FIGURE 5-18 Practitioner lunging while performing range-of-motion technique of the client's hip joint.

rocking forward on both feet. The horse stance can also be used rocking sideways on the feet, accompanied by stepping to make larger movements. Sometimes this side-lunging provides a more neutral positioning for hands than the lunge position does.

To change direction of movement during the application of techniques, the practitioner can move her pelvis and feet slightly to turn. If a greater change in movement is needed, the practitioner should use the lunge stance to prevent overstressing the paraspinal muscles of the back by twisting. Also, the elbows should not be raised laterally or above the practitioner's shoulders; these positions prevent the most advantageous leverage and weight transfer from the practitioner to the client.

Kneeling Stance

To address certain areas of the client's body, such as the feet, hands, or neck, the practitioner may choose to kneel on one knee, which is a **kneeling stance** (Fig. 5-20). In this case, the practitioner's center of gravity is dropped even lower into her abdomen. She is in balanced posture, and her entire body is facing the area of the client's body she is working on. Practitioners should avoid kneeling on both knees to

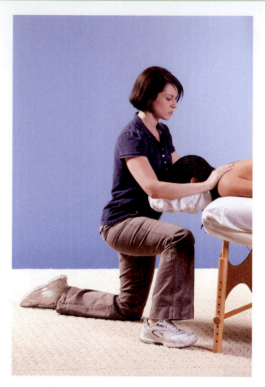

FIGURE 5-20 Practitioner in kneeling stance.

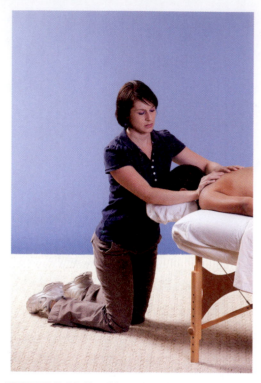

FIGURE 5-21 Practitioner kneeling on both knees.

apply techniques. As Figure 5-21 shows, kneeling on both knees is not as stable as kneeling on one knee, and the practitioner's center of gravity is no longer in her abdomen. There is increased strain on the deep paraspinal group and erector spinae muscles as they increase in tension to keep her upright. There is also added pressure on the practitioner's knees, because she cannot adjust her leg movements as she applies pressure. Her strength is coming mostly from her shoulder and arm muscles, increasing the risk of injury. The practitioner should also avoid sitting on the floor, because she may have to reach to apply the techniques, making them less effective and possibly straining her back muscles.

Body Awareness

How often do you wait until you feel pain before becoming aware of your body alignment and mechanics?

Using a Stool or Exercise Ball

Some practitioners choose to use a stool or exercise ball when applying certain techniques, such as those for the neck, face, hands, and feet (Fig. 5-22). An exercise ball is a more optimal choice because it allows the practitioner greater movement and his core muscles will be engaged. The stool or ball is placed close enough to the massage table so the practitioner is not reaching to work on the client. If the stool has wheels, it needs to stay firmly in place while working; this will, for example, keep the client's neck from being pulled suddenly should the practitioner find himself sliding on a moving stool. The practitioner has balanced posture while sitting on the stool or ball, and he is directly facing the area of the client's body he is working on.

STANCES FOR WORKING ON A FUTON

As with treatments performed on massage tables, the center of gravity for the practitioner performing treatments on a futon on the floor is her

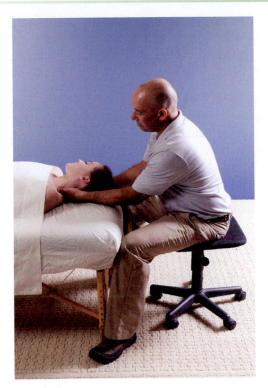

FIGURE 5-22 Practitioner using a stool.

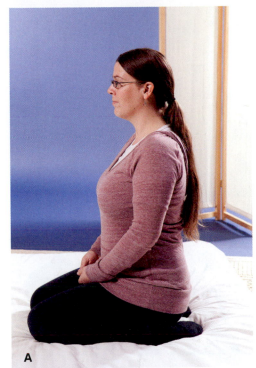

A

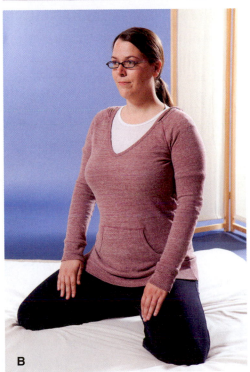

B

FIGURE 5-23 (A) Practitioner sitting on her heels.
(B) Practitioner sitting in a wider position.

abdomen. In Asian bodywork, this is the source of the practitioner's qi (the body's energy) and strength, providing direction for the treatment. The practitioner must keep her abdomen facing toward the area of the client's body. This helps direct qi flow from the practitioner to the client and qi flow within the client.

The practitioner must have balanced posture to prevent straining while working. To support the core and give effective treatments, the practitioner must have a stable stance. One way the practitioner can do this is by sitting with her gluteal muscles on her heels and knees (Fig. 5-23A). A variation of this is sitting in a wider position, with the practitioner's legs open at least 45 degrees (Fig. 5-23B). This position allows smooth pivoting so the practitioner can keep her abdomen aimed at the area she's working on. To reduce chance of injury to self or the client, the practitioner should never twist or apply techniques at an awkward angle.

From this position, the practitioner can rise to apply more pressure (Fig. 5-24). The strength for applying pressure and qi connection needs to come from the ground, up through the practitioner's

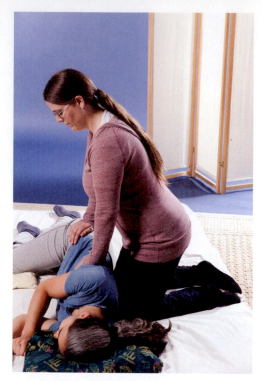

FIGURE 5-24 Practitioner rising up to apply more pressure.

abdomen, and then out through the practitioner's arms and legs. Muscling in from the shoulders or knees can put the practitioner at risk for injury and may hurt the client. The practitioner's shoulders and arms are relaxed throughout the treatment.

Other stances include crawling, squatting, and lunging. Crawling is a movement natural to children and is something that adults generally "forget" how to do. Crawling, however, is a natural way of moving around a client lying on a futon. If necessary, the practitioner can practice crawling until it becomes comfortable again. She can feel her weight shift from hand to hand, from knee to knee, and from hands to knees. While crawling, she uses her abdomen as the center of gravity and maintains a balanced posture. Feeling the connection to the earth and the flow of qi through her body will occur naturally. In time, crawling will be as effortless as walking (Fig. 5-25).

Squatting is also a natural position for children and is something that adults may need to relearn. Squatting provides a stable base from which to move into other positions easily (Fig. 5-26). This position may be difficult at first. The practitioner can practice sinking into a squat and rising from a squat without placing her hands on the floor for balance. She uses her abdomen as her center of gravity and maintains a balanced posture. Over time, her leg muscles will gain strength, and her balance will improve.

Lunging is modified squatting (Fig. 5-27A). Many stretches and ROM techniques performed on futons are done with the practitioner in a lunge position (Fig. 5-27B and C). Reaching certain parts of the client's body is also easier when lunging. Once squatting becomes comfortable, moving into a lunge is easy. As with crawling and squatting, the

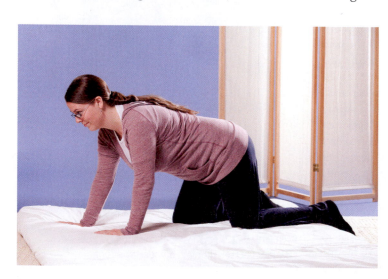

FIGURE 5-25 Practitioner crawling.

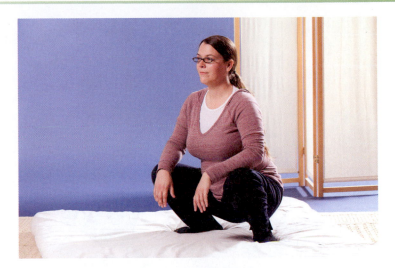

FIGURE 5-26 Practitioner squatting.

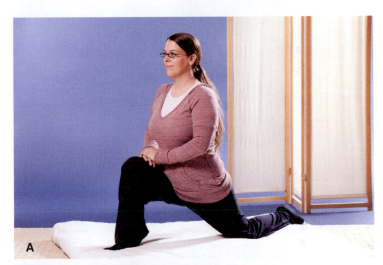

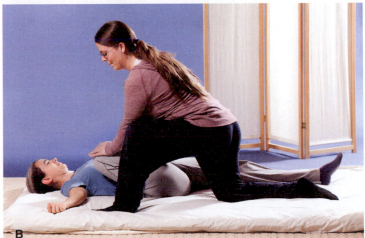

FIGURE 5-27 (A) Practitioner lunging,
(B) lunging while performing a hip stretch
on the client,

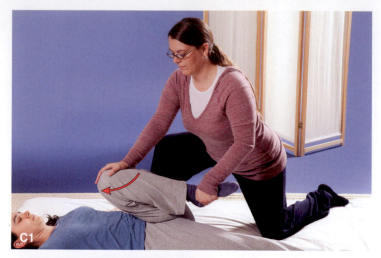

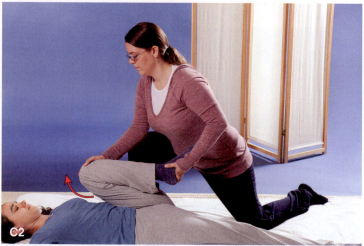

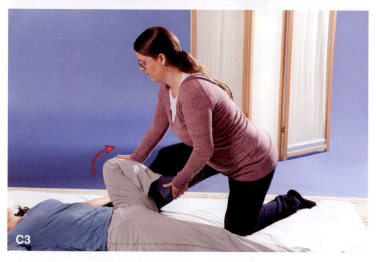

FIGURE 5-27 cont'd (C) lunging while performing a hip range-of-motion technique.

practitioner uses her abdomen as her center of gravity, and she keeps a balanced posture and steps one foot in front of the other, with toes of both feet parallel and the hips facing the same direction as the feet. Both feet, and the practitioner's entire body, are in alignment with the area she is working on. The practitioner can increase the width of her stance to enlarge her base of support.

The principles of the lunge stance while working on a massage table are the same as those for working on a futon. The practitioner's body weight is kept on the back leg and the client's body is in front of the practitioner. This position provides adequate leverage.

The practitioner's strength comes from the back leg; as she pushes forward off her back leg, the front knee flexes somewhat but the majority of the weight is transferred through the arms and hands to the client's body. The practitioner controls the amount of weight (pressure) she places on the client's body by adjusting the movements of her legs, not by increasing muscular strength from the shoulder and arm muscles. Practicing lunging helps build leg strength and improve balance.

Body Awareness

There are **archetypes**, or models, that describe common examples of inefficient body mechanics. An archetype is defined as the original pattern or model of all things of the same type.

The following archetypes show common body mechanic pitfalls and how to avoid them. Practitioners may even have combinations of these archetypes.

The Hunchback of Notre Dame
This posture is characterized by the practitioner attempting to somehow make her shoulders meet in front of her body while elevating them up to her shoulders (Fig. 5-28A). She is also bending so far forward she is unstable and risks falling onto her client. The Hunchback of Notre Dame can be avoided by keeping a balanced posture and your chest open, hinging from your hips, and lunging.

The Frightened Turtle
The practitioner can have this posture when standing, sitting, or kneeling. It is characterized by the practitioner projecting her chin upward and slumping her head into her torso until her neck disappears (Fig. 5-28B). The Frightened Turtle can be avoided by keeping a long, lean neck. Imagine a wire attached to the top of your head, pulling it upward.

The Lazy Lean
This posture is characterized by one of the practitioner's hips always touching the edge of the massage table (Fig. 5-28C). All of the practitioner's pressure must therefore come from her upper body muscles. The Lazy Lean can be avoided by standing with the weight on both your feet or lunging as needed.

The Tree and Long-Distance Hands
The Tree posture is characterized by the practitioner firmly planting her feet in one place on the floor and not moving them. She is essentially "rooted to the spot" no matter where on the client's body she is working. Often this is accompanied by Long-Distance Hands, which is characterized by the practitioner's hands seeming to be in a different time zone than the rest of her body (Fig. 5-28D).

The Tree can be avoided by simply moving around the massage table while working. Long-Distance Hands can be avoided by moving closer to the client and making sure your feet, torso, shoulders, and hands are always close to each other.

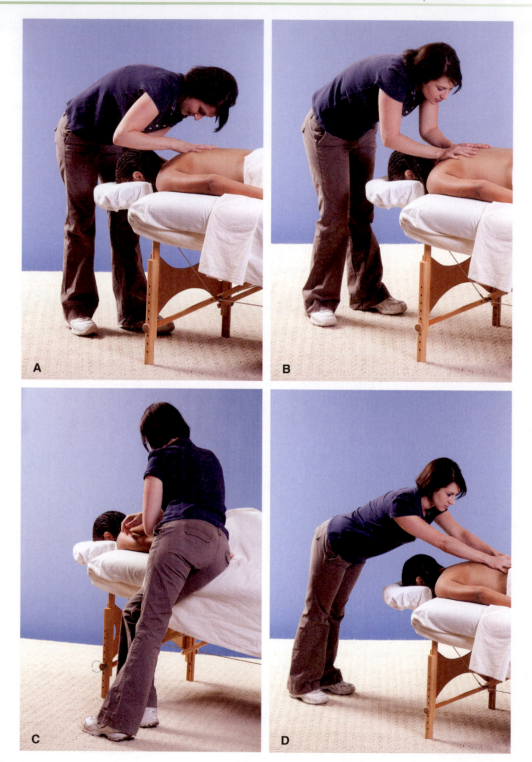

FIGURE 5-28 (A) Practitioner in the Hunchback of Notre Dame posture. **(B)** Practitioner in the Frightened Turtle posture. **(C)** Practitioner in the Lazy Lean posture. **(D)** Practitioner in the Long-Distance Hands and Tree posture.

Body Awareness

For practitioners of energy modalities, such as Reiki, Jin Shin Jyutsu, Healing Touch, and so forth, stance is important as well. Even though they may be applying little or no pressure to the client's body, these practitioners still need to make sure they are using appropriate body mechanics. This will decrease their risk of fatigue and injury and increase their stamina. They should be sure to use the stances as described for working on either a massage table or a futon. It is important the practitioners have a balanced posture and a head-to-tail connection, and they should keep their shoulders down and breathe efficiently.

Focus on Wellness

Here are key questions that you should ask yourself as you perform treatments:

- Is it obvious to someone watching you where you are getting the strength to perform the treatment?
- What is your position of strength? Are both your feet on the floor, your heart over your hands (or slightly behind), and your elbows toward your midline? Is your strength being drawn up from the floor through your feet and coming out through your hands onto the client?
- Are you remembering your body's midlines? Are you keeping your arms close to the midline of your body by keeping them close to your trunk? Are you keeping your fingers close to the midlines of your hands to brace them?
- Are you moving dynamically and not staying static?
- Are you using your body weight and not muscle strength to apply more pressure?
- Are you using a wide variety of techniques and avoiding repetitive movements?

WORKPLACE ERGONOMICS

Ergonomics is the science of devices and systems for humans at work. *Ergonomics* comes from the Greek word *ergon*, meaning "work" and *nomos*, meaning

Focus on Wellness

Here are online resources practitioners can use to find out more information about workplace ergonomics:

- Ergonomics Ideas Bank: www.LNI.wa.gov/wishe/ergoideas
- Human Factors and Ergonomics Society (HFES): www.hfes.org
- OSHA Training Institute (OTI): www.osha.gov/SLTC/ergonomics/index.html
- Ergoweb: www.ergoweb.com
- National Institute for Occupational Safety and Health (NIOSH): www.cdc.gov/niosh/topics/ergonomics

"laws of." Contributing factors to musculoskeletal disorders (MSD) are physical demands of bodywork exceeding the practitioner's capabilities or a poorly designed workplace putting the practitioner in awkward positions for hours at a time.

According to the Bureau of Labor Statistics (BLS), U.S. Department of Labor, "musculoskeletal disorders (MSDs), often referred to as ergonomic injuries, are injuries or illnesses affecting the connective tissues of the body such as muscles, nerves, tendons, joints, cartilage, or spinal disks. Injuries or disorders caused by slips, trips, falls, motor vehicle accidents, or similar incidents are not MSDs." (A more detailed definition can be found on the BLS website at www.bls.gov/iif/oshdef.htm.) Musculoskeletal disorders are the primary cause of injuries in the workplace and are the result of repetitive movement. The end result can be **repetitive stress injuries (RSI)**.

REPETITIVE STRESS INJURIES

RSI are also known as **repetitive movement injuries (RMI), occupational overuse syndromes (OOS), and cumulative trauma disorders (CTD)**. All of these are descriptions and not diagnoses. They are comprehensive terms that include a wide range of symptoms or syndromes. A *syndrome* is defined as "a group of signs and symptoms that occur together and characterize a particular abnormality or condition" (www.merriam-webster.com). An RSI develops slowly and can affect many parts of the body. Sometimes symptoms come and go before becoming chronic: aching, tenderness, swelling, pain, cracking, tingling, numbness, loss of strength, loss of joint movement, and diminished coordination of the injured area. These symptoms can then lead to a disorder. The many diagnosable disorders that RSI encompasses can include carpal tunnel syndrome, ulnar nerve entrapment, de Quervain syndrome, thoracic outlet syndrome, tennis elbow, and tendinosis or tendinitis. All of these are covered in more detail in Chapter 6.

The main cause of RSI is too much stress on a part of the body. Predisposing factors for RSI are a lack of physical fitness, muscle tension, individual work habits, stress, long hours, lack of breaks, bad ergonomics, and poor, static posture. Stress tends to worsen symptoms, mainly due to the accompanying muscle tension and, correspondingly, pain.

Recently injured tissue is already inflamed, and repetitive motion sets up a pain cycle that allows secondary inflammation to take hold in the area. This diminishes movement, and compensation patterns set in. The person then falls into movements designed to avoid pain. For chronically injured tissue, repetitive motion may or may not cause inflammation. However, a pain cycle that diminishes movement and creates compensation patterns also occurs.

WARNING SIGNS AND ADDITIONAL RISK FACTORS FOR RSI

Repetitive strain injuries usually affect the neck, shoulders, upper back, upper arms, elbows, forearms, wrists, thumbs, or fingers. However, they can also affect the hips, knees, ankles, and toes. Warning signs of RSI can appear in any of these areas and can include the following:

- Weakness
- Fatigue
- Lack of endurance
- Tingling, numbness, or loss of sensation
- A feeling of heaviness
- Difficulty opening and closing hands
- Stiffness
- Difficulty using hands (e.g., turning pages of books or magazines, turning doorknobs or faucets, holding a coffee mug, and so forth)
- Reluctance to shake hands because of the pain it will cause
- Difficulty carrying things or holding on to things
- Waking up with pain or numbness, especially during early morning hours

- Lack of control or coordination
- Cold hands
- Frequent self-massage
- Difficulty buttoning clothing or putting on jewelry
- Tremors
- Avoidance of activities or sports that were once enjoyable
- Pain or soreness (Eustice, 2010; Safe Computing Tips.com, 2010)

Additional risk factors for RSI include:

- Ignoring warning signs
- Spending over 2 hours on the computer or doing other repetitive hand movement per day
- Engaging in binge or marathon computer use (e.g., video games, report deadlines, and so forth)
- Not taking frequent, regular breaks
- Doing high-stress work
- Lacking time or workload management (e.g., rush work, meeting deadlines, filling quotas, and so forth)
- Being bored, angry, or lacking assertiveness
- Having unbalanced posture
- Sitting for long periods
- Doing **static loading**, which is holding still for long periods (e.g., holding the mouse while staring at a computer monitor)
- Keeping elbows flexed, extended or hyperextended for long periods
- Twisting or resting wrists, forearms, or elbows while using a keyboard or mouse
- Having an improper workstation setup (e.g., keyboard too high, monitor too high, low, or off to one side, and so forth)
- Having improper seating (e.g., chair too high, low, or lacking lumbar support)
- Having awkward positions (e.g., typing while using the telephone cradled on one shoulder, reaching for the mouse, and so forth)
- Having long fingernails
- Smoking
- Being obese
- Having **hypermobile** (overly flexible) joints
- Having weak or tight muscles
- Lacking regular exercise
- Having cold hands
- Having an improper eyeglass prescription or undiagnosed vision problem, causing the head to be held in awkward positions to see or read
- Having arthritis, diabetes, thyroid disease, pregnancy, menopause, and other medical conditions

- Having hand-intensive hobbies, such as playing a musical instrument, gardening, doing carpentry, doing needle crafts, bowling, throwing or racquet sports, playing video games, and so forth

ENVIRONMENTAL FACTORS FOR PRACTITIONERS TO CONSIDER

Sometimes the focus of body mechanics is entirely on how the practitioner uses his or her body when performing the treatment. However, that is really only half the story. The other half involves the equipment the practitioner uses, the space in which the practitioner performs treatments, and personal considerations such as the practitioner's attire and hygiene.

Other considerations include having the correct massage table height (how high or low to set the massage table was covered in the "Stances for Working on a Massage Table" section) and properly lifting and carrying the massage table, massage chair, or futon. This can be awkward because of the size, shape, and weight of the table, chair, or futon. If proper body mechanics are not used, undue stress can be placed on the hands and wrists and on the vertebral column.

Lifting and Carrying the Massage Table, Massage Chair, or Futon

If the practitioner lifts and carries the massage table, massage chair, or futon using just her arm strength and not her legs, and uses only one side of her body, this puts a great deal of stress on the body. In order for the body to compensate for the increased load on the one side, the muscles in the low back on the opposite side must contract more. This leads to an asymmetrical loading around the lumbar region, which can result in intervertebral disk damage (Fig. 5-29).

Practitioners need to lift the massage table, massage chair, or futon using balanced posture. As they get into position to lift, they can inhale; then as they lift the table or futon, they can slightly extend their

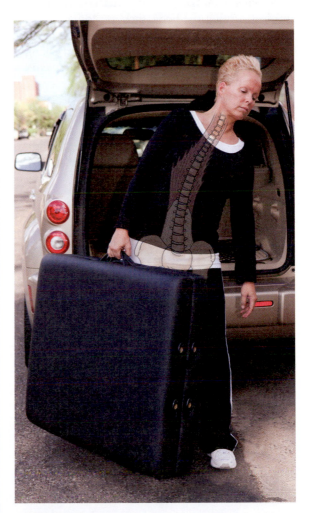

FIGURE 5-29 Practitioner lifting a massage table with one side of her body.

Voice of Experience

Good body mechanics and the power of healthy movement have always been important to me throughout my career as an instructor and a massage therapist. Our work is dynamic. If it hurts—change it, move it. Sometimes it's as easy as a micro change, perhaps taking that breath we remind our clients about. Pain or discomfort are not necessarily the cues to stop an activity; rather, these symptoms cue us to reevaluate our body mechanics, our physical fitness, our nutrition, and in general, a holistic consideration of the mechanics of our life. Is there a stressor elsewhere that distracts us from being present while performing our job? What do we need to do to draw us back to the present and be self-aware? To this day, in my 24th year of practice, I still self-evaluate during each and every massage, to be sure I am as comfortable as possible, knowing that my comfort ultimately delivers my best possible massage.

Jill Bielawski, BS, NCTMB, coauthor with Jerry Weinert of *Stretching for Health: Your Handbook for Ultimate Wellness, Longevity, and Productivity* and *Head to Toe: A Manual of Wellness & Flexibility*, Vodder certified in Manual Lymphatic Drainage and Combined Decongestive Therapy; licensed massage therapist since 1987.

knees and exhale. This way, the larger muscles of the hip joints and legs are providing the lifting power, not the smaller muscles of the low back (Fig. 5-30).

Practitioners should consider using a wheeled cart to transport the table or futon. For massage chairs, practitioners should consider using a massage chair with wheels on it or a carrying case with wheels. If this is not possible, at least use a carrying case with a longer shoulder strap and a shorter strap for maneuvering. The longer strap should cross over to the practitioner's opposite shoulder. This makes sure the weight of the table or chair is more evenly distributed on the body. The shorter strap can be used as a handle to maneuver the table or chair (Fig. 5-31A). Be sure to alternate the shoulder the table or chair is carried on to avoid overusing one side of the body. Figure 5-31B shows the improper way to carry a massage table in a case.

Moving a massage table or massage chair often involves turning the body, such as placing the table or chair into and taking it out of the trunk of a car. When placing the table or chair into and taking it out of the trunk, make sure the carrying strap crosses

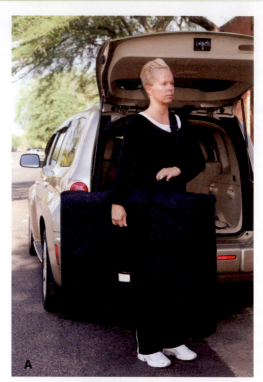

A

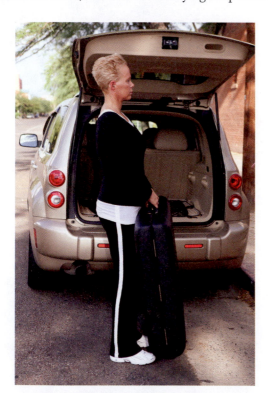

FIGURE 5-30 Practitioner lifting a massage table with appropriate biomechanics.

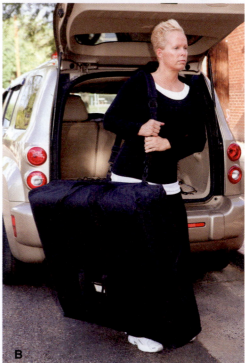

B

FIGURE 5-31 Practitioner carrying a massage table in a case **(A)** properly and **(B)** improperly.

over the body. Using a head-to-tail connection, keeping the vertebral column aligned and lifting with the legs, use the shorter strap as a handle to maneuver the table or chair. Figures 5-32A and B show the improper and proper ways to grip the case and lift it in and out of a car.

Many low back injuries involve twisting movements of the spine, so practitioners should take particular care when turning while handling their massage tables, massage chairs, or futons. Lift and then turn, pivoting on the feet; do not twist with the back. Figure 5-33 shows the improper way to turn while handling a massage table.

Myth: Work-related environmental factors do not play a role in the delivery of effective treatments.

FACT: Work surfaces, lighting, clothing, table height, music, and hygiene are just a few of the environmental factors involved in providing the best possible treatments to our clients. However, inadequacies in these environmental factors can hamper body mechanics. For example, a bodywork table that is set too low or too high or a hard, uncushioned floor can place stress on the practitioner's body.

FIELD NOTES

I stretch before and after each treatment that I give; do an alternate hot and cold hand dip (this is described in Chapter 6), especially after doing deep-tissue work; give myself a paraffin treatment once a week (paraffin treatments are presented in Appendix A); and receive regular massage, hot and cold stone, and craniosacral treatments. I use my fists, elbows, and forearms as much as possible to save overusing my thumbs. Most important, I use good body mechanics, pace myself, and try and schedule treatments with at least 30 minutes in between. I know my limits, and at this time in my life, I do not schedule more than three treatments a day.

Stretch, stretch, stretch! Pace yourself and utilize paraffin and other hydrotherapy self-care techniques regularly. If possible, have a mirror in your treatment room so you can check your body mechanics. Receive bodywork regularly. Make yourself a PRIORITY!

Ann L. Mihina, LMT, certified hydrotherapist, certified LaStone practitioner, continuing education presenter, and coauthor (with Sandra K. Anderson) of Natural Spa and Hydrotherapy. Massage therapist since 1994.

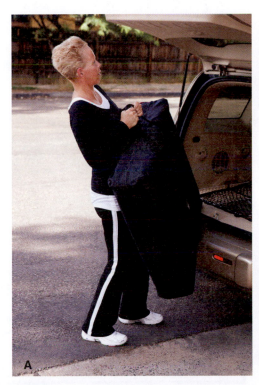
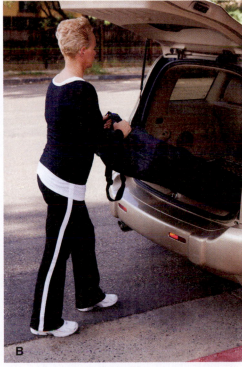

FIGURE 5-32 (A) Improper way to lift a massage table out of the trunk of a car. **(B)** Proper way to lift a massage table out of the trunk of a car.

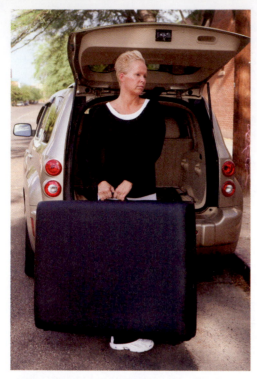

FIGURE 5-33 Improper way to turn while handling a massage table.

tight it restricts your movements. Both of these types of clothing will compromise your body mechanics.

- Keep your nails trimmed and filed smooth. It is uncomfortable for clients to feel your nails in their skin. If this happens, you will likely end up modifying your hand and finger positions, causing undue stress in your wrists and hands.
- It is important to have good hygiene. Bad hygiene promotes poor body mechanics. For example, if you are aware that you have bad breath or underarm odor, you might move your body in such a way to prevent the smell from being detected by your client. These body distortions are not likely to be within the parameters of balanced posture or efficient body mechanics. Be sure to have breath mints handy, and be free of bad smells. If you smoke, do not do this at least 2 hours prior to a treatment. After smoking, make sure to wash your hands, brush your teeth, and use mouthwash.
- If you use a holster for massage lubricant, its placement may be a cause for a repetitive injury if

Treatment Room Considerations

Here are treatment room ergonomic considerations to keep in mind:

- Be sure to have proper lighting. If the room lighting is too bright, it may detract from the therapeutic atmosphere; if the room is too dim, it may cause you to get too close to your work, as in the Hunchback of Notre Dame poor body mechanics archetype. Both of these situations can compromise your body mechanics.
- Be sure to have enough space to work around your table, chair, or futon comfortably. This allows you to move freely and maintain proper body mechanics.
- If possible, make sure you work on a cushioned floor. If your treatment room does not have carpeting with cushioning underneath, consider investing in cushioned mats. These decrease the fatigue that can be felt after working long hours on a hard surface.
- Be sure to wear comfortable clothing. It should not be so loose that it touches the client, nor so

---

Focus on Wellness

Complete this self-evaluation at the end of your treatment day. Do this for at least 2 weeks. Compare your answers from the beginning of the 2 weeks with your answers at the end of the 2 weeks.

1. On a scale of 1 to 10 (1 being "not aware at all" and 10 being "fully aware"), how would you rate your level of awareness of your body mechanics during your treatments today? Please comment on why you chose this rating.
2. Describe how your body feels after today's treatments.
3. Are you experiencing any soreness in your body? If so, where? If you are experiencing soreness, is it related to bodywork? If yes, how?
4. If you use a massage table, was it set at the correct height? If no, why and what did you do about it?
5. Were your hands and wrists relaxed and neutral throughout your treatments? If not, when did you notice this, and what did you do about it?

Case Profile

Isaac is 35 years old. He does 25 to 30 bodywork treatments each week. He runs 5 miles every day after work to decompress from work and to keep himself fit. Over the last 6 months, he has been having some difficulties sleeping. He has also noticed over the last couple of months that halfway through his treatments, he finds himself leaning against the table and, at times, reaching over, instead of staying behind, his work.

Isaac is now experiencing pain in his low back and gluteals. He also has persistent deep, aching back pain when he is at rest and it seems to get worse when he sits upright. On Sunday, he was in such pain he could barely move. He called into work and canceled all his treatments for the week.

- *What are the problems Isaac is experiencing and why?*
- *How do you think Isaac's work habits will impact his career longevity?*
- *What would you have done differently if you were Isaac?*
- *If you were Isaac's practitioner, what suggestions would you give him?*

you wear it on one side and consistently stretch to reach it. To prevent RSI, alternate the sides of your body you wear it on.
- Take a good look at how you have set up your office equipment. Make sure your computer, chair, keyboard, and monitor are all at heights that promote a balanced posture.

Wellness Profile Check-In

Looking at the Wellness Profile you completed at the end of Chapter 1, are there any challenge areas you could remedy through a plan for efficient body mechanics? If so, what are they? How would you like these areas improved? What methods or activities will you use to improve these areas? Write down a plan for improvement that includes the methods you will use, a timeline for implementing these methods, and ways you will assess your improvement along the way.

SUMMARY

A healthy lifestyle and efficient body mechanics are part of self-care and career longevity, and they help deliver the best care to clients. Practitioners must be relaxed and comfortable and must not strain when doing bodywork. Therefore, body mechanics involves good posture, balance, leverage, and use of the strongest and largest muscles to perform the work.

Compressive, pushing, pulling, lifting, and circular forces are used when performing techniques. The strength or energy for these forces is transferred from the practitioner's body to the client's body. Efficient body mechanics allow practitioners to apply the necessary forces for long periods of time without the risk of injury to themselves and to clients. Components of efficient body mechanics include stability, balance, coordination, and stamina. The keys to all of these are body awareness and mindful movement, balanced posture, an understanding of center of gravity, and core stability. Practitioners should also use a variety of techniques that are effective according to their muscles, body style, and the client. Additionally, they should maintain a technique as long as it is comfortable for their bodies and make sure they breathe efficiently throughout the treatment.

Basic principles of efficient body mechanics involve having proper body positions, movement, and awareness. Proper body positions include hinging from the hips; keeping the shoulders down and moving them rhythmically; keeping the arms close to the midline and not medially rotated or reaching; keeping the elbows soft; having the wrists in neutral position; bracing the hands and fingers; aligning the feet with the knees, which should be aligned with the pelvis, which should be aligned with the shoulders; keeping the knees soft; and having the feet at least shoulder-width apart.

The massage table should be at a width and height that allows practitioners to have their work centered around their core muscles. Stances for working on a massage table include the lunge (archer or bow), the straight (horse), and the kneeling. Practitioners can also sit on a stool or exercise ball to apply techniques. Stances for working on a futon include sitting with the gluteal muscles on the heels and knees together, sitting with the gluteal muscles on the heels with the legs open at least 45 degrees, crawling, squatting, and lunging.

Archetypes of poor body mechanics include the Hunchback of Notre Dame, the Frightened Turtle, the Lazy Lean, Long-Distance Hands, and the Tree. Practitioners should evaluate themselves to see if any of these archetypes apply to them. If so, improvement will ensure their career longevity.

Musculoskeletal disorders are the primary cause of injuries in the workplace and are the result of repetitive movement. The end result can be repetitive stress injuries (RSI), also known as *repetitive movement injuries (RMI), occupational overuse syndromes (OOS),* and *cumulative trauma disorders (CTD).* The many diagnosable disorders that RSI encompasses can include carpal tunnel syndrome, ulnar nerve entrapment, de Quervain syndrome, thoracic outlet syndrome, tennis elbow, and tendinosis or tendinitis. RSI is caused by many factors, including lack of physical fitness, muscle tension, individual work habits, stress, long hours, lack of breaks, bad ergonomics, and poor, static posture.

Repetitive strain injuries usually affect the neck, shoulders, upper back, upper arms, elbows, forearms, wrists, thumbs, or fingers. Symptoms include aching, tenderness, swelling, pain, cracking, tingling, numbness, loss of strength, loss of joint movement, and diminishing coordination of the injured area. Stress tends to worsen symptoms.

In order to decrease risk of injury, practitioners need to be mindful of how they lift and carry the massage table or futon. There are also treatment room ergonomic considerations practitioners should keep in mind. These include having the proper lighting, having enough space to work around the massage table or futon comfortably, working on a cushioned floor, wearing comfortable clothing, keeping the nails trimmed and filed smooth, having good hygiene, and setting up office equipment ergonomically.

Review Questions

MULTIPLE CHOICE

1. Massage therapists who consider themselves full-time workers perform treatments how many hours per week?
   a. 3 to 5
   b. 7 to 9
   c. 10 to 14
   d. 15 to 30

2. The application of pressure is really the application of what type of force?
   a. Compressive
   b. Pushing
   c. Lifting
   d. Circular

3. Without core stability, what will practitioners use to apply the forces necessary in bodywork treatments?
   a. Balance
   b. Center of gravity
   c. Muscular strength
   d. Awareness

4. Which of the following accurately describes a body position practitioners should have for efficient body mechanics?
   a. Arms far away from the midline
   b. Knee positioned past the foot when lunging
   c. Feet together when in the straight stance
   d. Hinging from the hips

5. As practitioners adjust the height of the massage table for different clients and their needs, they must always work at the level of their
   a. core.
   b. shoulders.
   c. elbows.
   d. midback.

6. The straight stance is best used for
   a. precise techniques requiring little pressure.
   b. stretches.
   c. range-of-motion techniques.
   d. applying deeper pressure.

7. A treatment room ergonomic consideration practitioners should keep in mind is
   a. having good hygiene.
   b. wearing comfortable clothing.
   c. working on a cushioned floor.
   d. All of the above

FILL-IN-THE-BLANK

1. Range of motion techniques involve using _____ force.

2. The components of efficient body mechanics include stability, balance, _____ and _____.

3. To avoid strain, the practitioner should use his or her eyes and not do _____ _____ to look at the client while working.

4. One foot stepped in front of the other, with toes of both feet parallel and the hips facing the same direction as the feet describes the _____ _____stance.

5. Pressure of bodywork techniques should be applied in a way that minimizes the _____ force on the shoulder and arm joints.

6. The practitioner should avoid kneeling on both knees to apply techniques because it is not as _____ as kneeling on one knee.

7. _____ disorders are the primary cause of injuries in the workplace and are the result of repetitive movement.

SHORT ANSWER

1. Explain why practitioners should pay attention to their body mechanics all the time, not just when they are providing treatments.

2. Describe where the strength or energy required for performing bodywork techniques comes from.

3. Describe the body positions for the vertebral column, hips, shoulders, elbows, wrists, hands, fingers, legs, knees, and feet in efficient body mechanics.

4. Briefly describe each of the archetypes of poor body mechanics and how they can be improved.

5. Briefly describe the stances used for performing bodywork on a futon.

6. Define *repetitive stress injuries* (RSI), and briefly describe the causes, symptoms, and risk factors.

7. Explain the optimal way to lift and carry a massage table or futon.

Activities

1. Review the archetypes of poor body mechanics. Does one of the archetypes fit you? If so, which one? What are you willing to do to improve your body mechanics?

2. Set up a large mirror in your treatment space. Look at it periodically during your bodywork treatments to check your body mechanics.

3. Ask a trusted colleague to observe your body mechanics as you perform a treatment. Have your colleague give you honest feedback on what he or she sees.

4. Videotape yourself as you perform a treatment. Review the recording to see your body mechanics.

Do they look different from what you thought you were doing? If so, how? Periodically videotape yourself while performing treatments so that you can see how your body mechanics change or you can identify areas needing further attention.

5. Perform 10 bodywork treatments while bringing your awareness to your body mechanics. Journal what you discover about your body mechanics during each of the treatments—what feels comfortable for you, what feels uncomfortable, what you find challenging, what you find successful, and so forth. Review your journals to see what awareness you are developing as you perform each treatment, how your body mechanics have changed, and what you still need to work on.

REFERENCES

Bureau of Labor Statistics. "Massage Therapists." In *Occupational Outlook Handbook,* 2010–11 edition. Retrieved 2 November 2010 from www.bls.gov/oco/ocos295.htm.

Eustice, Carol. What Are Repetitive Stress Injuries? (2010). Retrieved November 2010 from http://arthritis.about.com/od/arthritisbyanatomy/a/stressinjuries.htm.

Safe Computing Tips.com. Repetitive Stress Injury Warning Signs (2010). Retrieved November 2010 from www.safecomputingtips.com/repetitive-stress-injury-signs.html.

Injury Prevention and Management

Key Terms

Acute
Adhesions
Anesthesia
Annulus fibrosus
Anterior scalene syndrome
Aromatherapy
Avulsion
Chronic
Costoclavicular syndrome
Counterirritant
Crepitus
Double or multiple crush
   phenomenon
Hyperesthesia
Hypertonicity
Muscle guarding
Nerve compression,
   impingement, entrapment
Neuropathy
Nociceptors
NSAIDs
Nucleus pulposus
Paresthesia
Pectoralis minor syndrome
Phagocytosis
Radiculopathy
Rubefacient
Trigger point

Learning Objectives

After studying this chapter, the reader will have the information to:

1. Explain signs and symptoms of repetitive stress injuries (RSI).
2. Describe factors that contribute to RSI.
3. Delineate the phases of tissue healing.
4. Describe the types of injuries bodywork practitioners are likely to have in muscle, fascia, tendons, ligaments, joint capsules, nerves, and cartilage.
5. Identify what RSI he or she is at risk for developing.
6. Develop a plan to prevent or manage injuries.

> "Action is the foundational key to all success."
> — Pablo Picasso

INJURIES IN THE BODYWORK PROFESSION

As discussed in the previous chapters, most injuries that bodywork practitioners experience are due to inefficient body mechanics and not enough self-care.

As you think about the information presented, you may have figured out what your body mechanic concerns are and what changes you need to make in other aspects of your life so you can be healthier. Ideally, you are already working on these issues so you can enjoy a long and successful career in bodywork.

However, if practitioners do not use appropriate body mechanics or make necessary changes to enhance self-care, they may find themselves with an injury or some other condition as a result. If that is the case, then practitioners will lose income as they take time to heal, and they will need to spend time, effort, and, in many cases, money to find the best treatment options. They also need to reevaluate how they have been performing bodywork and make adjustments to avoid a recurrence of the injury or to help manage the condition. Some practitioners find this too much to deal with and leave the bodywork profession.

Despite their best efforts, sometimes practitioners do become injured. Perhaps it is because they are in a hurry and twist from the waist instead of lifting from the legs when moving a massage table. Or maybe they need extra money and so schedule more clients than usual and do not take breaks to rest their bodies, resulting in muscle and fascial tightness and pain. Maybe they have been using appropriate body mechanics for the most part but are unaware that there are one or two ways in which they can improve. They may have even come from other jobs in which they performed repetitive movements. These movements could either result in dysfunctions they now need to deal with or predispose them to injury as a bodywork practitioner. Perhaps they do not look at other lifestyle choices that can impact their health and career. Then, over time, dysfunction that has been unnoticeable builds up until, seemingly out of the blue, they are faced with an injury.

This chapter presents specific information about disorders and conditions that can arise from body mechanics dysfunctions and less-than-optimal lifestyle choices. The causes, symptoms, and treatments of these injuries are discussed. Also included are ways to prevent specific injuries, along with recommendations for overall health and well-being. It is important to realize that the physical demands of bodywork can lead to injury but that injury is not inevitable. Sometimes changing one or two minor things can mean the difference between having a long and successful bodywork career and having to leave the profession too soon.

REPETITIVE STRESS INJURIES (RSI)

There is no doubt that performing any type of bodywork involves repetitive motions. These motions place stress on practitioners' bodies, making them susceptible to repetitive stress injuries. Many bodywork practitioners experience signs and symptoms of repetitive stress and should use these as signals that they need to change something to ensure career longevity. Identifying symptoms early is essential to managing the injury and the condition. Otherwise, the injury or condition could become chronic, which can make it much more difficult to deal with.

To assist you in determining if you are experiencing an RSI, ask yourself if you have any of the following:

- Muscular tightness, weakness, fatigue, or spasms
- Areas of hypersensitivity or tenderness
- Areas of swelling or inflammation
- Pain or discomfort during and after performing bodywork
- Body aches
- **Paresthesia** (tingling, burning, or numbness sensations) in areas of the body. Do they wake you up at night?
- **Crepitus** (a crackling, grating, or grinding sensation caused by abnormal movement between two structures)?
- Uncoordinated movements or feeling clumsy while performing bodywork
- Areas of your body that no longer function as well as they should
- Hesitation to use certain parts of your body to perform bodywork, such as your forearms, hands, fingers, or thumbs?

If the answer is yes to any of these questions, then it is quite likely you have an RSI.

PAIN

Everyone has aches and pains from time to time. These can develop after working out too much, doing yard work, sleeping in awkward positions, or just having a really tough day at work. However, with RSI, pain is the most common symptom and is often the first to arise when injury occurs. Therefore, it is important to be able to distinguish whether the pain is from hard work or is an early indication of an injury.

Pain occurs when **nociceptors** become irritated or overstimulated. Nociceptors are nerve endings located in most of the body's tissues. They relay sensations that are usually interpreted by the brain as pain. Nociceptors can be stimulated by physical trauma, chronic muscular contraction, imbalanced posture, the stress of awkward movements, or disease. Additionally, pain can be made worse by many different factors—duration, the level of nervous tension a person carries, a negative attitude, stress, noise, pollution, and an unhealthy diet, just to name a few.

The musculoskeletal system has more sensory nerves and nociceptors than organs, with receptors located in muscles, fascia, tendons, ligaments, and joints. Therefore, pain caused by strained or damaged muscles, tendons, and joints is easily felt. Muscle and joint pain is probably the most common source of minor or nagging aches and is usually not life-threatening. The musculoskeletal system can undergo an enormous amount of abuse, including a long period of misuse, before it breaks down, although muscle and joint pain increases as the damage becomes more serious (Tortora and Derrickson, 2009).

The benefit of pain is that it forces practitioners to become aware of their bodies. They can use the pain to discover inefficient body mechanics, awkward body positions and movements, imbalanced posture, and body areas that they are overusing. Various types of pain sensations can provide clues about where the pain might be coming from.

The following are general guidelines for assessing pain. Note that these guidelines *are not given to diagnose a specific problem.* They are meant to alert practitioners to conditions that may require medical evaluation.

1. Pain caused by muscles tends to be deep, aching, and localized in the area.
2. Pain caused by muscle spasms tends to refer to other areas of the body. A muscle spasm is the body's way of protecting itself. Therefore, this tissue is in a contracted state, meaning that muscles can be locked long or locked short, and they can "pull on" or "refer to" surrounding tissue. Recall that because of fascia and tensegrity, everything in the body is connected to each other.
3. If there is pain in an area with active movement but the area is absent of pain when at rest, the pain may be coming from a strain in the muscles or tendons. Conversely, if there is pain with passive joint movement, the source may be in the joint structures, such as ligaments or joint capsules.
4. Pain caused by spinal facet joint damage generally feels sharp and pointed (like stabbing from a nail) and strong and piercing. It can be so intense it keeps the person awake at night.
5. Pain caused by nerve irritation radiates and may be sharp, stabbing, searing, burning, or itching.
6. Only nerves radiate pain. Every other body structure causes referred pain. Spinal nerve root pain radiates into all the surrounding tissues that this nerve innervates. The farther it radiates from the spine, the more serious the problem. A good sign of healing is when the pain centralizes—that is, when peripheral pain diminishes and the pain gradually moves closer to the spine.
7. Unrelenting, constant bilateral pain is very serious. It is almost always due to a damaged, herniated disk in the spine and requires medical attention (Let's Talk Pain, 2010; Lowe, 2009).

The more information practitioners have about pain or discomfort they may be feeling, the better equipped they will be in dealing with it. Also, the information can be invaluable in helping a physician make an assessment about the cause of the pain. It is important to realize that interventions done prior to an accurate assessment can mask the true cause of pain and may result in further damage and suffering.

Here are symptoms that require medical attention:

- Intense pain
- Pain lasting more than a week
- Prolonged numbness, tingling, or burning sensations
- Moderate to severe inflammation, especially if it lasts more than 5 days
- Unexplained awkward movements, weakness, or loss of physical abilities
- Changes in skin color and temperature
- Any other symptoms that do not improve over time

Once the source of the pain has been identified, whether it is due to illness, psychological issues, physical injury, or repetitive movement or overuse, the course of treatment can be established. This is another reason why it is important to address conditions immediately, before they become chronic.

Body Awareness

*O*ften pain and discomfort create a loud and noticeable signal. Although you need to pay attention to pain, becoming overly focused on it can actually increase the pain. In other words, if you perceive pain to be great, it will be. If you do not perceive the pain to be great, it will not be. Being overly focused on pain can also drown out your awareness of progress toward pain reduction, healing, and growth. If you are currently experiencing pain and want to counteract the tendency to focus on it, keep track of your progress with the following exercise (you can also use your Wellness Profile):

1. Keep a daily log of the degree of pain or discomfort you feel. You can use a scale of 1 to 10 (1 being the lowest amount of pain; 10 being the highest amount of pain) to quantify the intensity. Also log the location of the pain or discomfort, and what it feels like (sharp, dull, aching, shooting, and so forth). A helpful acronym to use is LID for *location*, *intensity*, and *duration*.

2. Log the activities you do that precede the pain or discomfort and those that reduce the pain or discomfort.

3. Study the log to identify which activities cause the pain or discomfort and which relieve it.

4. Create a plan to modify your activities accordingly to reduce your pain or discomfort. A good place to start is by using the information in Table 6.1 and the information in the "Types of Injuries Bodywork Practitioners Are Likely to Have" section.

FACTORS CONTRIBUTING TO RSI

There are, of course, specific causes for each RSI. However, there are other factors practitioners need to take into consideration that will help them stay injury-free and achieve career longevity. The four most common factors contributing to RSI are imbalanced posture, stress, injury, and movement habits. They are also responsible for the majority of all RSIs.

Imbalanced Posture

The human body is designed to work best when it is in balanced alignment. Using the example of a car, when the front wheels get out of alignment, the car starts to shimmy and shake. This can lead to front-end damage, uneven wear on the tires, steering difficulties, and problems throughout the entire car. In other words, the car's structures and systems start to break down, and it can cost a lot of money and time to get everything fixed.

The same is true of the human body. Everything in the body is suspended in a matrix of connective tissue called *fascia*. Fascia changes its consistency if stress is present. Normal fascia is quite strong and flexible. It shifts and gives with every movement. However, if movement patterns are stressful, as can happen, for example, in a slouched posture, fascia starts to become either shorter and tighter or longer and tighter, less resilient, and less flexible. It can even adhere to other tissues and structures, which prevents efficient movement and causes pain and discomfort. The body becomes stiffer. It becomes harder for the person to sit or stand up straight. Some movements may become uncomfortable or even painful.

If the fascia that is affected by the imbalanced posture covers a nerve, symptoms of nerve disorders can develop. If the fascia that is affected by the imbalanced posture is embedded in muscle, movements become more restricted, and symptoms of muscular disorders can develop.

Stress

At some point, everyone experiences stress. If practitioners pay attention to how they feel when they are under stress, they will probably notice that their bodies tighten up, their movements become restricted and more rigid, and their breathing slows down and becomes very shallow.

All of these responses place strain on the muscles, fascia, and joints. Once the body feels tight, the brain begins to associate it with feelings of stress, so the body continues to respond and adapt to the stress. Stress causes strain, which causes more stress, which leads to even more strain. After a while, it becomes difficult to know which came first—the stress or the feeling of strain. They actually go hand in hand; one perpetuates the other.

Sometimes it is hard to determine how stress is affecting the body because it may show up as symptoms of other conditions. For example, chronic headaches or digestive issues, depression, and being especially susceptible to colds and flu (due to a lowered immune system) have all been linked to stress. The fact is that too much stress can affect major body systems. Knowing how stress affects their bodies can give practitioners necessary information to change aspects of their lives to protect their health and career longevity.

Injury

All injuries, recent and older ones, are recorded in the body's fascial system. The fascia actually changes at the moment of injury and remains tighter and more restricted in an effort to support and protect the injured body. For example, those who have broken a bone probably noticed that once the cast came off, they had stiffness; had lost range of motion in the area; and had muscles that felt thicker, shorter, and less pliable. This is due to the changes in the fascia that permeates their muscles. All these changes occurred because of the stress caused by the injury and by the inactivity of being in a cast.

Other types of injury to fascia include surgeries, cuts, wounds, and the internal damage that happens with RSI. The fascia forms scar tissue and, in some cases, **adhesions** in response to these kinds of injuries. Adhesions are the abnormal joining of separate tissue surfaces. Scar tissue is thicker and denser than the surrounding tissue and can restrict movement, as can adhesions.

One way to think of this is to use the example of knitted fabric. If the fabric is pulled in any direction, it will give fairly easily in that direction. All the threads along the pathway are pulled; the movement caused by the pulling is transmitted equally throughout the fabric (Fig. 6-1A).

If a 2-inch opening is cut into the fabric, the hole must be stitched closed or the fabric will unravel because of the interconnectedness of the fabric's fibers (Fig. 6-1B). However, when the opening is stitched closed, the fabric can no longer stretch easily and equally in all directions. It is inhibited by the sewn-up area (Fig. 6-1C).

The same is true of fascia. When it is cut or torn, as happens in any surgery, wound, or rupture, it must stitch itself back together to maintain the integrity of the whole sheet of fascia. The result is that the repaired tissue, like the repaired fabric, no longer stretches easily and equally throughout the sheet of fascia. This now becomes a source of stress to the body, and it responds by building up more restricted tissue. Figure 6-2 shows scar tissue and adhesions restricting movements of pectoralis major (Lowe, 2009).

Movement Habits

Everyone has unconscious movement habits. For example, parents may always carry their babies on the same hip. Over time, they may not realize that their baby-carrying hip is higher than the other hip, causing structural stress inside their bodies.

People who often carry a heavy load, such as a backpack, have structural stress as well. Most of the time, people have the habit of carrying heavy loads with the same hand or on the same shoulder. Their bodies tend to slump in the direction of the load. Over time, their bodies tilt toward the side of the backpack.

For bodywork practitioners, a typical unconscious movement habit is looking down at their work and medially rotating the shoulders. The neck flexes forward and the shoulders may elevate, causing great

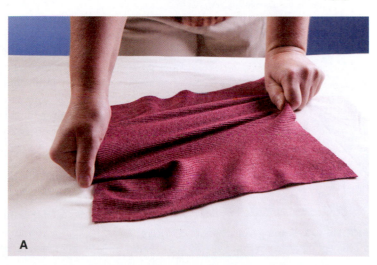

FIGURE 6-1 (A) Threads in the pathway of a pull in knitted fabric.

A

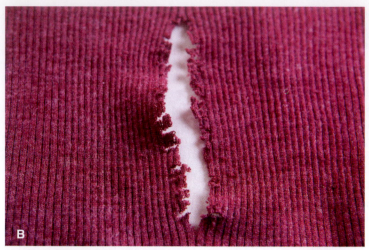

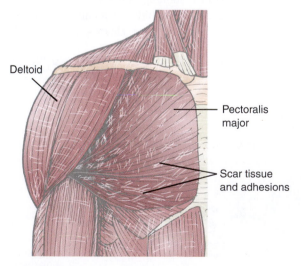

FIGURE 6-1 cont'd **(B)** Unraveling threads in a slit cut into knitted fabric. **(C)** Restitched slit causing restricted movement in the pull of knitted fabric.

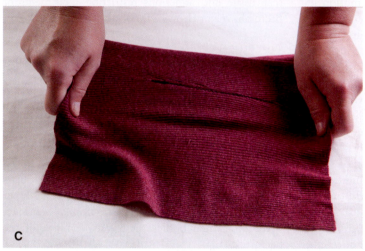

Deltoid

Pectoralis major

Scar tissue and adhesions

FIGURE 6-2 Scarring and adhesions restricting movement of pectoralis major.

stress in the neck and shoulders. This position can create a host of problems. The brachial plexus, a network of nerves that supply the shoulder, arm, and hand, passes through the lateral neck and shoulder region. This means that when the fascia changes in this area because of the stress, these nerves can become trapped in the thickening and tight fascia, and can be compressed by tightened muscles. The result is thoracic outlet syndrome, which we discuss in more detail in the "Types of Injuries Bodywork Practitioners Are Likely to Have" section.

Other Factors That Contribute to RSI

In addition to the four major contributing factors to RSI, there are several others to consider:

- How much attention you pay to your body when you are doing your work. The greater your body awareness during all your activities, especially

Body Awareness

1. *Identify your holding pattern.* Begin to sense the shape or quality of tension in areas of your body. Sense the chronically contracted or lengthened muscles. Feel what sensations this holding pattern creates, especially if it causes pain. What purpose does the holding pattern serve? How does it restrict movement? What unevenness does it create in your posture and movement?

2. *Feel the overall pattern.* You cannot release something you cannot feel. Sense the holding pattern as deeply as you can. Feel how it affects your whole body. This simple awareness can actually help to release the holding pattern. Use your intention and breathing to dissolve the pattern without actively trying to change it. Sometimes trying too hard to change a pattern can actually make it worse.

3. *Take conscious control with exaggeration.* Release holding patterns by actively contracting your muscles and going further into the pattern. As you hold it, sense the energy you have tied up in holding. Then release the holding as much as you can. Do this several times, tightening into it a little bit less each time, releasing it a little bit more each time. This process will deepen your awareness of the holding pattern and will teach you how to come out of it.

4. *Release the holding pattern while actively moving.* Explore micromovements, making the tiniest, slightest movements you can. This will help you to facilitate smaller, more intrinsic muscles and release chronic holding in the larger, more extrinsic muscles. Move slowly enough to give yourself the time and space to release chronic contractions as you move. Also, breathe easily and occasionally sense your body weight sinking into the ground.

while performing bodywork, the more likely you are to use efficient body mechanics and movements that reduce your chances of becoming injured.

- Whether your bodywork education program included sufficient information about RSI

prevention and management, how much attention you paid to it, and whether you currently use that information as you practice bodywork.

- Activities you do outside of work, such as playing sports, gardening, reading, and so forth, and how much attention you pay to how you use your body when doing them. Using efficient body mechanics and movements only while performing bodywork and not during your ADLs increases your chances of becoming injured.

- Your age and gender. As we age, we are more prone to certain conditions such as a loss of muscle strength or osteoarthritis. Additionally, older bodies take longer to heal than younger bodies. Generally, women have a smaller body size and less strength than men, so women may be more subject to injury if not using efficient body mechanics and movement while performing bodywork.

- Heredity. Did you inherit a slight build that is easily subject to wear and tear, or do you have a more robust build with strong muscles?

- Obesity. The more weight on the body, the greater the load on the joints and associated tissues such as ligaments, muscles, and tendons. This increases the chance of injury to these structures.

- Smoking. Smoking cigarettes can contribute to changes in breathing patterns and can limit the ability to take efficient breaths. Recall from Chapter 4 how important breathing is to overall health and wellness.

- Level of fitness. The higher our level of fitness, the less likely we are to get injured. This is discussed in more detail in Chapters 7 and 8.

- Physical flexibility. The more flexible we are, the more mobility we will have and the less likely we will become injured. When our soft tissues are pliable and healthy, they are less prone to injury. This is discussed in more detail in Chapters 7 and 8.

- Whether you warm up before doing treatments. When muscles are not warmed up before they are used for physical activity such as bodywork, they are more susceptible to injury. An athlete would never compete without the proper warm-up, because he knows it puts him at risk for injury. The same is true for bodyworkers. Warm up and stretching protocols are presented in Chapters 7 and 8.

- Whether you stretch and center yourself between treatments. This is a quick and easy way to rejuvenate and keep your body performing optimally.

Protocols for stretching in between treatments are presented in Chapter 7.

- How often you receive regular bodywork treatments. Bodywork practitioners need to receive regular bodywork in order to reap its benefits. It is also a good way to model wellness for your clients.
- Mental factors, such as depression and anxiety, versus a positive mental outlook. Psychological stressors interfere with our ability to be centered and focused, which can lead to using inefficient body mechanics and movements. This can result in injury.

When several of these factors are combined, unraveling them to discover the actual cause of an RSI can become tricky. In almost every case, an injury is due to several of these causes, affecting multiple parts of the body. Therefore, when designing a recovery system for an RSI, it should be approached from several directions and all possible causes should be investigated. To leave out one of the causes is an invitation to delayed results, poor results, or no results.

TISSUE INJURY AND HEALING

Recall from Chapter 5 that in hands-on bodywork modalities, the application of pressure is really the application of compressive force. The terms *force* and *effort* are often used interchangeably, but they are two different concepts. For example, when pressure is applied to a part of the client's body, force is the end result. Effort is what practitioners experience in their bodies as they generate that force.

There are many ways to reduce the effort practitioners experience when performing bodywork. By recruiting large, strong muscles, such as those in the legs and core, practitioners need much less effort to apply the same amount of force than if they use the smaller, weaker muscles in the arms, forearms, or hands. Also, when in a balanced posture, practitioners can apply force with less effort than when they

What Do You Think?

Have you ever worked at a job other than in bodywork where repetitive stress injuries occurred? How were symptoms or injuries dealt with there?

are in an awkward position. When practitioners have gained experience with a particular technique, they can often generate more force with less effort than when they were first learning that technique.

Emotional tension can also make practitioners use more effort than a task truly requires. For example, if a practitioner is apprehensive about working with a particular client, is nervous about impressing his boss, or is stressed about something going on outside of work, these feelings can generate a high level of overall muscular tension. When the practitioner is performing bodywork, that tension will increase her level of effort without actually generating any more force. If practitioners can remain relaxed, they will experience less overall effort while accomplishing the same amount of work.

TERMINOLOGY

There are specific signs and symptoms that characterize a particular condition. Signs and symptoms do not, of course, mean the same thing. A *sign* refers to a finding that is observed or that can be objectively measured as a result of the injury, such as swelling, discoloration, deformity, redness, or crepitus. A *symptom*, on the other hand, is a subjective complaint or an abnormal sensation that cannot be directly observed by someone else. Pain, nausea, altered sensation (e.g., numbness), fatigue, a loss of function, and so forth, are examples of symptoms.

Acute injuries are conditions that have a sudden onset and are of short duration, usually 6 months or less. They typically result from a one-time traumatic event. The individual clearly knows and recalls how the injury came about (e.g., stepping off a curb and spraining the ankle), and the signs and symptoms associated with the injury typically begin to surface immediately.

Chronic injuries usually have a gradual onset and are of prolonged duration, lasting longer than 6 months and sometimes for the rest of the person's life. The exact mechanism or time of injury is often not known. Chronic injury usually results from an accumulation of minor traumas or repetitive stresses that would not be sufficient to cause injury if they were an isolated event. Consequently, chronic injuries are primarily conditions in which the demands on the tissues exceed the ability to heal and recover before additional stress is applied.

Chronic injury often occurs following periods of inadequate rest or recovery, overuse of a muscle or body part, overactivity, repetitive overloading of a structure, or repetitive friction between two structures. As such, these injuries may also be referred to as *repetitive stress injuries* or *overuse injuries*. Chronic injuries are more difficult to treat than acute injuries, as the longer the injured state continues, the longer it takes for healing to occur and symptoms to subside. This is why practitioners need to keep their bodies healthy—injury prevention is one of the keys to career longevity (Cleveland Clinic, 2008).

PHASES OF TISSUE HEALING

Soft tissue injuries include burns, bruises, wounds, strains, sprains, and dislocations. Most of the injuries bodywork practitioners experience do not involve traumatic tissue injury. Instead, it is more likely they will have repetitive stress injuries. Recall from Chapter 5 that an RSI develops slowly and can affect many parts of the body. Sometimes symptoms come and go before becoming chronic: aching, tenderness, swelling, pain, cracking, tingling, numbness, loss of strength or function, loss of joint movement, and diminished coordination of affected limbs.

However, the healing process of damaged tissues from traumatic injury is the same as for RSI. The main difference is that with a traumatic injury such as a wound or burn, the tissue remains healed unless the person is wounded in exactly the same place again. With RSI, the tissue does not get a chance to fully heal as long as the repetitive stress is still occurring. This is one of the main reasons it takes so long to recover from RSI and why it is essential to modify habits and movements that contribute to it. This is

also why it is essential that bodywork professionals who have an RSI need to heal from the injury completely before returning to work. Performing bodywork or any other activity that aggravates the condition too soon not only delays the healing process, but it can also cause further tissue damage.

Generally, healing involves three physiological phases: inflammation (acute phase), regeneration (subacute phase), and remodeling (maturation phase).

Inflammation (Acute Phase; Fig. 6-3A)

- The purpose of inflammation is to contain the damage and prepare for tissue repair.
- There is increased blood flow to the area, and local capillaries become more permeable; these cause the cardinal signs and symptoms of inflammation, which can be remembered by the acronym SHARP: *S*welling, *H*eat, *A* loss of function, *R*edness, and *P*ain.
- Increased blood flow and capillary permeability bring oxygen and nutrients necessary for rebuilding tissue to the area, as well as white blood cells that phagocytize foreign particles and debris from damaged tissues. **Phagocytosis** is defined as the process by which certain white blood cells called *phagocytes* ingest and destroy microbes, cell debris, and other foreign matter.
- If blood vessels get damaged, platelets form a clot to stop the loss of blood through the damaged area.
- Duration varies depending on the severity of the initial trauma and the strength of the person's immune system.

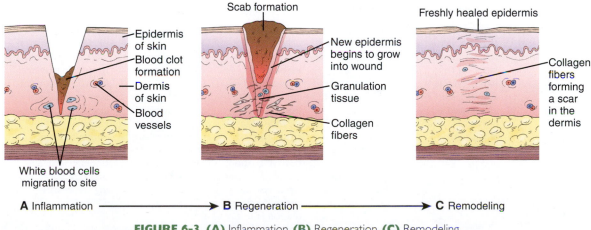

FIGURE 6-3 (A) Inflammation. **(B)** Regeneration. **(C)** Remodeling.

Regeneration (Subacute Phase; Fig. 6-3B)

- Damaged capillaries regrow; tissue structure is rebuilt and restored as collagen fibers are laid down, and granulation tissue forms to provide a framework for the new tissue to grow into. Granulation tissue is fragile and can be reinjured easily.
- Swelling reduces as excess interstitial fluid enters the lymphatic system.
- If the injury affects only the more superficial layers (the epidermis of the skin), no scarring will result.
- If the injury is deep enough into connective tissues (the dermis of the skin), scarring and adhesions may result. During regeneration, the collagen fibers are laid down haphazardly, which is why scar tissue looks and functions differently from normal tissue.

Remodeling (Maturation Phase; Fig. 6-3C)

- Inflammation is gone.
- Damaged blood vessels have regrown.
- Tissue is almost completely healed, and depending on the extent of the original damage, tissue function returns as much as is possible.
- Collagen fibers become more organized and scars diminish somewhat. (The purpose of the deep friction massage technique is to manually assist the collagen fibers in becoming more aligned and to loosen adhesions.)

Three main factors affect tissue repair: nutrition, blood circulation, and age. Nutrition is important because the healing process requires great amounts of nutrients. For example, dietary protein is important because most of the structural components of tissues are proteins. Vitamin C is necessary for the normal production and maintenance of tissue elements, especially collagen. It also strengthens and promotes new blood cell formation. Proper blood circulation is essential so that oxygen, nutrients, white blood cells, and platelets are transported to the injured site. Blood and lymph flow also remove excess tissue fluid, bacteria, foreign bodies, and debris. This removal helps the healing process.

Tissues heal faster and leave less obvious scars in people who are younger. The younger body is generally in a better nutritional state, there is a better blood supply to the tissues, and the body cells have a higher metabolic rate. This means the cells in a younger person's body can synthesize needed materials and divide more quickly to repair tissues (Tortora and Derrickson, 2009).

Table 6.1 shows the phases of healing. Included are the signs and symptoms, physiology, treatment goals, and treatment choices for inflammation (acute stage), regeneration (subacute phase), and remodeling (maturation phase) of tissue repair.

TABLE 6.1 The Phases of Healing

Phase	Description	Signs and Symptoms	Physiology	Treatment Goals	Treatment Choices
Inflammation (acute phase)	Inflammation is present; vascularized tissues respond to injury; pain is diffused; pain is aggravated by movement; pain is felt with passive ROM	Swelling, heat, a loss of function, redness, pain (SHARP); pain felt immediately upon movement; muscle spasm; muscle guarding; injury to deeper structures may show no visible signs of inflammation.	Local tissue changes First response: vasoconstriction; second response: vasodilation causes slowing of local circulation; edema; congestion; stagnation; possible damage to surrounding tissue if inflammation is not controlled.	Decrease pain, edema, and muscle spasm; maintain available mobility within limits of pain; maintain function of associated areas; stimulate circulation to the injured area.	Ice massage, cold plunge, cold packs, cold compresses;* lymphatic massage; elevation; compression; rest and reduce activity; passive range of motion within limits of pain; passive positioning techniques massage surrounding structures.

TABLE 6.1 The Phases of Healing—cont'd

Phase	Description	Signs and Symptoms	Physiology	Treatment Goals	Treatment Choices
Regeneration (subacute phase)	Healing stage; may have pain with no activity; aggravated by too much movement.	Same signs and symptoms as in the acute phase but less in intensity; pain is felt near the limits of movement at the end of ROM.	Inflammation decreases; repair of injured site begins; cell debris and waste products begin to be removed; regrowth of damaged blood vessels; granulation tissue develops; collagen fibers are produced and laid down; connective tissue is immature and fragile; adhesions form	Decrease pain, edema, and muscle spasm; maintain available mobility within limits; increase soft tissue mobility and ROM; align scar tissue; maintain function of associated areas; strengthen supporting or related musculature; stimulate circulation to the injured area.	Ice massage, cryokinetics cold plunge, cold packs, cold compresses, alternating plunges;* lymphatic massage; compression; reduce activity; deep tissue techniques on the affected area; massage surrounding structures; muscle energy techniques; passive positioning techniques.
Remodeling (maturation phase)	May have slight inflammation that lasts for weeks or months; no pain at rest; pain only with specific activity; has a specific pain site; poor healing response	Pain is felt beyond the limits of movement; adhesions; limited ROM and mobility; strength not fully returned; some loss of function and mobility; restoration of function begins.	Remodeling and maturation of scar tissue; collagen and connective tissue matures; collagen fibers become reoriented along the lines of stress; scar tissue shrinks; adhesions form if not prevented.	Decrease pain from adhesions; decrease trigger points and tender points; decrease hypertonicity; increase soft tissue mobility and flexibility; strengthen affected area and associated structures; return tissue to normal function.	Ice massage, cryokinetics cold plunge, cold packs, cold compresses, alternating plunges, hot plunge, hot packs, hot compresses;* myofascial stretching and release; trigger point therapy; deep specific friction; muscle energy techniques; active ROM; massage surrounding structures; remedial exercises; stretching.

*See Focus on Wellness Box on pages 179–181. Also, see Appendix A.

Myth: You should always rub the spot that hurts.

FACT: Rubbing a painful area feels soothing, especially when we bump an elbow or a knee. However, when the pain is caused by inflammation, rubbing this area can make the problem worse. You should avoid rubbing inflamed tissues. Also, to keep from irritating damaged tissues, techniques that manipulate tissues (such as massage techniques) should not be applied during the first 24 to 72 hours after the injury, when the area is in an acute phase of healing.

TYPES OF INJURIES BODYWORK PRACTITIONERS ARE LIKELY TO HAVE

The types of work-related injuries bodywork practitioners are most likely to have involve the musculoskeletal system. Recall from Chapter 2 that the musculoskeletal system is composed of the bones, skeletal muscles, joints, and associated structures such as tendons, ligaments, and intervertebral disks.

The most common types of injuries bodywork practitioners experience are to these soft tissues.

MUSCLE

Skeletal muscle makes up 40% to 45% of the adult body's total weight. Body motions result from the alternating contraction and relaxation of muscles. Additionally, muscle tissues stabilize body position, regulate organ volume, generate body heat, and move fluids and food through various body systems (Tortora and Derrickson, 2009).

Several factors can cause muscle injuries and conditions. These include overuse, lack of proper strength training, metabolic stress (e.g., oxygen debt), and fatigue.

Common Muscle Injuries and Conditions

HYPERTONICITY

Another term for tight muscles is **hypertonicity**

> *Signs and symptoms:* Hypertonic muscles feel tight, are resistant to stretching, may have limited movement or cause limited range of motion in joints, and usually feel painful when palpated or stretched.
> *Causes:* It frequently develops due to an increased amount of nervous stimulation to muscles to make them contract. As a result, the muscles have a higher degree of resting tone than they normally would. Stresses cause the increased muscular tone. It could be a mechanical stress such as postural distortion, a chemical stress such as excessive intake of caffeine, or a psychological stress.
> *Treatment:* One of the best methods to reduce hypertonicity is to receive bodywork on a regular basis and to increase flexibility. Ways to increase flexibility are discussed in Chapter 7.

ACUTE MUSCLE SORENESS

This is usually accompanied by fatigue.

> *Signs and symptoms*: Transient muscle pain; occurs during and immediately after exercise or when performing bodywork.
> *Causes*: Lack of oxygen to the muscles and buildup of metabolic waste that results from oxygen debt (which is why it is important to pay attention to the breath when performing bodywork).
> *Treatment*: Dissipates as oxygen is restored to the muscle tissue and metabolic waste is removed. Receiving bodywork can assist with this.

DELAYED ONSET MUSCLE SORENESS (DOMS)

This becomes most intense after 24 to 48 hours and then gradually decreases so that the muscles become symptom-free after 3 or 4 days.

> *Signs and symptoms:* Increased muscle tension, swelling, stiffness, and resistance to stretching.
> *Causes:* Can be very small tears (microtrauma) in the muscle tissue that result in inflammation. It is more likely to occur with eccentric isotonic or isometric contractions, which overload the muscles. (Recall from Chapter 2 that during eccentric isotonic contractions, the muscle lengthens in a controlled manner while it continues to contract. In isometric contractions, the muscle does not change in length while the tension within it increases.) Other contributing factors can be microtrauma in the connective tissue that holds muscle tendon fibers together, and increased interstitial fluid, which presses on pain receptors.
> *Treatment:* Receiving regular bodywork can assist in alleviating DOMS. Also, applying ice on the affected muscles within the first 24 to 48 hours may help. More information about applying ice can be found in Appendix A.

Muscle soreness can be limited by engaging in regular weight training or muscle building exercise (also known as *weight-bearing exercise*) and by increasing flexibility. The key is to begin exercising at a moderate level and gradually increase the intensity of the exercise over time. Exercising regularly builds strength for performing treatments, and over time it increases stamina, efficiency of breathing, energy levels, and flexibility, while decreasing psychological stressors. More information about increasing flexibility is found in Chapter 7; more information about building strength is found in Chapter 8.

MUSCLE STIFFNESS

Muscles are not pliable and are not easily stretched.

> *Signs and symptoms:* Not usually accompanied by pain; occurs when a group of muscles have been worked hard for a long period. The muscles become swollen and shorter and thicker; therefore, they are less able to be stretched.
> *Causes:* Fluids collect in the muscles during and after exercise (these are absorbed into the bloodstream slowly); situations in which connective tissue becomes less pliable, such as during stress.

Treatments: Hydration, light exercise, flexibility training, and regular bodywork treatments (Jones, 2007; Quinn, 2010).

The Focus on Wellness box has hydrotherapy methods that can be useful for tight, sore, and stiff forearm and hand muscles. Also, see Appendix A for cold compresses, cold packs, ice massage (cryotherapy), hot compresses, alternating (contrast) compresses, and paraffin applications.

TRIGGER POINTS

Janet Travell, MD, defined a myofascial **trigger point** as "a hyperirritable spot in skeletal muscle that

Focus on Wellness

If you experience tight, sore, and stiff forearm and hand muscles after a day of performing bodywork, hydrotherapy may help alleviate your symptoms. One type of hydrotherapy that can be particularly helpful is plunges. This involves plunging your forearms and hands into basins of hot, warm, or cold water. An alternating plunge involves alternately placing your forearms and hands in hot and cold water.

The supplies needed for plunges are one or two basins (at least 10 to 12 inches deep and long enough to fit your forearms and hands); hot, warm, or cold water (depending on which type of plunge you want to do); ice for the cold plunge to make the cold water the appropriate temperature; a thermometer (one that is easy to read, such as a pool thermometer); and two or three towels (approximately 18 in. × 30 in.; Fig. 6-4).

Cold Plunge

Cold plunges can provide relief from muscle tension, pain, and spasms and can help alleviate inflammation. Cold plunges should not be done by those who are physically frail, have heart conditions, have untreated high blood pressure, or are intolerant to cold.

The forearms and hands can be plunged into the cold water for anywhere from 10 seconds to 3 minutes. Repeated plunges can be done for as long as is tolerable.

The water temperature for a cold plunge should be between 40° and 55°F, depending on your tolerance for cold.

In addition to cold water, make sure you have ice handy in case you need to cool the water to your desired temperature.

The following are the steps for a cold plunge:

1. Unfold one towel and place it on a flat surface.
2. Place an empty basin on top of the towel.
3. Pour cold water into the basin until it is approximately two-thirds full. Check the temperature of the cold water using the thermometer (Fig. 6-5). Add ice until the desired temperature is reached.
4. Plunge your forearms and hands into the water for the desired length of time (Fig. 6-6). Repeat the plunges for as long as you desire.

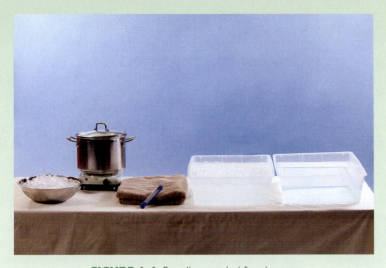

FIGURE 6-4 Supplies needed for plunges.

Continued

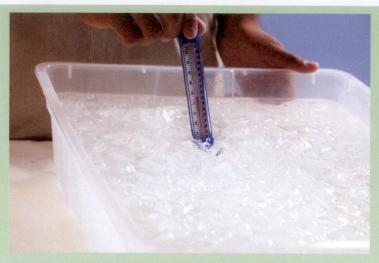

FIGURE 6-5 Check the temperature of the cold water.

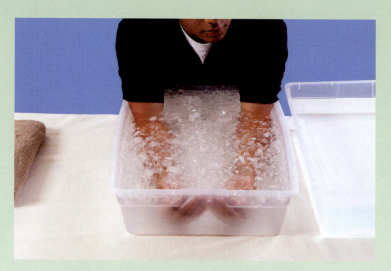

FIGURE 6-6 Plunge your forearms and hands into the water.

5. After the plunge, dry your forearms and hands with a towel.

Hot Plunge

Hot plunges can provide relief from muscle tension, pain, and spasms and from noninflammatory joint pain. Other benefits are overall relaxation and stress relief. Hot plunges should not be done if there are areas of inflammation on the forearms or hands or by practitioners who have an intolerance to heat.

The forearms and hands can be plunged into the hot water for anywhere from 2 to 45 minutes. A short plunge (2 minutes) is stimulating to the muscles; a longer plunge (30 to 45 minutes) is sedating.

The water temperature for a hot plunge should be between 98° and 108°F, depending on your tolerance for heat.

The following are the steps for a hot plunge:

1. Heat the water. For a long plunge, make sure to have more hot water handy, as the hot water in the basin will cool off over time.
2. While the water is heating, unfold one towel and place it on a flat surface.
3. Place an empty basin on top of the towel.
4. When the water is hot, pour it into the basin until it is approximately two-thirds full. Check the temperature of the hot water using the thermometer. Add more hot water, or cool water, until the desired temperature is reached.

5. Plunge your forearms and hands into the water for the desired length of time (Fig. 6-7). After the plunge, dry your forearms and hands with a towel.

Warm Plunge

Warm plunges can provide relief from muscle tension, pain, and spasms and from noninflammatory joint pain. Other benefits are overall relaxation and stress relief. Warm plunges should not be done if there are areas of inflammation on the forearms or hands.

The forearms and hands can be plunged in the warm water for anywhere from 2 to 45 minutes. The water temperature for a warm plunge should be between 92° and 98°F, depending on your tolerance for heat. The steps for a warm plunge are the same as for a hot plunge.

Alternating Hot and Cold Plunge

Alternating hot and cold plunges can provide relief from muscle tension, pain, and spasms. Alternating plunges should not be done by those who are physically frail, have heart conditions, have untreated high blood pressure, have areas of inflammation on the forearms or hand, or are intolerant to heat or cold.

The forearms and hands can be plunged in the basin of heated water for 3 minutes or longer, depending on your tolerance for heat, and in the basin of cold water for 30 to 60 seconds, depending on your tolerance for cold. A general rule of thumb is a 3:1 ratio—for every 3 minutes of heat, follow it with 1 minute of cold. Always place the forearms and hands in the heated water first and end the treatment with the forearms and hands in the cold water. The hot water causes the blood vessels to vasodilate, increasing blood flow into the tissues. Oxygen and nutrients are distributed to the cells, and the blood picks up metabolic wastes. The cold water causes the blood vessels to vasoconstrict, decreasing blood flow into the tissues. Blood travels away from the area, taking the wastes with it. Because the overall effect is a pumping of blood into and out of the tissues, it is important that vasodilation happens first. For optimal results, alternating temperature plunges should be done in rapid succession five times.

The water temperature for the hot water should be 98° to 108°F, and the cold water should be 40° to 55°F, depending on your tolerance for heat and cold.

In addition to cold water, make sure you have ice handy in case you need it to cool the water to your desired temperature.

The following are the steps for an alternating hot and cold plunge:

1. Heat water. While the water is heating, unfold two towels and place them on a flat surface.
2. Place an empty basin on top of each towel.
3. Pour cold water into one basin until it is approximately two-thirds full. Check the temperature of the cold water using the thermometer. Add ice until the desired temperature is reached.
4. When the water is hot, pour it into the other basin until it is approximately two-thirds full. Check the temperature of the hot water using the thermometer. Add more hot water, or cool water, until the desired temperature is reached.
5. Plunge your forearms and hands into hot water for 3 minutes or longer, depending on your tolerance for heat. Take them out of the hot water and immediately plunge them into the cold water for 30 to 60 seconds, depending on your tolerance for cold.
6. Take them out of the cold water and immediately plunge them back into the hot water for 3 to 5 minutes. Repeat the alternating plunges five times.
7. After the plunges, dry your forearms and hands with a towel.

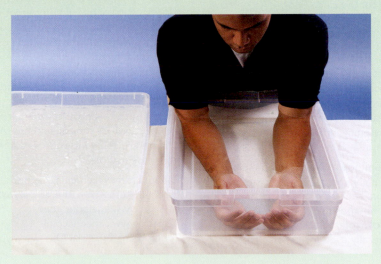

FIGURE 6-7 Plunge your forearms and hands into the hot water.

Focus on *Wellness*

Topical analgesics are applied directly to the skin for temporary relief of muscle aches and pains. They come in a variety of forms:

- Creams
- Gels
- Lotions
- Sprays
- Patches

When used moderately, and according to the directions on the label, topical medications are relatively safe. However, they should not be used long-term or in excessive quantities. It is also important to realize that many of these medications mask or suppress the natural pain signals of the body. Ignoring pain can increase your risk of further muscle or joint injury. If you do use these medications for temporary pain relief, it is important to rest the affected muscles, so try to avoid intense activity until soreness subsides.

There are several categories of topical analgesics:

Non-Steroidal Anti-Inflammatory Drugs (NSAIDs)

- Salicylates (methyl salicylates), the same ingredients found in aspirin, are effective pain relievers that also reduce inflammation. The use of salicylates is contraindicated for those who are allergic to aspirin.
- Other NSAIDs are diclofenac, felbinac, ibuprofen, ketoprofen, piroxicam, naproxen, and flurbiprofen.
- These are generally used for acute conditions such as sprains and strains, as well as for chronic conditions such as arthritis.
- Brand name products include Bengay, Aspercreme, and Sportscreme.

Rubefacients

A **rubefacient** is a substance for external application that produces redness of the skin through vasodilation. It is believed to relieve pain through *counterirritant* effects. A counterirritant is a substance that creates inflammation in one location with the goal of lessening inflammation, and the accompanying pain, in another location.

- Capsaicin is a commonly used rubefacient. It is the compound in chili peppers that causes a hot, burning sensation. The use of capsaicin is contraindicated for those who are allergic to it or who have a low tolerance to heat sensations.
- Capsaicin is generally used for chronic pain conditions.

- Brand name products include Arthricare, Capzasin, and Zostrix.

Other Counterirritants

- These products contain ingredients such as menthol, wintergreen, or eucalyptus oil that make the skin feel hot or cold. Wintergreen contains methyl salicylate; salicylates are both NSAIDs and counterirritants.
- These are generally used for acute and chronic pain.
- They are commonly used in bodywork.
- Brand name products include Flexall 454, Icy Hot, JointFlex, Sombra, CryoDerm, ActivOn, Prossage, Tiger Balm, and Biofreeze.

Other Natural Remedies

- Lavender is a popular essential oil used for its calming properties. However, it also acts as an analgesic and anti-inflammatory with potency comparable to NSAIDs. It can be used in aromatherapy or added to a bath or an aroma burner, and it can be applied topically for muscle, bone, and joint pain.
- Marjoram, basil, and black pepper essential oils ease soreness and promote muscle healing.
- Mountain arnica (arnica montana) is an herb used in topical creams to treat bruising and pain, especially for minor injuries and arthritis. The active ingredient, helenalin, has anti-inflammatory and antibacterial properties.

It is important to buy only pure, organic, good-quality essential oils. True essential oils will have the botanical name and the common name on the label and will say that it is a "pure essential oil" or a "100% essential oil." If you cannot tell from the label whether it is a true essential oil, do not buy it.

Other ways to distinguish true essential oils from synthetic fragrance oils is by price and by the bottle containing the oil. Pure, organic oils cost more than synthetic oils or synthetic oil blends. The best-quality oils will always be in dark bottles, such as blue or brown glass. This protects them from sunlight exposure, which can cause them to deteriorate.

Here are some Internet resources for purchasing pure essential oils:

Enfleurage: www.enfleurage.com
Essential Aura Aromatherapy: www.essentialaura.com
Kneipp: www.kneippus.com
Oshadi: www.oshadhi.co.uk
Young Living Essential Oils: www.youngliving.com

The effects of essential oils can be so powerful that practitioners should attend formal courses in **aromatherapy** to learn how to use them appropriately. Aromatherapy is the therapeutic use of fragrant essential oils that have been extracted from plants. The National Association for Holistic Aromatherapy (www.naha.org) is a valuable source of information. This is an educational, nonprofit organization dedicated to enhancing public awareness of the benefits of true aromatherapy.

Precautions for Using Topical Analgesics
- Side effects from these products often include burning, stinging, or irritated skin.
- Never use these products on broken or irritated skin.
- Do not apply heat or ice to the area on which you have used a topical medication. This can injure the tissue.
- Always wash your hands thoroughly after applying creams, lotions, or gels. Another option is to wear protective gloves, such as those made of latex, when applying topical analgesics. If you are allergic to latex, consider using gloves made of nitrile.
- While it is extremely rare, it is possible to overdose on these topical pain relievers. Always carefully follow the instructions for product use.

is associated with a hypersensitive palpable nodule in a taut band. The spot is painful on compression and can give rise to characteristic referred pain, referred tenderness, motor dysfunction, and autonomic phenomena" (Travell and Simons, 1998)

Signs and symptoms: Active trigger points refer to sensations of pain, tingling, numbness without being pressed. *Latent trigger points* refer to sensations of pain, tingling, and numbness upon being pressed. Other symptoms include muscle tightness, weakness, and loss of function.

Causes: Lack of exercise, muscle overload, imbalanced posture, traumatic injuries, metabolic issues, and sleep disturbances. For example, sleeping in awkward positions can cause trigger points to develop in the affected muscles. Or if an individual does not get enough sleep, the muscles tend to respond by increasing in tension, which can result in trigger points (Travell and Simons, 1998).

Treatment: The best remedy is receiving regular bodywork, especially deep tissue massage techniques, such as trigger point therapy, deep friction, stripping, and myofascial stretching. Getting regular exercise, increasing flexibility, not overexerting muscles, and working to gain or maintain balanced posture can also help alleviate trigger points.

MUSCLE STRAIN (PULL)

Muscle strain is a stretch or tear in the muscle; it may also include the fascia surrounding the muscle. Muscle strains usually occur at the musculotendinous junction. The strain can involve a few muscle fibers or a large area of the muscle. Muscle strains typically occur during eccentric contractions, because force is greater on a muscle in eccentric contraction than during isometric or concentric contractions. However, an explosive concentric contraction can also result in muscle strain. It is this increased load on the fibers that results in strain injury. The muscles that are most susceptible to strain injury are those crossing more than one joint such as the hamstrings, the erector spinae group, biceps brachii and the quadriceps femoris group. These muscles are not designed to become fully lengthened over all the joints at the same time. This makes them vulnerable to reaching their limits with abnormal stress, and injury can result.

Signs and symptoms: Pain and loss of muscle function.
- First-degree strain (Grade 1, or mild): Only a few muscle fibers are torn (less than 25%). There is some local pain, mild tenderness, minor loss of strength, and mild swelling. The individual is usually back to normal levels of activity rather quickly. Healing time is about 5 to 14 days.
- Second-degree strain (Grade 2, or moderate): More fibers are involved in the injury (25% to 75%). There is likely to be a greater level of pain and area of tenderness in the muscle tissue, swelling, bruising, and impaired muscle function. The individual needs longer to heal; the average length of time is 2 to 4 weeks.
- Third-degree strain (Grade 3, or severe): Severe tear or complete rupture of the muscle and tendon unit (75% or more). There is severe pain at the time of the injury and an audible pop or snap, with loss of muscle

function that results in joint instability. Commonly, there is a palpable defect in the muscle because the muscle may curl up from being torn. On the other hand, pain may be minimal if the muscle ends are completely separated (because moving the limbs does not put additional stress on the separated ends of the muscle) or if there has been damage to the nerves supplying the muscle. Surgery is usually required to repair the ruptured muscle. In some cases, the muscle may not be solely responsible for a joint's movement, and the potential dangers of surgery do not outweigh the loss of partial muscle action. For example, a rupture in the rectus femoris is commonly left as is, since the other three quadriceps muscles can usually make up for the strength deficit. Healing time is about 2 to 12 months.

Inflammation (Acute Phase) Signs and Symptoms
- Lasts several hours up to 3 or 4 days
- SHARP
- Possible loss of function, depending on the severity
- Possible pain while at rest
- Possible hematoma and bruising, depending on the severity

Regeneration (Subacute Phase) Signs and Symptoms
- Minimal heat, redness, and swelling
- If bruising occurred, change in bruise color from purple to yellow
- Aching pain after activity, but not while at rest
- Trigger points can appear in affected muscles and their antagonists
- Increased active ROM and strength

Remodeling (Maturation Phase) Signs and Symptoms
- Mild to no redness, heat, or swelling. If they do occur, it is usually after activity.
- Compensation patterns have set in.
- Goals should be to strengthen the muscle and increase mobility.

Causes: Usually an abnormal muscle contraction during abrupt movement, such as lifting with the small muscles of the back instead of the large muscles of the legs, and twisting while lifting. Other causes include not warming up the muscles before activity, limited flexibility, strength imbalances, and previous injuries.

Treatments: The PRICE protocol (see below), analgesics, and anti-inflammatory medications such as NSAIDs. Massage the accessory muscles to encourage circulation and lymphatic drainage, which can support healing.

PRICE protocol:
- P = Protect the area from further injury.
- R = Rest the area for a chance to heal.
- I = Ice the area to decrease inflammation and swelling, vasoconstriction, and pain. See "Ice Massage (Cryotherapy)" in Appendix A.
- C = Compress the area to decrease or control swelling; this provides stability and reduces the chance of secondary injury.
- E = Elevate the area to decrease swelling (Lowe, 2009; Tortora and Derrickson, 2009; Werner, 2009).

FASCIA

Recall from the "Factors Contributing to RSI" section that fascia is a connective tissue that is found throughout the body and is composed mainly of elastic collagen fibers. It lines the body wall and limbs, and it supports and surrounds muscles and other organs of the body. Fascia is wrapped around every individual muscle fiber and around every individual muscle (Fig. 6-8), and it holds together muscles with similar functions (e.g., all the quadriceps are held together by fascia; Fig. 6-9). Fascia allows free movement of muscles, carries nerves, blood vessels and lymphatic vessels, and fills the spaces between muscles.

FIELD NOTES

Because of a previous auto accident injury, I experience flare-ups of pain and limited movement in my left shoulder. These flare-ups can be prevented as long as I keep up my self-care routine and bring awareness to my whole body, especially my weaker areas such as my left shoulder. I always use correct body mechanics. If I do experience a flare-up, I follow the PRICE protocol.

By using a wide range of modalities, I have remained injury-free in my practice as a bodyworker. Prevention is key, in my opinion, incorporating it into all aspects of a healthy lifestyle. This includes eating right, exercising regularly, stretching, strengthening the core, knowing your physical limitations, receiving various types of bodywork, making time for yourself, and, most important, *listening to your body* and *staying connected!*

Jesseca Maglothin, LMT, Reiki master, craniosacral therapist, instructor and continuing education presenter. Massage therapist since 2004.

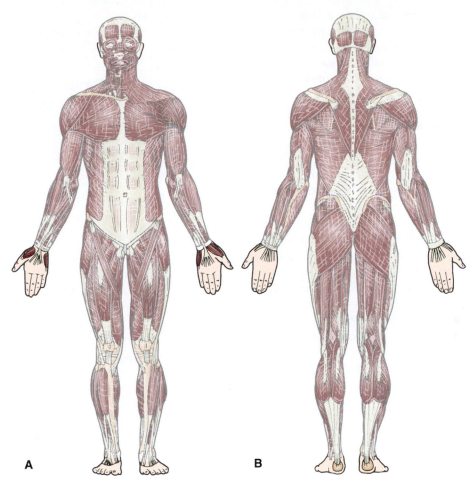

FIGURE 6-8 Fascial system of the body. **(A)** Anterior view. **(B)** Posterior view.

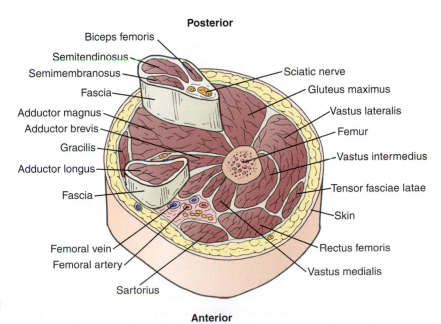

FIGURE 6-9 Cross section of the thigh showing the muscles and associated fascia.

There is a special interdependent relationship between muscle tissue and fascia, both structurally and functionally. Often the term *myofascia* or *myofascial tissues* (*myo* meaning "muscle") is used when discussing them. Modalities involving myofascial release and myofascial stretching use the relationship between muscle tissue and fascia.

Fascia can be injured in several ways. It has a great deal of elasticity, but extreme tensile stress can cause it to tear or perforate. Many injuries that involve damage to fascia also affect the tissues it envelopes, such as muscle. An example is trigger points, which are sometimes referred to as *myofascial trigger points*. When fascia remains in a shortened position for prolonged periods, it tends to stay in that shortened position. Tensions in associated muscle fibers also cause contractile fibers within the fascia to maintain the shortened position. Long periods in a shortened position may even lead to fibrous cross-linking within the fascial tissue, which can result in limited or painful movement and trigger points (Travell and Simons, 1998).

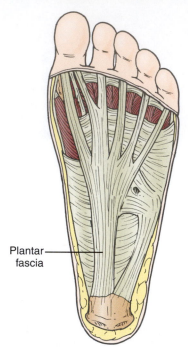

FIGURE 6-10 Plantar fascia.

PLANTAR FASCIITIS

Plantar fasciitis involves pain at the plantar fascia; it may or may not also involve inflammation.

Signs and symptoms: Sharp or aching pain in the arch of the foot and sometimes the fascial attachment at the heel or calcaneus. The pain occurs when assuming activity after a period of rest. It lessens as the tissue warms and then begins to hurt again with continued use.

Causes: The plantar fascia is on the sole of the foot and stretches from the calcaneus to the proximal phalanges (Fig. 6-10). It supports all the arches of the foot, especially the medial longitudinal arch. Repetitive excessive biomechanical force causes the connective tissue fibers to unravel and become disordered, and the collagen in the fascia breaks down. When the foot has been immobile for some time, the fascial fibers begin to reweave as part of the healing process. Then when activity resumes, the fibers become irritated again, causing pain.

The excessive biomechanical force can come from being overweight (placing more stress on the feet), wearing shoes without good arch and lateral support, having legs of unequal length, having flat or pronated feet, having excessively tight calf muscles, having a dysfunction elsewhere in the body that causes a postural distortion, and sleeping with the ankles plantarflexed so that the feet are pointed downward. Other underlying causes can include diabetes, rheumatoid arthritis, and gout.

Treatment: Decreasing activities that aggravate the symptoms; warming and massaging the foot with broadening techniques that spread the plantar fascia; using shoes that prevent strong dorsiflexion of the foot (this prevents excessive stretch on the plantar fascia); using shoe inserts; using night splints that hold the foot in a slightly dorsiflexed position so that the collagen fibers reweave in a healthy, elongated position; not going barefoot until the fascia can stretch without tearing; rolling a golf ball along the bottom of the foot from the base of the toes to the heel (for more severe conditions, a tennis ball can be used to start with); using anti-inflammatory medications or steroid injections; applying ice; stretching; using deep tissue techniques such as deep friction; stripping; using trigger point therapy; and performing myofascial stretching on the calf muscles and the area of pain; undergoing surgery (Lowe, 2009; Werner, 2009).

TENDON

In order to create movement, tendons transmit the force of skeletal muscle contractions to bones. Tendons are dense connective tissues that have some "give." In tendons, collagen fibers are arranged in parallel bundles, which give them the greatest amount of strength in a longitudinal direction. Surrounding many tendons are tendon sheaths that contain a gelatinous substance; tendon sheaths reduce friction as the tendons slide back and forth (Fig. 6-11).

Recall from Chapter 3 that a tendon's tensile stress (ability to withstand tension along its length) can be more than twice that of its associated muscle. Because tendons have tensile strength, they can withstand a lot of tension when stress is placed on them, specifically the stress from contracting muscles. This means that tendons do not stretch when the muscles contract and pull on them. Instead, the bones that the tendons are attached to move (Fig. 6-12).

Overloading a muscle usually results in muscle strain or a severe tear or rupture in the muscular fibers near the musculotendinous junction rather than in the tendon. Sometimes, because tendons are so strong, if the muscle is greatly overloaded, a piece of the bone the tendon is attached to is pulled off instead of the tendon rupturing. This is called an **avulsion,** which is considered a fracture (Lowe, 2009; Tortora and Derrickson, 2009).

Tendon injuries are not usually due to abrupt trauma. Instead, most are RSIs. Tendon injuries usually progress slowly over a long period, and repeated acute injuries can lead to chronic conditions such as tendinosis, tendinitis, and tenosynovitis.

TENDINOSIS, TENDINITIS, AND TENOSYNOVITIS

Tendinosis is the most common condition involving tendons. It is caused by repetitive mechanical loads placed on the tendon. Originally it was thought that the tendon fibers tore and subsequently led to inflammation in the tendon, resulting in the term *tendinitis* (also spelled *tendonitis*). However, recent research shows that in this condition, no cells become inflamed in the tendon.

Therefore, the term *tendinosis* is more accurate, describing a degenerative condition in which tendon fibers are not torn. Instead, the collagen fibers break down. This collagen breakdown leads to chronic pain, since the tendon loses tensile strength. It takes a long time to heal from tendinosis; rebuilding damaged collagen is a very slow process. Therefore, tendinosis can become chronic or recurrent if measures are not taken to alleviate the cause. The collagen continues to be broken down faster than the body can repair it. While any tendon can develop tendinosis, tendons in the extremities are more susceptible.

Tendinitis involves injuries to a tendon that involve an inflammatory response. True tendinitis involves tendon fiber tearing with inflammation, which can occur but is quite rare. Inflammation requires blood circulation, and tendons have a limited blood supply. The tendon fiber tear would need to occur near the blood supply or within the periosteum

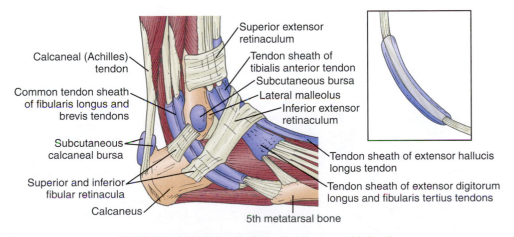

FIGURE 6-11 Structure of a tendon in a synovial sheath.

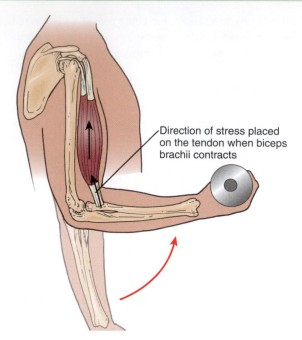

FIGURE 6-12 Force of muscle contraction transmitted through a tendon, causing a bone to move.

Direction of stress placed on the tendon when biceps brachii contracts

(the membrane surrounding bone, which has a high blood supply).

Physicians and rehabilitation practitioners often diagnosis tendinosis as tendinitis. In many cases, they continue to focus on anti-inflammatory treatment strategies rather than on collagen rebuilding. In some cases, NSAIDs can be detrimental for healing collagen degeneration. If practitioners are concerned they may have been misdiagnosed based on this information, they should speak with their health-care providers. Getting a second opinion can be helpful as well.

Tenosynovitis affects the synovial sheath that surrounds some tendons, such as those in the distal extremities and certain other locations. The sheath reduces friction between the tendon and the retinaculum that binds the tendon close to the joint. The tendon must be able to glide freely within the synovial sheath.

In tenosynovitis, chronic overloading or excessive friction causes inflammation or irritation between the tendon and its synovial sheath. The inflammation causes the tendon's surface to become rough, and as a result, fibrous adhesions can develop between the tendon and the sheath (Fig. 6-13). The roughened tendon surface may cause crepitus when the joint is moved through its range of motion.

> *Signs and symptoms:* Symptoms of tendinosis and tenosynovitis are similar and include pain or swelling (in the acute stage). Pain and tenderness can extend into the surrounding muscles. If the tendon has a synovial sheath, tenosynovitis is most likely. If there is no sheath, tendinosis is probably the issue.
>
> *Causes:* Trauma, repetitive use, lack of flexibility, and inflammatory diseases such as rheumatoid arthritis (Lowe, 2009; Werner, 2009).

Common Tendon Disorders

LATERAL EPICONDYLITIS/EPICONDYLOSIS (TENNIS ELBOW)

Lateral epicondylitis/epicondylosis is an overuse injury affecting the attachments of the wrist extensors, usually extensor carpi radialis brevis at the lateral

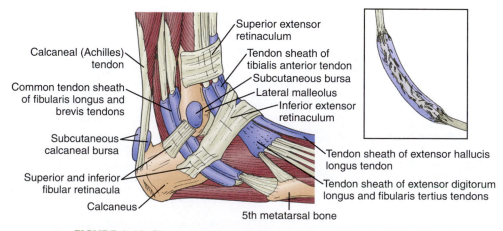

Calcaneal (Achilles) tendon

Common tendon sheath of fibularis longus and brevis tendons

Subcutaneous calcaneal bursa

Superior and inferior fibular retinacula

Calcaneus

Superior extensor retinaculum

Tendon sheath of tibialis anterior tendon

Subcutaneous bursa

Lateral malleolus

Inferior extensor retinaculum

Tendon sheath of extensor hallucis longus tendon

Tendon sheath of extensor digitorum longus and fibularis tertius tendons

5th metatarsal bone

FIGURE 6-13 Fibrous adhesion between a tendon and its synovial sheath.

epicondyle of the humerus. It has been called *tennis elbow* due to the frequency seen in tennis players. However, this condition is seen quite often in people who have never picked up a tennis racket. Repetitive stress at the musculotendinous junction at the epicondyle is the most common cause of lateral elbow pain; this leads to tendinitis in its most acute form and to tendinosis in its more chronic form.

Signs and symptoms: Pain and tenderness at the lateral epicondyle of the humerus, weakness in the wrist, difficulty doing simple tasks such as turning a door handle or shaking hands, pain at the lateral elbow when the wrist is extended against resistance, pain on the lateral elbow when trying to straighten the fingers against resistance, and tenderness under the lateral epicondyle.

Causes: Overuse or repetitive strain, repeated extension and hyperextension of the wrist during activities such as tennis, the performance of bodywork, and ADL.

MEDIAL EPICONDYLITIS/EPICONDYLOSIS (GOLFER'S OR PITCHER'S ELBOW)

Medial epicondylitis/epicondylosis is an overuse injury affecting the attachments of the wrist flexors, usually the flexor carpi radialis at the medial epicondyle of the humerus. It has been called *golfer's* or *pitcher's elbow* due to the frequency seen in golfers and baseball pitchers. However, this condition is seen quite often in people who have never done these activities. Repetitive stress at the epicondyle attachment is the most common cause of medial elbow pain; this leads to tendinitis in its most acute form and to tendinosis in its more chronic form.

Signs and symptoms: Pain and tenderness at the medial epicondyle of the humerus, with wrist flexion or forearm pronation. Range of motion of the elbow and wrist is usually within normal limits.

Causes: Overuse or repetitive strain, repeated flexion of the wrist during activities such as performing bodywork and ADL, traumatic injury, an improper golf swing, improper pitching in baseball.

Treatments of tendon disorders: Analgesics, NSAIDs, hydrotherapy (see Appendix A), the PRICE protocol, braces, and gradual return to activities. If the tendinitis or tenosynovitis is chronic and in an inflammatory stage, deep tissue massage techniques are contraindicated. If it is in a noninflammatory stage, the area can be addressed with deep specific friction on the involved tendons in the musculotendinous junction, and a 20-minute follow-up treatment with ice is recommended (see Appendix A for ice massage; Holland and Anderson, 2011; Lowe, 2009; Werner, 2009).

BURSITIS

A bursa is a small sac or pouch made of connective tissue filled with synovial fluid that has the consistency of an egg yolk. Bursae decrease friction by cushioning the movements between muscles and bones, tendons and bones, tendons and ligaments, and in areas where skin moves over bony prominences. Figure 6-14 shows bursae of the shoulder

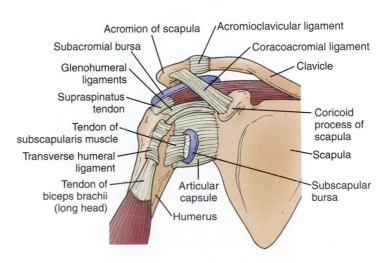

Acromion of scapula
Subacromial bursa
Glenohumeral ligaments
Supraspinatus tendon
Tendon of subscapularis muscle
Transverse humeral ligament
Tendon of biceps brachii (long head)

Acromioclavicular ligament
Coracoacromial ligament
Clavicle
Coricoid process of scapula
Scapula
Subscapular bursa
Articular capsule
Humerus

FIGURE 6-14 Bursae of the shoulder joint.

joint. The body can generate new bursae in areas that need additional protection. Bursitis is inflammation of one or more bursae. There are approximately 160 bursae throughout the body. Often bursitis occurs where tendons are located, such as at the ischial tuberosity and in the knee, shoulder, hip (at the greater trochanter), elbow, and heel.

Signs and symptoms: Swelling and sometimes heat, pain with any movement, redness limited range of motion, and sometimes loss of function. Repeated trauma can lead to calcification and degeneration of the inner lining of the bursa.

Causes: Sudden irritation can cause acute bursitis. Overuse of muscles or tendons (repetitive stress), as well as constant external compression or trauma, can result in chronic bursitis.

Treatments: Short-term use of anti-inflammatory medications and NSAIDs, steroid injections, drainage of excess fluid, surgery (bursectomy), massage therapy, rehabilitative exercise. Some cases of bursitis respond well to ice application. In other cases, warm, moist heat is effective in the acute stage, and dry heat is

effective in the subacute and chronic stages (Lowe, 2009; Tortora and Derrickson, 2009; Werner, 2009).

LIGAMENT

Ligaments are thick, tough, fibrous tissues that connect adjacent bones, creating a stable skeletal structure and preventing abnormal movements. Like tendons, most of the collagen fibers in ligaments are arranged in parallel bundles, which give them the greatest amount of tensile strength in a longitudinal direction. However, within the ligament

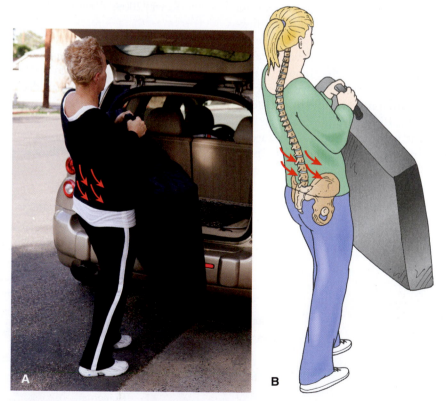

FIGURE 6-15 (A) Spraining the low back while lifting a massage table and twisting. Arrows show direction of force. **(B)** Forces on the low back leading to sprain.

there are also fibers that are oriented in other ways. These give pliability, strength, and a certain amount of stretch to the ligament as the joint moves in various directions.

Ligament injuries usually occur from sudden high-tensile loads on the fibers, such as a sudden blow to a joint or an abrupt wrenching of a joint (e.g., lifting a massage table while twisting the trunk may sprain the intervertebral joints of the low back; Fig. 6-15A and B). The severity of the injury depends on how much force is applied to the ligament. If the tensile stress is minimal, the ligament can usually absorb the force with minor stretching of the fibers. If the force is greater, the ligament fibers may stretch slightly.

SPRAIN

Sprains are joint traumas that stretch or tear the ligaments of a joint, but there is no dislocation of the bones. A first-degree sprain involves stretching of the ligaments without tearing; a second-degree sprain involves partial tearing of the ligament; a third-degree sprain involves complete tearing of the ligament.

Signs and symptoms: A sprain causes blood and synovial fluid to pour into the joint cavity, producing joint swelling, heat in the area, mild to severe pain and tenderness, bruising, and skin discoloration. Ligaments and joint capsules heal slowly because of their relatively poor blood supply. They can, in fact, take 3 to 6 months, or longer, to heal fully.

Causes: Overuse (especially without proper recovery time), lack of flexibility, an underlying cause such as a history of hypermobility, and a history of corticosteroid injections. Low back sprains are usually caused by lifting with the small muscles of the back instead of the large muscles of the legs and twisting the torso at the same time. The joints most vulnerable to sprains are the ankles, knees, wrists, fingers, low back, sacral ligaments, and shoulders because these joints are used more frequently and absorb the stress of movement. Therefore, they are more vulnerable to being twisted, wrenched, or receiving a direct blow.

If the ligament is stretched greatly enough or often enough, it can become permanently lengthened. The ligament tissue can be stretched, but it does not recoil back to its original length. This leads to unstable and hypermobile joints that can be injured or reinjured easily. Repeated joint twisting can also result in chronic inflammation, degeneration, and arthritis.

Treatments: Analgesics, anti-inflammatory medications such as NSAIDs, and the PRICE protocol. Bodywork modalities that involve tissue manipulation, such as massage therapy, are contraindicated on the area until the inflammation has subsided or until 72 hours after the initial injury, whichever comes first. At this point, lymphatic massage can manage swelling outside the joint capsule. Light gliding strokes and light friction around the area can be helpful to increase blood circulation and support healing. Once healing is fully completed, deep friction in the area to loosen adhesions may be helpful (Lowe, 2009; Tortora and Derrickson, 2009; Werner, 2009).

JOINT CAPSULE

The outermost layer of a joint capsule is a fibrous capsule made up of mostly ligament tissue, and it stabilizes and supports the joint. The inner layer is synovial membrane, which secretes synovial fluid (Fig. 6-16). Synovial fluid lubricates the joint, supplies it with nutrients, and removes metabolic wastes from the area. The fibrous capsule is highly innervated, so even minor injury can cause a great deal of pain and discomfort.

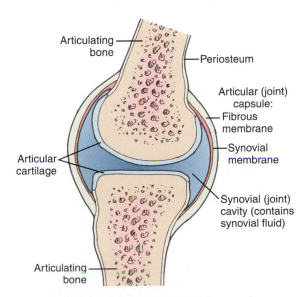

FIGURE 6-16 Structure of a joint capsule.

FROZEN SHOULDER AND ADHESIVE CAPSULITIS

Frozen shoulder and adhesive capsulitis involves restricted range of motion of the glenohumeral joint due to inflamed and stiffened surrounding connective tissue and adhesions. **Muscle guarding** also occurs. *Muscle guarding* is the term for involuntary muscle contractions that occur in response to pain after musculoskeletal injury. These signs and symptoms can last from approximately 5 months to 3 years or more and may resolve, at least partially, spontaneously. It usually occurs in people 50 to 70 years of age, but can occur in people of any age who use this joint in repetitive motions. Frozen shoulder can include not only adhesive capsulitis, but also bursitis, tendinosis (to the point that the tendon is becoming calcified), and rotator cuff muscle and tendon problems. Adhesive capsulitis results in loss of shoulder joint motion due to adhesions within the glenohumeral joint capsule and is usually the end result of frozen shoulder.

Signs and symptoms: Severe restricted range of motion, chronic pain characterized as diffuse, dull, and aching in the shoulder. Certain movements can cause sudden onset of pain and muscle cramping that can last several minutes.

Causes: Unclear in some cases. In other cases, it results from rotator cuff tears, muscle guarding in the area due to some other injury, arthritis, tendinosis or tenosynovitis in the biceps brachii tendon (as it travels through the bicipital groove), surgery, shoulder separation, or diabetes. Scar tissue from these problems causes the axillary folds of the joint capsule to adhere together. The shoulder joint loses movement because of chronic inflammation, the formation of adhesions, and a decrease of synovial fluid.

Treatments: Can be painful; consists of physical therapy, various medications, massage therapy,

and, in severe cases, surgery (Fritz, 2009; Lowe, 2009; Tortora and Derrickson, 2009; Werner, 2009).

NERVE

Nerve injuries that result from nerves being trapped against ligaments or bones are called **nerve compressions. Impingement** or **entrapment** is compression on the nerves by soft tissues such as muscle. Injury can also occur due to direct blows, acute swelling of tissue within an enclosed space, imbalanced posture, or any condition that compromises the tissue spaces through which nerves travel.

Compressive pressure can occur anywhere along a nerve, but several sites are most vulnerable for nerve damage. These include lumbar and cervical regions of the vertebral column. **Radiculopathy** is the term for nerve pathology that occurs at the nerve root. A common radiculopathy is a herniated disk in which the disk presses on a nerve root, resulting in sciatica-like symptoms (see the "Sciatica" section later in this chapter).

Neuropathy is a pathology farther along the length of the nerve. The term *peripheral neuropathy* is also used to indicate that the pathology is farther along the peripheral nerve, far from the nerve roots and spinal cord. Impingements such as thoracic outlet and carpal tunnel syndrome (also discussed later in this chapter) are examples of peripheral neuropathies.

Sometimes there can be multiple areas of pathology along a nerve. This is called the **double or multiple crush phenomenon**. For example, brachial plexus compression near the thoracic outlet can inhibit nerve function distally on the arm. As a result, symptoms of both thoracic outlet syndrome and carpal tunnel syndrome can develop.

Signs and symptoms of nerve compression include pain and other sensations. Sensory impairment can range from **anesthesia** (no sensation) to paresthesia to **hyperesthesia** (hypersensitivity). Motor function can also be impaired. It can range from no loss in muscle strength or function to weakness to complete loss of muscle function (paralysis). Loss of motor function can lead to muscular atrophy, or wasting away of the muscle.

THORACIC OUTLET SYNDROME (TOS)

Thoracic outlet syndrome is compression or entrapment of one or more of the structures of the neurovascular bundle (brachial nerve plexus and associated

---

What **D**o **Y**ou **T**hink**?**

A fellow practitioner comes to you complaining of chronic pain in the anterior aspect of her shoulder. Given the anatomical structures in this area, what types of chronic inflammatory conditions might you suspect? Do you think you can differentiate which structure is involved based on the signs and symptoms? Why or why not?

blood vessels) in the lateral neck. The brachial nerve plexus arises at the lateral neck, travels through the anterior and middle scalene, under the clavicle, under pectoralis minor, through the axilla, and down into the arm and hand (Fig. 6-17A). TOS can affect the muscles of the shoulder, upper chest, arm, and hand and can affect blood supply of the arm.

Signs and symptoms: Arm swelling; shooting (radiating) pain, sometimes down into the hand and first three digits; sensitivity to temperature change; weakness; and numbness in the shoulder and scapular regions, down the arm, and sometimes in the chest and neck (Fig. 6-17B).

Causes: Compression or impingement of the brachial plexus. Generally, the most medial nerve, the ulnar nerve, is impinged.

Pectoralis minor syndrome involves impingement of the neurovascular bundle between pectoralis minor and the ribs. **Anterior scalene syndrome** involves impingement between anterior and middle scalenes. **Costoclavicular syndrome** involves impingement between the clavicle and the first rib (Fig. 6-17C). The impingement can be due to excessive arm movements, or chronic tight scalene muscles such as from cradling a telephone receiver on the shoulder. Other causes include herniated cervical disks or cervical spondylosis (stiffening of the vertebral joints), improper breathing, and smoking. Smoking can impair efficient breathing, placing a greater load on the accessory breathing muscles such as the scalenes.

Treatments: Postural changes, physiotherapy, massage therapy, chiropractic adjustments or osteopathic manipulation, and strengthening the muscles that stabilize the shoulder (Lowe, 2009; Tortora and Derrickson, 2009; Werner, 2009).

CARPAL TUNNEL SYNDROME (CTS)

Carpal tunnel syndrome is a painful repetitive stress injury of the wrist and hand. The carpal tunnel is formed where the transverse carpal ligament connects across carpal bones in the anterior wrist, creating a narrow passageway. The tendons of the wrist flexors and the median nerve pass through this tunnel into the hand (Fig. 6-18A). Tendinous sheaths may become swollen and irritated through overuse and not keeping the wrist neutral. The swelling can compress the median nerve (Fig. 6-18B). Chronic inflammation can also cause the tendon sheath to thicken, compounding the problem.

Signs and symptoms: Tenderness, hypertonicity, fascial restrictions, pain, numbness, paresthesia along the median nerve pathway into the hand (Fig. 6-19), and weakened muscles in the hand and first three digits.

Causes: Repetitive movements of the wrist and hand. Some additional risk factors are rheumatoid arthritis, osteoarthritis, certain hormonal disorders, diabetes, thyroid disorders, and menopause. CTS can result from overuse or strain in certain jobs involving repetitive move-

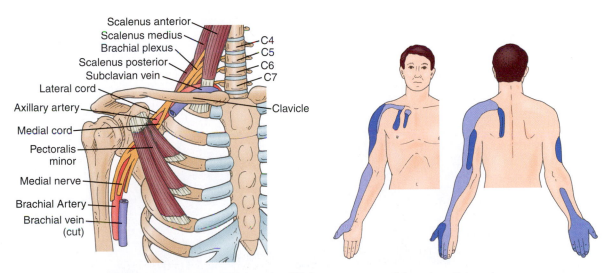

FIGURE 6-17 (A) The thoracic outlet. **(B)** Sensory pattern of thoracic outlet syndrome.

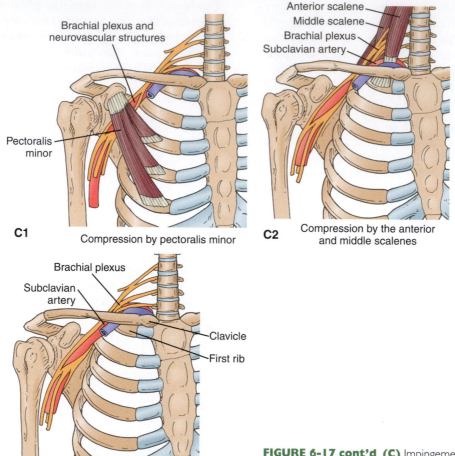

C1 Compression by pectoralis minor

Brachial plexus and neurovascular structures

Pectoralis minor

C2 Compression by the anterior and middle scalenes

Anterior scalene
Middle scalene
Brachial plexus
Subclavian artery

C3 Compression by the clavicle and first rib

Brachial plexus
Subclavian artery
Clavicle
First rib

FIGURE 6-17 cont'd (C) Impingement of the brachial plexus by pectoralis minor, the scalene muscles, and the clavicle and first rib.

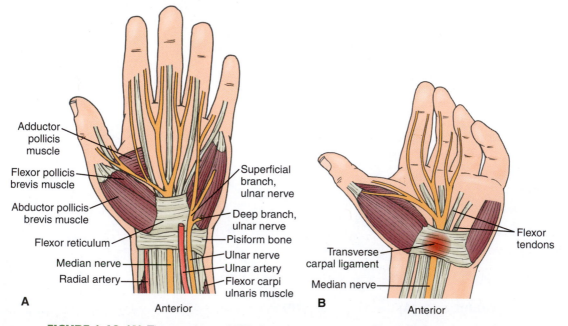

Adductor pollicis muscle
Flexor pollicis brevis muscle
Abductor pollicis brevis muscle
Flexor reticulum
Median nerve
Radial artery
Superficial branch, ulnar nerve
Deep branch, ulnar nerve
Pisiform bone
Ulnar nerve
Ulnar artery
Flexor carpi ulnaris muscle

A   Anterior

Flexor tendons
Transverse carpal ligament
Median nerve

B   Anterior

FIGURE 6-18 (A) The carpal tunnel. **(B)** Compression of the median nerve in the carpal tunnel.

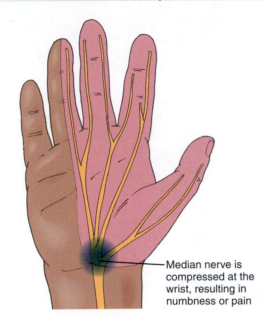

Median nerve is compressed at the wrist, resulting in numbness or pain

FIGURE 6-19 Pathway of sensations along the median nerve.

Signs and symptoms: Mild or moderate aching in the forearm; sharp, shooting pain; numbness or paresthesia along the median nerve pathway into the hand (see Fig. 6-19); and weakened muscles in the hand and first three digits.

Causes: In most people, the median nerve passes between the two heads of pronator teres (Fig. 6-20A), which is where the compression occurs. In some people, the median nerve runs deep to both heads of pronator teres (Fig. 6-20B), and the compression occurs when pronator teres presses the median nerve against the ulna. If pronator teres becomes excessively tight or has trigger points, it can entrap the median nerve. Repetitive motions of the flexed elbow or pronation of the forearm are usually the cause of tightness and trigger points in the pronator teres.

Another cause of median nerve compression is a fibrous band called the bicipital aponeurosis that connects from biceps brachii to the forearm. The median nerve passes underneath it and can be compressed by it (Fig. 6-20C), causing the same signs and symptoms as pronator teres syndrome. This can occur from repetitive, strong contractions of biceps brachii.

A way to distinguish pronator teres syndrome from carpal tunnel syndrome is that prolonged wrist flexion during sleep aggravates carpal tunnel syndrome. That position compresses the median nerve in the tunnel. Since pronator teres is not involved in wrist flexion, it does not increase compression on the median nerve at night while the wrists are in this position.

Treatments: Decreasing the activities that aggravate the symptoms; using splints or braces; undergoing surgery on pronator teres or the bicipital aponeurosis to relieve the compression; receiving deep tissue techniques such as trigger point therapy; stripping; performing myofascial stretching and deep friction on pronator teres, biceps brachii, and the forearm flexors and extensors (Lowe, 2009; Tortora and Derrickson, 2009; Werner, 2009).

ments, or from forceful, awkward, or stressed motions of the hand and wrists such as using power tools, driving for long periods of time, or performing bodywork.

Treatments: Modifying habits that contribute to the symptoms is essential. If there is acute inflammation, bodywork modalities that manipulate the tissues, such as massage therapy, over the wrist are contraindicated. Otherwise, massage techniques such as deep specific friction can loosen scar tissue. Passive movements of the elbow, wrist, and finger joints maintain joint range of motion. Addressing the neck, shoulders, and arms can also be helpful to reduce muscle spasms, lengthen shortened muscles, and soften and stretch surrounding connective tissue. Other treatments include wrist splinting, NSAIDs, and surgery. If surgery has been done, the area is contraindicated for massage until healing is complete—the stitches have been removed and inflammation is gone, approximately 8 to 12 weeks after the surgery. Deep specific friction in the area can help reduce adhesions from surgery.

PRONATOR TERES SYNDROME

Pronator teres syndrome is compression of the median nerve by pronator teres; it is often mistaken for carpal tunnel syndrome.

SCIATICA

Sciatica is a set of symptoms that may be caused by general compression or irritation of one of five nerve roots that give rise to the sciatic nerve or by compression or irritation of the sciatic nerve itself.

Signs and symptoms: Weakness and pain in one leg that often feels better with movement. There is

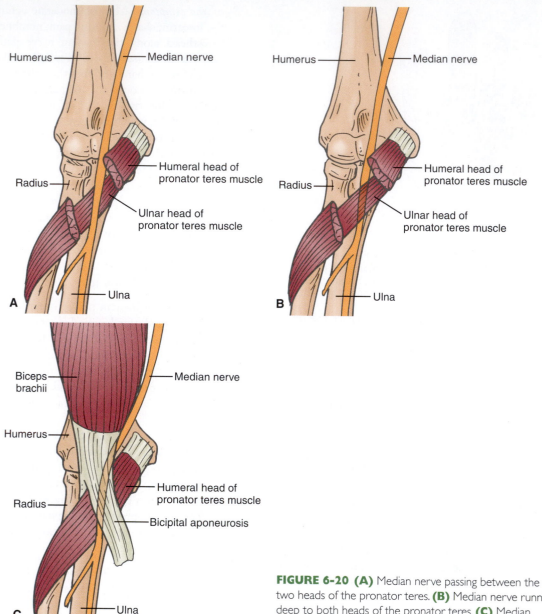

FIGURE 6-20 (A) Median nerve passing between the two heads of the pronator teres. **(B)** Median nerve running deep to both heads of the pronator teres. **(C)** Median nerve passing underneath the bicipital aponeurosis.

dull pain and tenderness in the gluteal region; sharp, radiating pain; numbness; tingling; or a sensation of pins and needles down the leg along the path of the sciatic nerve down the posterior leg and into the foot (Fig. 6-21). With increased inflammation, leg movement can become impaired and the knee may become unstable. Sciatica can involve either one or both legs.

Causes: Compression of lumbar nerves L4 or L5 or sacral nerves S1, S2, or S3, or less commonly, by compression of the sciatic nerve itself. The compression can be from a herniated disk, dislocated hip, or spinal stenosis. Other causes are inflammation, irritation, osteoarthritis of the lumbosacral spine, overuse (repetitive stress), or even excessive emotional stress.

Treatments: Because sciatica is a set of symptoms rather than a diagnosis, treatment for sciatica or sciatic symptoms will often be different, depending upon the underlying cause of

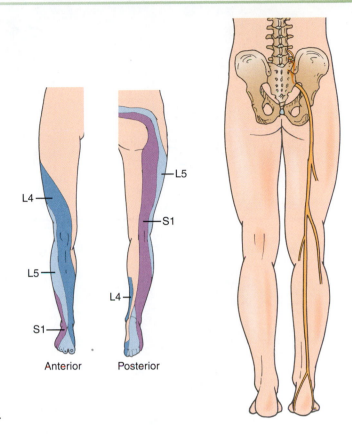

L5

S1

L4

L4

L5

S1

Anterior   Posterior

FIGURE 6-21 Pathway of symptoms of sciatica.

the symptoms. Treatments include anti-inflammatory medications, analgesics, physical therapy, stretching exercises, nonsurgical spinal decompression, massage therapy, chiropractic adjustments, ultrasound, acupuncture, weight loss if excess weight is placing pressure on the spinal nerve roots, and surgery. Sometimes the sciatica will resolve itself with no intervention.

PIRIFORMIS SYNDROME

Piriformis syndrome is compression of the sciatic or superior gluteal nerve by piriformis. The sciatic nerve travels from the anterior sacrum through the sciatic notch of the ilium. In most people, the nerve then passes inferior to piriformis and over the other deep hip rotator muscles (Fig. 6-22A). In some people, the sciatic nerve splits so that one branch goes through piriformis and the other branch travels below it (Fig. 6-22B), one branch travels above piriformis and one branch travels below it (Fig. 6-22C), or both branches travel through piriformis (Fig. 6-22D). The superior gluteal nerve also exits through the greater sciatic notch and travels

superiorly to piriformis to the gluteal muscles (see Fig. 6-22A).

Signs and symptoms: Similar to those of sciatica—dull pain and tenderness in the gluteal region; sharp, radiating pain; numbness; tingling or a sensation of pins and needles down the leg along the path of the sciatic nerve—the posterior lateral leg and into the foot (see Fig. 6-21). Pain may be experienced when getting out of bed and then lessen with movement. The symptoms get worse when sitting for long periods because this increases compression on the nerves.

Causes: Tightness and trigger points in the piriformis can entrap any or all parts of the sciatic nerves. Sitting with a wallet in the back pocket is a common aggravator of the nerve compression, as is walking and squatting. Piriformis syndrome can also result from an acute injury from a direct blow or fall onto the gluteal area.

Treatments: If piriformis syndrome is caused by certain habits such as sitting on a wallet, it

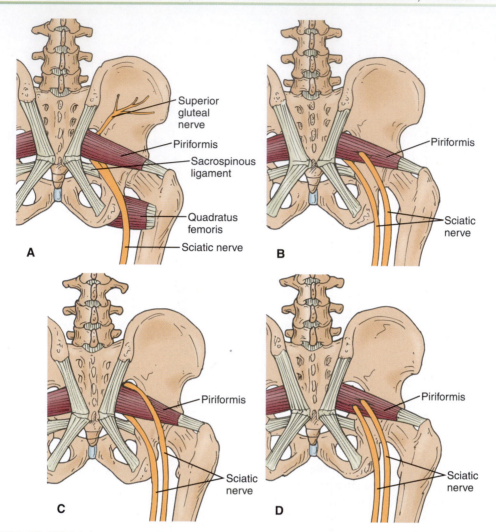

FIGURE 6-22 (A) Sciatic nerve passing inferior to piriformis and over the other deep hip rotator muscles. **(B)** Sciatic nerve with one branch through piriformis and the other branch below it. **(C)** Sciatic nerve traveling above and below piriformis. **(D)** Both branches of the sciatic nerve traveling through piriformis.

may be alleviated by simply changing the habit. Stretching; hip joint mobilization techniques; and deep tissue techniques such as trigger point therapy, myofascial stretching, and deep friction on the gluteals and into the deep lateral rotators can also be helpful. Sometimes anti-inflammatory medications are prescribed, and surgery may be performed to reposition the nerve if other treatments do not relieve the symptoms. Hydrotherapy treatments such as heat are beneficial, as is strengthening the adductor muscles and the posterior thigh muscles (Lowe, 2009; Tortora and Derrickson, 2009; Werner, 2009).

What Do You Think?

If you have a colleague who complains of pain, paresthesia, and muscle weakness in the right arm, what conditions would you suspect he or she has? Can you give examples of acute and chronic injury mechanisms that may cause these symptoms? How would you address these signs and symptoms through bodywork? What recommendations would you give your colleague?

CARTILAGE

There are several different types of cartilage in the body. Hyaline cartilage is located on the ends of long bones and is also known as *articular cartilage*. It provides a smooth gliding surface for movement at the joints and aids in joint flexibility and support. Elastic cartilage provides strength and elasticity and maintains the shape of certain structures such as the external ear.

Fibrocartilage is the strongest type of cartilage, providing strength, rigidity, and support. It is located in areas of high compressive force between bones such as the intervertebral disks and the menisci of the knee. The most common type of injury to fibrocartilage involves high levels of compressive stress that cause it to break down. These compressive forces can come from carrying heavy loads over a long period of time. Another example is imbalanced posture that increases compressive load on the intervertebral disks in the lumbar spine.

Intervertebral disks are in between the bodies of the vertebrae, from C-2 to the sacrum. Each disk has an outer fibrous ring of fibrocartilage called the **annulus fibrosus** (*annulus* means "ringlike"). Inside the disk is a soft, pulpy, highly elastic material called **nucleus pulposus** (*pulposus* means "pulp like"; Fig. 6-23A). The disks create strong joints, allow certain movements of the vertebral column, and absorb shock.

DISK HERNIATION (SLIPPED DISK)

In disk herniation, the fibrocartilage surrounding the intervertebral disk ruptures, releasing the nucleus pulposus (Fig. 6-23B). The disk can be thought of as similar to a jelly doughnut. The doughnut itself is the annulus fibrosus and the jelly is the nucleus pulposus. If the doughnut is compressed, the jelly will bulge outward. This condition most often occurs in the lumbar region, involving the L4 or L5 disks.

Symptoms: Resulting pressure on spinal nerve roots may cause pain and damage to surrounding nerves. There is weakness and pain in one leg. The pain radiates from the gluteal area down the lateral or posterior thigh, through the calf, and sometimes into the foot. It often feels better with movement. See the "Sciatica" section for more information.

Causes: Because intervertebral disks act as shock absorbers, disk herniations can occur from general wear and tear, such as occurs with jobs that require constant sitting; for example, at a desk or during truck driving. Traumatic injury to lumbar disks commonly occurs through lifting with the small muscles of the back (trunk extension) instead of with the large muscles of the legs, and using head-to-tail connection and an aligned vertebral column. Minor back pain and chronic back fatigue indicate general wear and tear; these can make disks susceptible to a traumatic herniated disk from doing something simple like bending to pick up a light item off the floor such as a face cradle cover or picking up heavier items such as massage tables and futons. Cumulative stresses

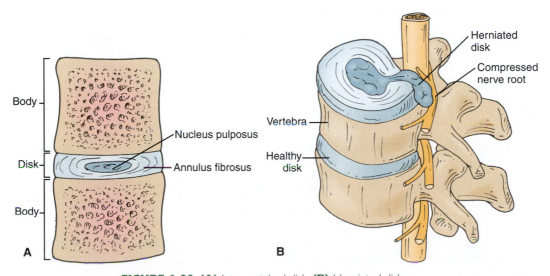

FIGURE 6-23 (A) Intervertebral disk. **(B)** Herniated disk.

caused by inefficient postures, sustained muscle contractions, ligament adhesions, or muscle imbalances can also be culprits.

Treatments: Analgesics, ice massage, surgery, bed rest, traction, physical therapy, and exercise, especially for the core muscles (Lowe, 2009; Tortora and Derrickson, 2009; Werner, 2009).

IDENTIFYING RSI

Certain areas of the body are more commonly affected by repetitive movements. Practitioners should be aware of which areas these are, what types of movements and techniques can lead to

RSI, how they can lead to RSI, and what injuries and conditions can result. Table 6.2 is a compilation of this information. You can use this table to

Body Awareness

Identify an area of your body in which you may be experiencing some discomfort. Using Tables 6.1 and 6.2, what condition might you be feeling, and how could you remedy or manage it? Could the information in these tables assist you with preventing an injury? If so, how?

TABLE 6.2 RSI That Can Develop in Various Parts of the Body

Area	Common Injuries and Conditions	Bodywork Movements That Cause These Injuries and Conditions	How to Prevent/Manage These Injuries and Conditions
Neck and shoulders	Hypertonicity, muscle soreness, stiffness, strain, trigger points; rotator cuff tears; frozen shoulder; tendonitis; tendinosis; bursitis; thoracic outlet syndrome; herniated disk	Forward head posture; lateral tilt of the head; elevated or medially rotated shoulders; repetitive techniques that involve pushing; lifting a client's body part or lifting equipment	Use balanced posture and keep the head in alignment with the spine; keep shoulders down, back, and relaxed; receive bodywork regularly to relieve tight, sore, stiff muscles and trigger points in the muscles; do not do any sudden twisting motions of the neck or upper back; use proper lifting and carrying techniques
Arms and forearms	Hypertonicity, muscle soreness, stiffness, strain, trigger points; tendinitis, tendinosis; carpal tunnel syndrome; pronator teres syndrome	Repetitive movements such as overpronating and over-supinating or applying vibration; hyperextending; reaching; holding one position for long periods of time; lifting a client's body part or lifting equipment	Vary the techniques you use; receive bodywork regularly to relieve tight, sore, stiff muscles and trigger points in the muscles; use hydrotherapy (see Body Awareness box on pages 179–181 and Appendix A); keep arm and forearm muscles relaxed; use proper lifting and carrying techniques
Wrists and hands	Hypertonicity, muscle soreness, stiffness, strain, trigger points; tendinitis, tendinosis; carpal tunnel syndrome	Repetitive movements such as ulnar and radial deviation; hyperextending; holding one position for long periods of time; maintaining force such as gripping and holding, or applying downward pressure	Vary the techniques you use; receive bodywork regularly to relieve tight, sore, stiff muscles and trigger points in the muscles; use hydrotherapy (see Body Awareness box on pages 179–181 and Appendix A); keep the wrists and hands aligned with the forearms; keep the wrists and hand relaxed

TABLE 6.2 RSI That Can Develop in Various Parts of the Body—cont'd

Area	Common Injuries and Conditions	Bodywork Movements That Cause These Injuries and Conditions	How to Prevent/ Manage These Injuries and Conditions
Fingers and thumbs	Tendinitis, tendinosis	Repetitive movements such as flexion, hyperextension, and abduction; holding one position for long periods of time; maintaining force such as gripping and holding or applying downward pressure	Vary the techniques you use; keep the fingers and thumbs aligned; support them when using them to apply pressure; use hydrotherapy (see Body Awareness box on pages 179–181 and Appendix A)
Back	Hypertonicity, muscle soreness, stiffness, strain, trigger points; low back sprain; disk degeneration; herniated disk; sciatica	Bending, twisting, reaching, hyperextending; repetitive techniques that involve pulling; lifting a client's body part or lifting equipment	Use balanced posture and keep the spine aligned; never lift and twist with the back; always lift with the legs; instead of reaching or hyperextending, move your entire body down so you can stay on top of your work; receive bodywork regularly to relieve tight, sore, stiff muscles and trigger points in the muscles; keep the back muscles relaxed; use proper lifting and carrying techniques
Hips	Hypertonicity, muscle soreness, stiffness, strain, trigger points; sacroiliac joint sprain; piriformis syndrome	Keeping the knees locked; keeping the hip muscles tight; bending, twisting, reaching, hyperextending; holding one position for a long period of time; lifting a client's body part or lifting equipment	Use balanced posture and keep the center of gravity over the hips; keep the hips relaxed; instead of reaching or hyperextending, move your entire body so you can stay on top of or just behind your work; incorporate movement into your work; receive bodywork regularly to relieve tight, sore, stiff muscles and trigger points in the muscles; keep the hip muscles relaxed; use proper lifting and carrying techniques
Thighs, legs, knees, and ankles	Hypertonicity, muscle soreness, stiffness, strain, trigger points; tendinitis, tendinosis; bursitis; sprain	Keeping the knees locked; keeping the leg muscles tight; bending, twisting; holding one position for a long period of time; moving awkwardly while carrying a heavy load such as a massage table	Use balanced posture and keep the center of gravity over the hips; keep the leg muscles relaxed; instead of reaching, move your entire body so you can stay on top of or just behind your work; incorporate movement into your work; receive bodywork regularly to relieve tight, sore, stiff muscles and trigger points in the muscles; keep the hip muscles relaxed; use proper lifting and carrying techniques
Feet	Tendonitis, tendinosis; plantar fasciitis	Repetitive movements such as pronation or supination; holding one position for a long period of time; not wearing proper footwear	Wear supportive footwear; incorporate movement into your work; receive bodywork regularly to alleviate plantar fasciitis

Voice of Experience

Bodywork is a fascinating and highly rewarding field to pursue. Yet, it is also highly demanding on each person's physical body. It should be approached like any serious physical activity that you would train for. Consequently, conditioning to take care of your body is an essential part of your practice. One of the most common reasons for people to leave this profession is physical burnout and inability to keep up with the physical demands of their daily work. Yet, there are also people who are not highly trained athletes who easily keep their work going for decades. What makes the difference? The key is in using good body mechanics during your daily work and paying attention to the numerous things you need to do to keep your body in good physical health. This highly rewarding career is not to your benefit if you can't stay in it for a long time. Taking good care of yourself will help you stay an active therapist for a long and prosperous career.

Whitney Lowe, director, Orthopedic Massage Education and Research Institute (OMERI), author of Orthopedic Massage, Theory and Technique and Orthopedic Assessment in Massage Therapy. Member of the editorial advisory board of the Journal of Bodywork and Movement Therapies and continuing education presenter. Massage therapist for over 20 years.

identify what areas of your body are at risk for developing an RSI, and use this information to prevent or manage injuries, especially if the injuries are in the early stages.

PREVENTION

As discussed in previous chapters, staying ahead of the game is imperative in injury prevention. Maintaining wellness and having body awareness and mindful movement, balanced posture, efficient breath, and efficient body mechanics are all essential components to preventing injury. Identifying potential and current problems, as outlined in this chapter, and taking the necessary steps to prevent or treat injuries early will also ensure career longevity.

Ask yourself what changes you can make to ensure complete wellness and career longevity.

For example, how do you use your body for ADL such as:

- Brushing your teeth
- Combing your hair
- Doing the laundry
- Cooking
- Cleaning
- Sleeping habits (including getting enough rest and bolstering yourself appropriately)
- Driving
- Writing
- Reaching and bending

Are there ways you can do all of these activities using better posture and without repetitive motions? Are there ways to do these activities without stress and strain on your body? Other useful suggestions for preventing injury are:

- Receiving regular bodywork.
- Protecting your hands *every day*. These are the tools of your trade; treat them with care. If possible, avoid straining or causing trauma to your hands when performing such activities as opening stuck jars, lifting heavy objects, and hammering nails.
- Avoiding other hand-intensive activities, if possible; for example, playing an instrument or working as a typist in addition to your bodywork practice might set you up for an injury.
- Protecting your joints at all times. Make sure you stack your joints and use efficient body mechanics.
- Getting in shape. Plan on working out at least three times a week. In addition to strengthening your body, your blood circulation will improve. Maintaining good circulation will help you heal any early injuries and keep them from developing into more serious ones. (Stretching exercises are discussed in Chapter 7; strengthening exercises are discussed in Chapter 8; nutrition and proper hydration are discussed in Chapter 9.)
- Integrating wellness and self-care into your everyday life. This is discussed more in Chapter 10. Included is looking at your treatment schedule and the number of sessions you do each day and each week, as well as how learning other bodywork modalities can place less stress on your body.

Case Profile

Chelsea has been a massage therapist for 3 years and recently completed certification in neuromuscular therapy. She is excited about practicing her new modality since it is exactly the type of work she has always dreamed of doing. To perform neuromuscular therapy to as many clients as she can, she decided to provide treatments 5 days a week instead of the 2.5 days she had been working when she offered general massage therapy. She also decided to give six treatments a day instead of the maximum of four she had decided on when she was doing solely general massage.

For the past month, Chelsea has been experiencing numbness and tingling in her right hand and fingers. Because of this, she has begun to notice just how often she uses her hands and fingers to apply the techniques during treatments. Upon visual assessment and tissue inspection, Chelsea finds that her forearm muscles are extremely tight and tender, but no swelling or heat is present.

■ *What condition could Chelsea have?*

■ *What actions might be causing Chelsea's signs and symptoms?*

■ *What else could be contributing to Chelsea's symptoms?*

■ *What treatments may be effective in alleviating Chelsea's symptoms? What do you think the outcome would be if Chelsea sought treatment immediately?*

■ *What recommendations would you give Chelsea to prevent further injury?*

- Using your Wellness Profile as a guide.
- Using the information in Tables 6.1 and 6.2 as guides.

Additionally, minor problems can turn into major injuries if you:

- Ignore symptoms you are feeling.
- Do not attempt to figure out what is causing your symptoms.

- Delay treatment.
- Try to "work through the pain."
- Continue to do the same techniques or carry the same workload that is causing your symptoms.
- Do not take time off to recover.
- Make no changes in ADLs that aggravate your symptoms.

Wellness Profile Check In

Looking at the Wellness Profile you completed at the end of Chapter 1, are there any challenge areas you could remedy through a plan for preventing or managing any injuries you have? If so, what are they? How would you like to improve these areas? What methods or activities would you use to improve these areas? Write down a plan for improvement that includes the methods you will use, a timeline for implementing these methods, and ways you will assess your improvement along the way.

SUMMARY

Performing any type of bodywork involves repetitive motions. If practitioners do not use appropriate body mechanics or enhance their self-care, the result can be injury or some other condition. This will require time, effort, and money to find the best treatment options, and often income is lost as practitioners take time to heal.

Many bodywork practitioners experience signs and symptoms of repetitive stress such as muscular tightness, weakness, fatigue or spasms, areas of swelling or inflammation, paresthesia, crepitus, and uncoordinated movements. Identifying symptoms early is essential to managing the injury and the condition. Otherwise, the injury or condition could become chronic, which can make it much more difficult to deal with.

The four most common factors contributing to RSI are imbalanced posture, stress, injury, and movement habits. Examples of other factors include body awareness while performing bodywork and ADLs, age, gender, heredity, obesity, low fitness levels, and whether a warm-up protocol is done before performing bodywork. Pain is the first and most common symptom of RSI. It forces practitioners to become aware of their bodies. They can use it to discover inefficient body mechanics, awkward body positions and movements, imbalanced posture, and body areas that they are overusing.

The healing process of damaged tissues from traumatic injury is the same as for RSI. With RSI, the tissue does not get a chance to fully heal as long as the repetitive stress is still occurring. This is one of the main reasons it takes so long to recover from RSI and why it is essential to modify habits and movements that contribute to it. Generally, healing involves three physiological phases: inflammation (acute phase), regeneration (subacute phase), and remodeling (maturation phase). The three main factors affecting tissue repair are nutrition, blood circulation, and age.

Common muscle injuries and conditions include hypertonicity, acute and delayed onset muscle soreness, muscle stiffness, trigger points, and muscle strain. Fascia can be torn or can stay in a chronically shortened or lengthened condition that can result in limited or painful movement and trigger points. A common fascial disorder is plantar fasciitis. Tendinosis is the most common condition involving tendons. Other conditions are tenosynovitis, lateral and medial epicondylitis/epicondylosis, and bursitis. Ligaments can be sprained, and joint disorders include frozen shoulder and adhesive capsulitis. Nerve injuries include thoracic outlet syndrome, carpal tunnel syndrome, pronator teres syndrome, sciatica, and piriformis syndrome. The most common cartilage disorder is herniated disk.

Practitioners should be knowledgeable about the signs, symptoms, causes, treatments, and prevention of all these injury types. They need to be able to identify what areas of their bodies are at risk for developing an RSI, and they need to use this information to prevent or manage injuries, especially if the injuries are in the early stages.

Review Questions

MULTIPLE CHOICE

1. Which of the following is a symptom of RSI?
   a. Pliable muscles
   b. Coordinated movements
   c. Functioning joints
   d. Swelling and inflammation

2. A factor that contributes to RSI is:
   a. balanced posture.
   b. stress.
   c. lack of previous injuries.
   d. efficient movement habits.

3. Conditions that have a sudden onset and are of short duration are considered:
   a. acute.
   b. chronic.
   c. signs.
   d. symptoms.

4. In what stage of tissue healing does function return as much as possible?
   a. Subacute inflammation
   b. Acute inflammation
   c. Remodeling
   d. Regeneration

5. Hypertonicity means:
   a. tight muscles.
   b. delayed onset muscle soreness.
   c. herniated disk.
   d. nerve impingement.

6. The most common issue involving tendons is:
   a. tendinitis.
   b. sprain.
   c. avulsion.
   d. tendinosis.

7. What condition is usually the end result of frozen shoulder?
   a. Nerve impingement
   b. Adhesive capsulitis
   c. Pronator teres syndrome
   d. Thoracic outlet syndrome

FILL-IN-THE-BLANK

1. The nerve endings that detect pain are called _____.

2. Scar tissue is _____ and _____ than surrounding tissue.

3. A _____ refers to a finding that is observed or that can be objectively measured.

4. Severe tearing or complete rupture of the muscle and tendon unit is a _____ degree strain.

5. Medial epicondylosis is an overuse injury resulting from repeated wrist _____ _____.

6. Compression or entrapment of one or more of the structures of the neurovascular bundle in the lateral neck is the cause of _____ _____.

7. Piriformis syndrome is compression of the _____ nerve by the piriformis.

SHORT ANSWER

1. List and explain at least five guidelines for assessing pain.

2. Describe at least seven causes of RSI other than imbalanced posture, stress, injury, and movement habits.

3. Explain the three factors affecting tissue repair.

4. Explain what each of the letters in PRICE in the PRICE protocol stand for.

5. Briefly explain what happens during tendinosis.

6. Describe carpal tunnel syndrome, including the signs and symptoms, causes, and treatments.

7. Explain at least five ways to prevent injury while working as a bodywork practitioner.

Activities

1. Contact at least three professional practitioners. Ask them how they have remained injury-free, or if they have had an injury, what they have done to treat and manage it.

2. Choose a condition or disorder presented in this chapter. Write down how you would talk to a fellow therapist who has the condition or disorder, what your treatment approach would be, and suggestions to prevent or manage the condition or disorder. Write down what treatment options you would like if you had the condition or disorder, and what you would do to manage it.

3. Contact a fellow student or colleague and exchange ideas on how to prevent or manage injuries for yourselves.

REFERENCES

Cleveland Clinic. Acute vs. Chronic Pain (2008). Retrieved November 2010 from http://my.cleveland-clinic.org/services/Pain_Management/hic_Acute_vs_Chronic_Pain.aspx.

Fritz, Sandy. *Fundamentals of Therapeutic Massage,* 4th ed. St. Louis, MO: Mosby Elsevier, 2009.

Holland, Patricia M., and Sandra K. Anderson. *Chair Massage.* St. Louis, MO: Mosby Elsevier, 2011.

Jones, J.C. Muscle Stiffness Health Article (2007). Retrieved November 2010 from www.healthline.com/hlc/muscle-stiffness.

Let's Talk Pain. Pain Definitions (2010). Retrieved November 2010 from www.letstalkpain.org/real_story/definitions.html.

Lowe, Whitney. *Orthopedic Massage*, 2nd ed. St. Louis, MO: Elsevier Mosby, 2009.

Quinn, Elizabeth. Muscle Pain and Soreness After Exercise—What Is Delayed Onset Muscle Soreness (2010). Retrieved November 2010 from http://sportsmedicine .about.com/cs/injuries/a/doms.htm.

Tortora, Gerard J., and Bryan Derrickson. *Principles of Anatomy and Physiology*, 12th ed. Hoboken, NJ: John Wiley & Sons, 2009.

Travell, Janet G., MD, and David G. Simons, MD. *Myofascial Pain and Dysfunction: The Trigger Point Manual.* Baltimore, MD: Lippincott, Williams & Wilkins, 1998.

Werner, Ruth. *A Massage Therapist's Guide to Pathology*, 4th ed. Baltimore, MD: Lippincott Williams & Wilkins, 2009.

Stretching: Why, How, When, and Where?

Key Terms

Active flexibility
Active-isolated stretches
  (AIS)
Ballistic stretches
Dynamic (kinetic) flexibility
Dynamic stretches
Endomysium
End point
Epimysium
Fascicles
Flexibility deficit
Flexibility reserve
Kinetic chain
Myofibrils
Neuromuscular efficiency
Passive (relaxed) stretches
Passive flexibility
Perimysium
Proprioceptive
  neuromuscular
  facilitation (PNF)
Sarcolemma
Sarcomeres
Seiza
Sliding filament mechanism
Static stretches
Target muscle

Learning Objectives

After studying this chapter, the reader will have the information to:

1. Explain the importance of flexibility in performing bodywork.
2. Describe the relationship between inflexibility and injury, the factors that affect flexibility, and the benefits of stretching.
3. Explain the physiological effects of stretching on the joints, muscle tissue, and proprioceptors.
4. Perform specific types of stretches.
5. Explain the six rules of successful stretching.
6. Evaluate when to stretch, what overstretching is, and how to prevent overstretching.
7. Integrate a stretching protocol into daily life.
8. Explain what stretches to avoid and why.

“Challenges make you discover things about yourself that you never really knew. They’re what make the instrument stretch—what make you go beyond the norm.”

— Cicely Tyson

THE IMPORTANCE OF FLEXIBILITY

Everyone, even the most inactive individuals, needs a certain level of mobility and strength. Human beings are designed to move. As discussed in previous chapters, joints are where movement occurs, and muscles provide the movement. Therefore, muscles must be strong enough to create the desired movement, and the joints need to be both mobile and stable enough to cope with the movement.

Along with muscular strength is the need for flexibility. Healthy muscle is flexible and pliable. Its blood supply is plentiful so it receives adequate amounts of nutrients and oxygen, and it has wastes removed efficiently. It does not expend excess energy remaining in a chronically contracted state. Flexible joints work more effectively as well and have a greater range of motion (ROM) than tight joints. Movement takes less effort and therefore less energy. There is an overall better sense of well-being when the body is flexible.

It is impossible to place too much emphasis on how physical the bodywork profession is. The major key to career success and career longevity is taking care of the single most important piece of bodywork equipment—the practitioner's body. Because your body is irreplaceable, it is essential that you keep it in the best shape possible. This means having optimal physical fitness that is balanced. Balanced physical fitness requires a blending of three basic components: flexibility, aerobic activity, and strength training. All of these are necessary to have true balanced fitness.

It is important to develop functional strength while in the stretched position as well. Significantly improving joint range of motion without also improving the strength of surrounding musculature, especially at its new range of motion, can cause injury. For example, when flexibility is improved in a given joint or group of joints to the point where an additional 5 degrees of motion is gained, the affected muscles need to work less to produce the same amount of strength. For this reason, strength and flexibility programs must occur at the same time.

This chapter assists you in increasing your flexibility, and Chapter 8 focuses on strengthening your muscles. Both chapters are equally important for increasing your strength, stamina, and ease of movement. For those practitioners who are hesitant about beginning a stretching and strengthening program, improving flexibility is usually an easier way to start.

The methods presented in this chapter are simple and require little time, effort, or specialized equipment.

Before beginning any stretching and strengthening program, you should consult with your physician to see if you have any contraindications for the exercises and to find out what levels of activity are best for you to start with.

WHAT IS FLEXIBILITY?

The terms *loose, lengthened, stretched, extended,* and *elongated* can all be used to describe the quality of any of the soft tissues. *Flexibility* refers only to a joint's mobility and how muscles, ligaments, tendons, or other soft tissues affect it. A more complete description of flexibility is the ability to move joints through their full intended range of motion.

The question many practitioners have is, "How flexible should I be?" Many people mistakenly believe that extreme flexibility, such as that of an Olympic gymnast, is what is necessary. In fact, the majority of individuals already have an adequate level of flexibility. They are flexible enough to easily meet the demands of their daily activities and have room to spare for life's little emergencies. For instance, they can have a minor slip on ice or trip while going upstairs and have enough flexibility to not become seriously injured. This is called **flexibility reserve**. Conversely, if a person has inadequate flexibility, the difference between what he has and what he needs is called **flexibility deficit**. An example of flexibility deficit is when an individual new to yoga finds it difficult and uncomfortable to do even the simplest poses.

Flexibility training is used to help correct muscle imbalances (e.g., if a muscle is disproportionally stronger than its antagonist or if one side of the body is stronger than the other), increase joint range of motion, relieve abnormal joint stress, maintain normal functional length of muscles, and improve **neuromuscular efficiency**. Neuromuscular efficiency is the ability of the neuromuscular system to allow agonists, antagonists, and stabilizers to work synergistically to produce, reduce, and dynamically stabilize the entire **kinetic chain**. The kinetic chain is an integrated functional unit made up of the myofascial systems (muscles, ligaments, tendons, and fascia), the articular system (bones and their joints), and the nervous system. These systems work interdependently for structural and functional movement efficiency.

INFLEXIBILITY AND INJURY POTENTIAL

Repetitive, limited ROM activities performed over a prolonged period of time can create shortened muscles or hypertonic muscles that are lengthened. For example, the hip flexors such as the rectus femoris, psoas, and iliacus can become shortened due to long periods of sitting or bending at the waist. These are activities in which the hip flexors contract repeatedly but over a reduced ROM. Likewise, the trunk extensors such as the erector spinae can become lengthened due to long periods of bending over. Even weight-training exercises, if habitually performed in a shortened ROM (e.g., without full extension or flexion, rotation, and so forth), can lead to shortening or lengthening of muscles.

Chronically shortened (locked short) or lengthened (locked long) muscles can be the first step in a series of events leading to injury. For instance, over time, shortened hip flexors can reduce the normal lordotic curve of the lumbar spine, which can, in turn, impair the spine's load-bearing and shock-absorption capacity. Overly tight hamstrings have the same effect on the lumbar spine. When the spine cannot function normally, a wide range of injuries, from acute to chronic, can result.

Another example involves tight quadriceps muscles. They can pull the patella upward proximally, causing it to track abnormally high on the femoral groove. Such a condition can impair the ability to lunge properly or evenly, resulting in the underside of the patella becoming rough. This condition is called *chondromalacia patellae* and is characterized by pain; inflammation; and eventually restricted movement, which can lead to inefficient body mechanics. Inefficient body mechanics can, of course, lead to decreased flexibility. As you can see, a repetitive cycle is created. One way to break the cycle is to receive an injury severe enough to force the individual to stop working. Another, more optimal, way is to engage in a stretching program.

FACTORS AFFECTING FLEXIBILITY

As with all other motor abilities, the potential to increase joint flexibility is genetically predetermined, to a certain point. In addition, younger people are generally more flexible than older people, and women are usually more flexible than men. Flexibility is affected by past injuries; length of the individual's bones; childhood nutrition; strength levels; core temperature; time of day; and even mood, stress levels, and personality types. In fact, sometimes a subjective association can be drawn between inflexible personalities and physical inflexibility.

On a structural level, flexibility is usually limited by the structure and shape of the joint, the joint ligaments and tendons that cross the joint, adhesions from past injuries or surgeries, too much muscle around a joint, too much fat around a joint, highly toned but shortened muscles, fascial binding, and shortened muscles due to inactivity. Contrary to popular belief, muscle length is not the primary limiting factor in developing great ROM. In fact, normal, healthy muscle tissue can be stretched to about twice its resting length.

Lack of flexibility may also be due to:

- Muscle imbalance. If one of a group of synergistic muscles is much stronger than the other, or if an agonist is greatly stronger than the antagonist for a particular joint action, the result can be impaired flexibility.
- Paralysis, neurological disease, injury, or joint immobilization. All of these affect the normal functioning of tissues and joints.
- Overuse of a muscle without maintaining a complete ROM. For example, in an individual wearing high heels much of the time, the calf muscles become chronically shortened with the ankles in plantarflexion.
- Aging. With aging, the soft tissues decrease in elasticity and muscles tend to atrophy.
- Periods of rapid growth, as occurs during puberty. Typically, if an individual's body is growing quickly, there is a chance flexibility is hindered because the body has not adjusted to changing ROM at the joints. Accordingly, the body's soft tissues have not had time to adapt to the rapid growth either (Run the Planet, 2010).

BENEFITS OF STRETCHING

Stretching offers these benefits:

- Decreases risk of injury by preventing joint sprains, muscle strains or tears, and reinjury to previous joint and muscle trauma.
- Increases ROM.
- Increases joint health by decreasing the viscosity (thickness) of synovial fluid so it can lubricate the joint better. This increases nutrition to the joint.

- Increases flexibility. A flexible joint requires less energy to move; a lengthened muscle requires less energy, whereas tight and contracted muscles waste energy.
- Increases mobility, which can potentially increase physical performance and efficiency.
- Increases blood supply and nutrients to muscles, joints, and connective tissue. This allows for greater elasticity and reduction in muscle soreness.
- Relieves muscle and joint stiffness associated with the aging process.
- Improves muscular balance and postural awareness.
- Increases neuromuscular coordination.
- Increases muscular relaxation, which decreases stress (Andersen, 2005; MayoClinic, 2009).

Myth: I am older and inflexible, so stretching will not work for me.

FACT: Flexibility decreases with lack of use. Age combined with a history of inactivity means that the process of becoming flexible may take longer, and more caution must be used. However, it is never too late to begin a regular flexibility program.

PHYSIOLOGICAL BASIS OF STRETCHING

To truly understand flexibility and how stretching works, it is important to understand the anatomy and physiology of all the structures involved. These include the joints, muscle tissue, and proprioceptors.

JOINTS

Recall from Chapter 2 that the joints that provide the most amount of movement in the body are synovial joints or diarthroses. They have a space between the bones called a *synovial cavity*. This gap allows quite a bit of movement at the joint; joints that do not have this gap have very little or no movement. Recall from Chapter 6 the structure of a synovial joint. The bones in the joint are joined by an articular capsule made of dense irregular connective tissue, and they often have accessory ligaments surrounding them for support (see Fig. 6-16). Figure 7-1A shows the hip joint with its ligaments, and Figure 7-1B shows the knee joint with its ligaments and associated structures such as muscles and bursae. As seen in these figures, synovial joints are quite complicated. That is because they need to be both mobile and stable.

Ligaments are thick, tough, fibrous tissue. Most of the collagen fibers in ligaments are arranged in parallel bundles, which give them the greatest amount of tensile strength in a longitudinal direction. However, within the ligament, there are also fibers that are oriented in other ways. This gives pliability, strength, and a certain amount of stretch to the ligament as the joint moves in various directions. Stretching improves the flexibility and health of ligaments. Also, even though ligaments can stretch only minimally, stretching the surrounding soft

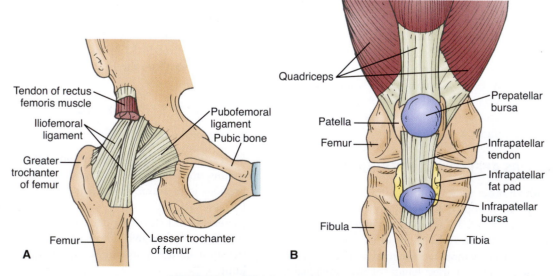

FIGURE 7-1 (A) Hip joint. **(B)** Knee joint.

tissues will improve the joint's flexibility. Therefore, the ROM of a joint can be increased and maintained through a regular stretching program.

MUSCLE TISSUE

Each skeletal muscle is a separate organ composed of thousands of cells. Muscle cells are also called *muscle fibers* because of their elongated shape. A typical muscle fiber is about 4 inches long. Skeletal muscle also has fascia that surrounds individual muscle fibers and the entire muscle. Three layers of connective tissue extend from the fascia to protect and strengthen muscle tissue. The outermost layer is called **epimysium**, and it surrounds the entire muscle. **Perimysium** surrounds groups of 10 to 100 or more muscle fibers that form bundles called **fascicles**. Within each fascicle, **endomysium** surrounds individual muscle fibers. All three connective tissue layers extend beyond the muscle fibers to form a tendon that attaches to bone. Muscle tissue also has a rich blood and nerve supply. Figure 7-2 shows skeletal muscle tissue and its connective tissue coverings (Muscolino, 2011; Tortora and Derrickson, 2009).

The plasma membrane of a skeletal muscle fiber is called the **sarcolemma**. The sarcolemma has thousands of inward folds called *transverse (T) tubules* that tunnel toward the center of each muscle fiber.

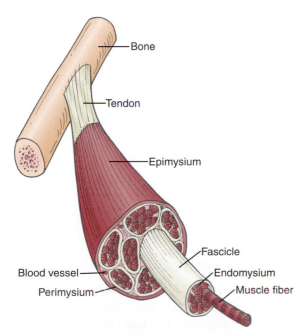

FIGURE 7-2 Skeletal muscle tissue and its connective coverings.

T tubules open to the outside of the fiber and are filled with interstitial fluid. Nerve impulses travel along the sarcolemma and through the T tubules, quickly spreading throughout the muscle fiber. This is how a nerve impulse excites all parts of the muscle fiber at once.

Within the muscle fibers are tiny, threadlike structures called **myofibrils**. These are the contractile organelles of skeletal muscle, and they extend the entire length of the muscle fiber. Within myofibrils are even smaller structures called *thin filaments* (made of a protein called *actin*) and thick filaments (made of a protein called *myosin*). They do not extend the entire length of a muscle fiber. Instead they are arranged in compartments called **sarcomeres**, which are the basic function units of a myofibril. Figure 7-3 shows the microscopic structures of skeletal muscle tissue.

Muscles can change length because of the overlapping thin and thick filaments. The boundaries of the sarcomere are called *Z disks*, to which the thin filaments are attached. In the center of the sarcomere are the thick strands, which, during contraction, pull the Z disks closer together by attaching to the thin filaments with specialized links called *cross bridges*. These cross bridges function much like boat oars as they reach out to attach and pull on the thin filaments, causing the Z disks to move toward one another. In turn, the Z disks pull on neighboring sarcomeres, and the whole muscle fiber shortens. Therefore, there is an overall shortening or contraction of the muscle in response to a nerve impulse. This is referred to as the **sliding filament mechanism**, shown in Figure 7-4. When the nerve impulse stops, the filaments slide back to their habitual resting positions (Muscolino, 2011; Tortora and Derrickson, 2009).

Microscopic Effect of Stretching a Muscle

During a stretch, muscle fibers elongate as each sarcomere extends to the point where no overlap between the thick and thin filaments exists. At this point, the tension of the stretch is taken up by the sarcolemma and endomysium (Fig. 7-5). If the stretch tension escalates beyond this point, microscopic tears can develop both in the connective tissue and within the sarcomere itself. Such microtraumatic injuries eventually heal, but there may be minute scarring and microadhesions that will leave the muscle fiber less capable of contracting and lengthening.

Each sarcomere has a habitual resting length. Correct stretching lengthens the muscle by causing the thin and thick filaments to adopt a new habitual

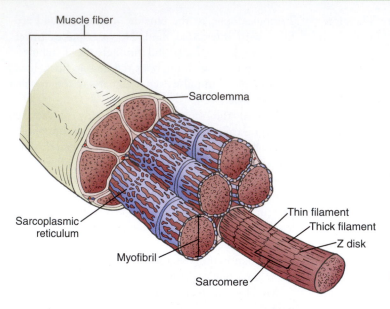

FIGURE 7-3 Microscopic structures of skeletal muscle.

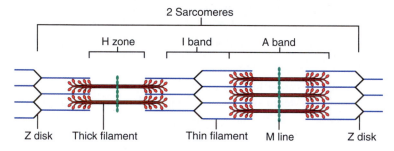

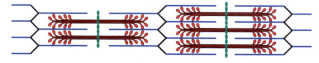

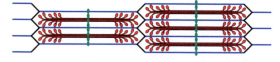

FIGURE 7-4 Sliding filament mechanism.

resting position that lengthens the sarcomere. Regular stretching will cause the myofibrils to become longer by growing new sarcomere segments. These new sarcomere segments increase the muscle's ROM and increases the power the muscle can generate. Therefore, stretching increases the muscle's pliability and its strength (McAtee and Charland, 2007).

PROPRIOCEPTORS

The neuromuscular system has built-in safeguards against severe muscular injury. These safeguards take the form of proprioceptors that can sense changes in muscle tension and muscle length. Recall from Chapter 2 that proprioceptors are embedded in

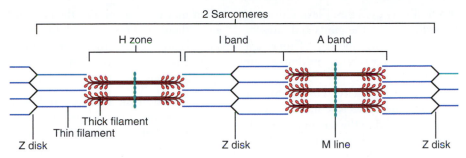

FIGURE 7-5 Sarcomere during a stretch.

muscles (especially postural muscles) and tendons. They tell the nervous system the degree to which muscles are contracted, the amount of tension on tendons, and give information about the pressure on the joint, the positions of joints, and the acceleration and deceleration of joints during movement.

The proprioceptors involved in stretch reflexes are muscle spindles, which are found in the bellies of muscles (see Fig. 2-10). Muscle spindles monitor changes in the length of skeletal muscle fibers. When a muscle has stretched far enough during a particular movement, the muscle is stimulated to contract, relieving the stretching. This is the stretch reflex. It prevents injury by preventing overstretching, and possible tearing, of muscle tissue (Muscolino, 2011; Tortora and Derrickson, 2009). Resetting the muscle spindle is the mechanism of proprioceptive neuromuscular facilitation (PNF) and contract-relax (CR) stretching methods that are discussed in the "Specific Types of Stretches" section.

It is believed that the stretch reflex is activated when a muscle is stretched too long, when it is stretched to the point of pain, or when the muscle is not flexible enough to tolerate the stretch. Thus, the muscle has a rebound contraction to prevent injury. To prevent this, always begin stretches slowly and within the tolerance of the muscle tissue. This can be thought of as meeting the tissue where it is and encouraging it to stretch itself a bit farther. Forcing a stretch will result in overstretching, and it can cause injury (McAtee and Charland, 2007; Muscolino, 2011).

The proprioceptors involved in tendon reflexes are tendon organs, which are found in the musculotendinous junction (see Fig. 2-10). Tendon organs measure tension applied to tendons from muscle contraction. The tendon reflex protects tendons and associated muscles from damage by causing the muscle to relax in response to excessive tension placed on tendons by muscle contraction.

Joint kinesthetic receptors are found in and around the articular capsules of synovial joints. They respond to pressure and acceleration and deceleration of joints. Articular ligaments contain receptors similar to tendon organs that cause adjacent muscles to relax when excessive strain is placed on the joint (Muscolino, 2011; Tortora and Derrickson, 2009).

TYPES OF STRETCHES

Flexibility can be developed at any age given the appropriate training. Rather than short, intense bouts of stretching that tend to trigger the proprioceptors, practitioners should opt for longer, frequent periods of stretching where less tension is used. Joint flexibility is optimized if the stretching methods are specific to the desired results.

These principles are crucial to increasing flexibility:

- Joint specificity. Stretching in one area of the body does not increase flexibility in another area. For example, a flexibility program for the hips will not improve flexibility in the shoulders. However, the joint-specific nature of flexibility training does not necessarily mean that all joints must be

Body Awareness

Have you ever given or received a stretch that was performed too quickly or was taken too far? Did you notice how that body part contracted quickly, without you even thinking about it? That is because the muscle spindles were activated and caused shortening of the muscle to prevent tearing.

targeted with flexibility exercises. Flexibility exercises can be performed on the joints and muscles that need them the most, especially if there are time constraints. This way you can maximize your flexibility training.

- Position and speed specificity. For maximum effectiveness, stretching exercises must be very similar in form and speed to the technique or skill you are trying to improve. Slow, static stretching, for example, will not improve fast movements such as those involved in performing the massage therapy techniques percussion or vibration nearly as well as will dynamic stretching movements. On the other hand, dynamic stretching methods have limited ability to improve a static skill, such as the slow pace involved in techniques like myofascial release or trigger point work in massage therapy. The same is true for the stillness involved in the qi connection in Asian bodywork techniques and craniosacral therapy. To be able to perform a full range of bodywork techniques, it is ideal to do both: slow and static stretching and dynamic stretching.

- Resistance training contributes to increased joint flexibility. Efficient and effective resistance training programs can improve flexibility levels. In fact, whatever your level of flexibility, the primary concern is to have adequate strength throughout any given joint's full ROM. Two key points are to perform resistance exercises through the involved joint's full ROM and to work antagonistic pairs of muscles equally. This is discussed in more detail in Chapter 8.

SPECIFIC TYPES OF STRETCHES

There are two terms to keep in mind for stretching. The muscle that is to be stretched is the **target muscle**. The limit at which the stretch is comfortable is the **end point**. During a stretch, there should be slight discomfort, and perhaps even a light, gradual sensation of "pins and needles." However, if the sensations become sudden, sharp, or uncomfortable, then you are past the end point and could potentially tear muscle or connective tissue. Therefore, the stretch should be eased up immediately.

Dynamic stretches involve swinging the arms or legs in a controlled manner. This can be combined with other movements, such as a trunk rotation, but the dynamic stretches involve only the arms and legs. The arms and legs can swing in various patterns (e.g., out to the sides and back or in large circles). However,

when moving dynamically, the current ROM of the joints should not be exceeded. Dynamic stretches are a good choice for warm-ups or cool-downs.

To ensure the safety of this type of movement, use these methods:

1. Establish an even, controlled rhythm, with swinging movements that are initially well within the current ROM (Fig. 7-6A). Gradually increase the size of the movements until you reach a comfortable level of tension at the end point of the stretch (Fig. 7-6B).

2. Prevent the stretch reflex by stopping the moving limb before the target joint reaches the end of its ROM. For example, during a standing dynamic hamstring movement, you can swing or kick your leg and stop it just before you reach the end limit of your hip joint's ROM (Fig. 7-6C). Your nervous system will anticipate this and will minimize or eliminate the stretch reflex.

Static stretches are the most commonly practiced form of stretching and an excellent method to use after a long treatment day, after exercise, or for recovery purposes. Do this form of stretching only after your body has been thoroughly warmed up. Static stretching consists of low force and long duration, holding for 20 seconds or more. Many of the movements or stretches found in various forms of yoga are static stretches. Static stretching can activate the stretch reflex if you continue the stretch beyond comfort or if you do not hold the stretch for at least 20 seconds. A possible rebound contraction can occur before that time, creating a tug-of-war between the desire to stretch and the target muscle resisting overstretching to avoid injury. This is why it is important to maintain focus while stretching and to pay attention to signals your body is giving.

Passive or **relaxed stretches** are similar to static stretches. A position is assumed and held with some other part of the body, with the assistance of a partner, or a piece of equipment. Movements should be slow, steady, and gentle to lengthen the soft tissues effectively. An example is shown in Figure 7-7A in which the quadriceps muscles are stretched by flexing the knee and holding the foot with one hand while holding on to the back of a chair for support with the other hand. In Figure 7-7B, a passive stretch of the deep lateral hip rotator muscles is performed with the assistance of a partner who places the leg across the body and holds it. Communication with the stretching partner is extremely important to ensure the stretch is not performed too quickly and

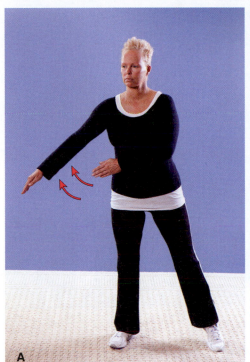

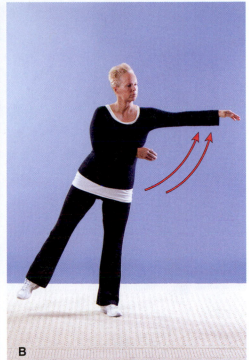

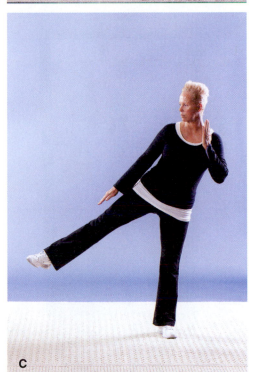

FIGURE 7-6 (A) Even, controlled swinging movements. **(B)** Increasing the size of the movements. **(C)** Stopping the leg during a standing dynamic hamstring stretch.

does not go too far. In Figure 7-7C, a passive stretch for pectoralis major is performed using a door frame.

Slow, passive stretching is useful in relieving spasms in muscles that are healing after an injury. Passive stretching is also good for cooling your body down after a long treatment day or after a workout, and it helps reduce muscle fatigue and soreness after the workout.

Ballistic stretches use the momentum of a moving body or limb in an attempt to force it beyond its normal end point. These stretches are of high

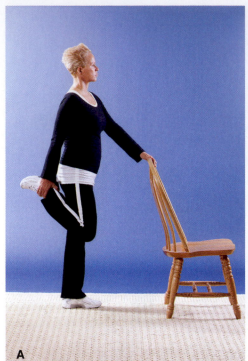

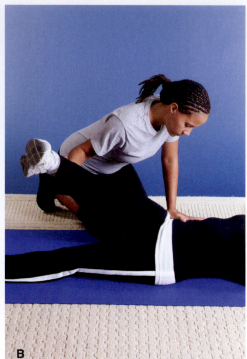

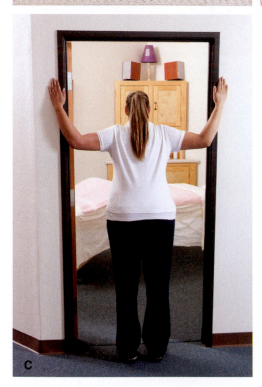

FIGURE 7-7 (A) Passive stretch of the quadriceps muscles using the hand. **(B)** Passive stretch of the deep lateral hip rotator muscles with the assistance of a partner. **(C)** Passive stretch for pectoralis major using a door frame as a piece of equipment.

force and short duration. This type of stretching is not considered safe and can lead to injury by aggravating muscle and connective tissue. The stretched target muscles are used like springs to pull the individual out of the stretched position. An example is

bouncing down repeatedly to touch the toes. It does not allow the muscles to adjust to and relax into the stretched position. Instead, it may cause them to tighten up by repeatedly activating the stretch reflex, often producing small muscle tears that result in scar tissue. It should be noted that ballistic stretching may be beneficial for athletes who, for specific events, require a quick power start. However, these athletes really have to be in tune with what their bodies are doing in order to prevent injury (Mattes, 2006; McAtee and Charland, 2007; Muscolino, 2011).

Active-isolated stretches (AIS) may be more appealing to those who find static stretching boring. The Mattes Method was developed by Aaron Mattes (see the Voice of Experience box). These stretches are useful for warming up cold muscles when time is limited and for stretching in between client treatments. This is the only method that is safe to use as a warm-up or cooldown or for training for performance or rehabilitation. Active-isolated stretching involves contracting muscles that are opposite the target muscles, using the principle that when the agonist contracts, the antagonist relaxes. The target muscles should be identified and isolated by using precise, localized movements.

Important components of this type of stretch are the following:

- Identify the target muscles and isolate them by using precise, localized movements. Figure 7-8A shows localized movements that isolate the lateral neck muscles.

- Hold the stretch 2 to 5 seconds, then relax. The muscle or muscles should be stretched only to the end point to prevent activating the stretch reflex. Figure 7-8B shows the lateral neck muscles being stretched.
- Return to starting position.
- Perform 3 to 10 repetitions (if time allows).
- Exhale while doing the stretch (this is true of any stretch).
- Inhale while returning to start position (this is true of any stretch; Mattes, 2006).

Voice of Experience

The Mattes Method has developed over a 40-year period and has become an outstanding modality for thousands of soft tissue workers. AIS enables the therapist to isolate the deepest tissues in the body without irritating the area. The secret is the opposite side antagonist contracting to move the reciprocally relaxing muscles and fascia. This work enables the bodyworker to maintain better posture and help prevent overstressing key joints and tissues that break down and become painful. This is an ideal approach for bodyworkers and subjects alike for greater quality of life.

Aaron L. Mattes MS, RKT, LMT; www.stretchingusa.com

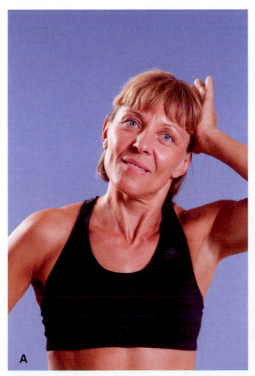 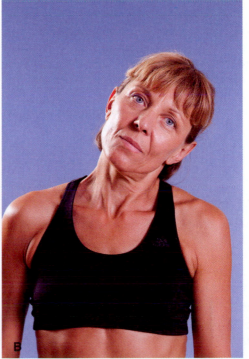

FIGURE 7-8 (A) Localized movement to isolate the lateral neck muscles. **(B)** Stretching the lateral neck muscles.

Proprioceptor neuromuscular facilitation (PNF) was originally developed by Dr. Herman Kabat and then later refined by physical therapists Dorothy Voss and Margaret Knott. PNF is defined as "methods of promoting or hastening the response of the neuromuscular mechanism through stimulation of the proprioceptors." It uses the body's neuromuscular responses to facilitate and enhance stretching results. *PNF* is an umbrella term for several types of contract-relax stretches.

PNF stretching is currently the fastest and most effective way known to increase flexibility. It follows the normal use patterns of the body, is a good option to use for rehabilitating and strengthening, and is more effective than passive stretching. It is the stretch of choice of many bodywork practitioners, including sports massage therapists. It is also used by physical therapists. However, to maintain flexibility gained from PNF (or any flexibility program), a regular daily regimen of training is required. PNF stretching is not recommended for those whose bones are still growing, like children or adolescents (Voss, Ionta, and Myers, 1985).

A typical contract-relax sequence involves the following:

- Actively move target muscle into a fully lengthened position or its end point.
- Isometrically contract the target muscle against the resistance of a piece of equipment like a doorway or with a partner (Fig. 7-9A). Only slight resistance should be used. Communication with the stretching partner is extremely important to ensure the stretch is not performed too quickly or does not go too far. Hold this contraction for 7 to 10 seconds.
- Slowly relax this resisted contraction for 2 to 3 seconds (you will feel the muscle "let go"). If using a partner, have him relax his resistance (Fig. 7-9B). The key is to relax the muscle before bringing it into another stretch.
- Then bring the target muscle into a farther stretch. If using a piece of equipment like a doorway, move closer to it. If using a partner, have him stretch the target muscle to a new end point (Fig. 7-9C).
- Repeat the contract-relax stretch cycle three or four times, holding the final passive stretch for at least 20 seconds (the same as for a static stretch).

What Do You Think?

What types of stretches do you think will be the most beneficial to you? Why do you think these stretches will be the most beneficial? How do you think you might incorporate these into your activities of daily living?

ELEMENTS OF STRETCHING

Stretching methods can be as simple as the intuitive limbering up, like the stretching done when first waking up (just watch what cats and dogs do every time they get up from a nap). This helps release adhesions and microscopic tissue bonding that occurs during periods of inactivity. At the other end of the scale are dynamic stretching regimens designed to radically increase a joint's ROM.

Engaging in an entire flexibility program will bring balance and symmetry to your body if done daily. Think of stretching as a sort of primer for other activities; it helps you get prepared for the effort you will expend. If your time is limited, stretching the muscles most in need will be sufficient. However, if all you do is "spot" stretching, then you will likely develop another set of imbalances over time. Later in this chapter are stretching routines that focus on various regions of the body and, through the use of different stretching methods, can fit into anyone's schedule.

The following are considerations and contraindications for stretching. If you have issues with any of these, you need to consult with your physician before starting any stretching regimen.

- Joint integrity. The integrity of the joints should be maintained throughout the entire stretch. This means that joints should be stretched in alignment with their movements and that awkward positions should not be used. Otherwise, there is a great risk of injury.
- Pain. Stretching should not be painful. In fact, stretching should feel rejuvenating and centering. Soreness after a stretching session is a sign that hydroxyproline, an amino acid found in connective tissue, and other biochemicals have been released into the muscle fiber to help repair damaged tissues. It is a sign that the stretching has been too vigorous.

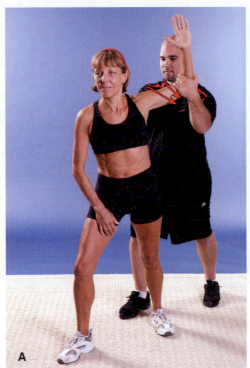
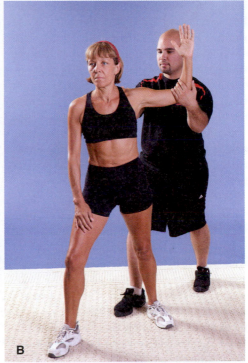
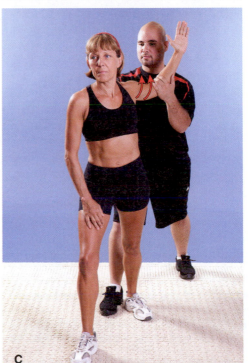

FIGURE 7-9 (A) Partner resisting pectoralis major (target muscle). **(B)** Relaxing the contraction. **(C)** Partner bringing pectoralis major into a further stretch.

- Joint inflammation. Any type of joint inflammation, including rheumatoid arthritis in the acute phase, is a contraindication. Stretching and ROM techniques will likely increase inflammation, be painful, and cause further damage to the affected joints.
- Neuropathy. Neuropathy is a contraindication for stretching and ROM techniques. It interferes with the body's ability to detect sensations, which means the individual will not receive accurate feedback from his or her body about the length and strength of the stretch. This increases the risk of injury.
- Bone disease. Diseases such as later stages of osteoporosis are a contraindication for stretching and ROM techniques. They increase the risk of injury. However, in the early stages it can be beneficial.
- Joint hypermobility. Stretching and ROM techniques may possibly cause the joints to become dislocated, so caution is warranted.
- Prolonged use of steroids. This can cause brittle bones and fragile skin, so caution is warranted when performing stretches.
- Untreated hypertension. Untreated hypertension is a contraindication for stretching. Because of the demands placed on blood vessels during stretches, there is a danger of increasing blood pressure.
- Nerve root damage or radiating pain. These are contraindications for stretching. Stretching can cause further damage and pain along the nerve pathways.
- Pregnancy. Pregnancy is a caution for stretching. The hormone relaxin that is secreted during pregnancy causes tendons and ligaments to loosen. This prepares the pelvis to open for birth of the baby. As a result, all joints and associated connective tissue structures become more pliable, increasing the risk of displacement during stretching and ROM techniques (American College of

Sports Medicine, 2009; Johnson, 2007; National Strength and Conditioning Association, 2008).

RULES FOR SUCCESSFUL STRETCHING

In order to stretch successfully, there are several rules to keep in mind. These assist the stretching process and enhance results. The rules involve relaxation, warmth, minimum force, breathing, duration, and patience.

Relaxation

Other than stretching itself, relaxation is probably the most important factor in developing flexibility. Relaxation is the opposite of tension. Tension originates in contracted muscles, which result in inflexibility, insufficient oxygen supply due to decreased circulation, and fatigue.

If a muscle is contracted at the time of stretching, the thin and thick filaments cannot slide to a longer resting position. This is asking the filaments to do opposing actions at the same time. All that is happening is that the tendons are being strained. A stretch can cause a muscle to remain elongated after being stretched *only* if the muscle is relaxed while it is being stretched.

The hamstrings provide a good example. Often, standing hamstring stretches are shown as simple toe touches all the way to extreme one-leg ballet bar stretches (Fig. 7-10A). However, unless the individual has had extensive yoga or ballet training to relax the muscles, none of these stretches work to elongate the hamstrings. When you flex the trunk while standing, the hamstrings automatically contract to pull on the pelvis to stabilize it (Fig. 7-10B). They cannot stretch because they are not relaxed. All you are doing is straining the hamstring tendons and overstretching low back ligaments. A more effective way to stretch the hamstrings is to be in a reclining position. The pelvis is now in a neutral position so the hamstrings can relax (Fig. 7-10C and D). Depending on your flexibility, you can start with your gluteal muscles 1 to 2 feet away from the wall, then move them closer as your hamstrings become more flexible.

Warmth

Temperature is an important consideration when working to improve joint flexibility. Warm muscles help facilitate increases in ROM, while cool muscles tend to remain shortened. Prior to stretching, your

Body Awareness

Have you ever stretched to the point of pain? How did you feel immediately afterward? How did you feel the next day? What do you think you should have done differently, if you feel soreness for a day or two after stretching?

body needs to be warmed. The warm-up can be passive such as by taking a hot bath or shower, or active such as a brief session of muscular activity. The latter is more effective because it raises core temperature, whereas the former may only elevate surface temperature.

Warm-ups are discussed in more detail in the "Stretching Protocols" section later in this chapter.

Minimum Force

Discomfort and pain are subjective experiences, and everyone has varying tolerances to both. It is recommended to stretch only to the point of mild to moderate discomfort if the goal is to improve ROM. Stretch only to that point, back off until the muscle relaxes, and then stretch again. If the primary objective is to speed up the removal of waste products during or after a bodywork treatment or a workout, then stretching should stop before reaching the end point. Using too much force during the stretch may injure the area at the end point. In response, the affected muscle would contract, inhibiting the removal of waste products. Using less force in a stretch makes muscles act like a mechanical pump that aids in venous return—wastes are pumped out and nutrients are pumped in.

Breathing

Proper breathing control is important for a successful stretch. Recall from Chapter 4 that efficient breathing assists in overall relaxation, increases blood flow throughout the body, and helps to facilitate the movement of lactic acid and other by-products of exercise from the muscle cells into the bloodstream.

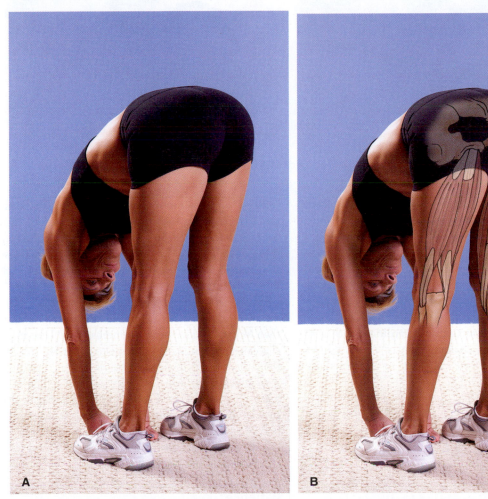

FIGURE 7-10 (A) Standing toe touches. **(B)** Hamstrings contracting to stabilize the pelvis when standing and flexing the trunk.

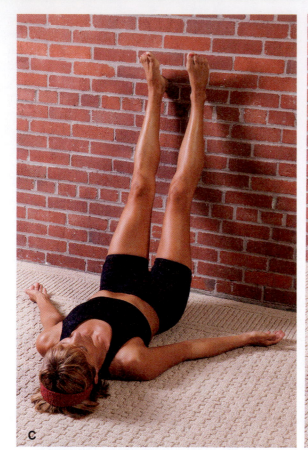
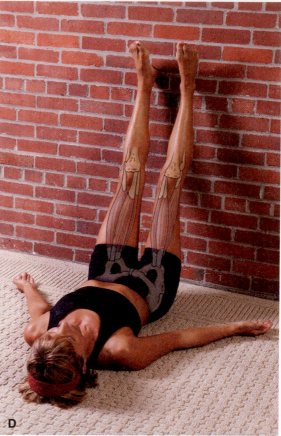

FIGURE 7-10 cont'd **(C)** Reclining hamstring stretch. **(D)** Hamstrings are relaxed in the reclining position.

There are many different schools of thought about proper breathing patterns while stretching. However, the most effective method is to breathe normally with efficient breaths, and visualize the muscles, tendons, and ligaments lengthening during the stretch. Avoid holding your breath, because this increases blood pressure and general muscular tension. Breathing efficiently should enhance your relaxation while stretching.

The general rule of thumb regarding breath is to exhale on the most challenging part of an activity and inhale on the easiest part of that activity. Therefore:

- Inhale before the stretch
- Exhale into the stretch
- Breathe normally during the stretch
- Inhale while returning to start position

Duration

Stretching duration can vary, and it depends on many factors. Foremost is the type of stretching being done. Dynamic stretching, for example, involves several "swings" or gross motor movements of the extremities that last only a few seconds each. Static and contract-relax methods involve longer periods lasting from 7 seconds to 1 minute. Ideally, stretching sessions would not last more than 20 minutes, with each muscle normally taking 1 to 3 minutes at the most.

Short, agonizing stretching sessions are no more effective (and may actually result in scar formation) than longer sessions of lesser intensities. Major muscles can stretch in a relaxed state to about 50% longer than their usual resting length if patience is used. This gives fascia time to relax as well, which it is often reluctant to do. Fascia, in general, is reluctant to relax due to the postural stressors placed on the body. Just as the stressors did not cause fascia to be in shortened state overnight, fascia does not relax and become more elastic instantly.

Patience

Depending on your level of flexibility, your body may be extremely tight when you first begin a stretching program. You need to be patient. If you force a stretch, you will inhibit your progress, and this could possibly be discouraging. However, just as chronic tension does not develop overnight, flexibility cannot be gained overnight either. If you perform stretches regularly, though, your results could be amazing.

WHEN TO STRETCH

The best time to stretch is when your muscles are warmed up. If they are not already warm before stretching, then you can warm them up by taking a hot shower or performing some type of brief aerobic activity. If the weather is cold, or if your muscles are more stiff than usual, it is important to take extra care to warm up before stretching in order to reduce the risk of injury.

People have an internal body clock, or *circadian rhythm*. Circadian rhythms are patterns of biological activity, such as the sleep-wake cycle that occurs in a 24-hour period. Some people are early risers while others are late-nighters. Being aware of your circadian rhythm should help you decide when it is best for you to stretch or perform any other type of activity. Interestingly, it seems that most people are more flexible and have the most strength in the afternoon than in the morning, with a peak time from about 2:30 to 4:00 p.m. Accordingly, you may consider performing your stretching and strengthening workouts during this time frame, if it fits in your schedule.

If you need or want to perform movements requiring considerable flexibility with little or no warm-up, consider a routine of early morning stretching, if it fits in your schedule. In order to do this properly, you need to first do a general warm-up, described under "Stretching Protocols" later in this chapter. This includes dynamic stretches or movements, followed by some light static, passive, or AIS stretches. Basically, an early morning stretching regimen should be identical to the complete warm-up described.

What Do You Think?

Why do you think that we would be more flexible in the afternoon than in the morning? Do you think our bodies are moving more during this time of day? Tomorrow, pay attention to how your body is feeling between 2:30 and 4:00 p.m.

STRETCHING WITH A PARTNER

When done properly, stretches performed with a partner can be more effective than stretches performed alone. This is especially true of PNF stretches. However, note that your partner will not feel what you feel. Therefore, partners cannot respond as quickly to any discomfort that might prompt you to immediately reduce the intensity, length, or position of the stretch. This can greatly increase your risk of injury while performing a particular exercise.

If you do stretch with a partner, choose someone you trust to pay close attention during the stretches. Make sure to have clear communication with your partner. This person also needs to be willing and able to respond appropriately when you signal that you are feeling pain or discomfort.

STRETCHING TO INCREASE FLEXIBILITY

A stretching routine to increase overall flexibility should accomplish at least these two goals:

- Train stretch receptors to become accustomed to greater muscle length
- Reduce resistance of connective tissues to muscle elongation

Before designing a particular stretching routine, it is important to first decide which types of flexibility you want to increase and which stretching methods are best for achieving them:

- **Dynamic flexibility**, also called **kinetic flexibility**, is the ability to perform dynamic (or kinetic) movements of the muscles in order to move a limb through its full ROM in the joints. The best way to increase dynamic flexibility is by performing dynamic movements, supplemented with static stretches.
- **Active flexibility** is the ability to assume and maintain extended positions using only the tension of the agonists and synergists while the antagonists are being stretched. An example is lifting the leg and keeping it extended without any support other than the leg muscles. The best way to increase active flexibility is by performing AIS stretches, supplemented with static stretches.
- **Passive flexibility** is the ability to assume extended positions and then maintain them using only body weight, the support of the limbs, or some other piece of equipment such as a chair or wall. The fastest and most effective way currently

known to increase passive flexibility is by performing PNF stretches.

Overall flexibility can be increased by following these guidelines:

- Perform stretches every day.
- Warm up properly before any athletic activity, including the performance of bodywork. A general warm-up routine is presented in "Stretching Protocols" later in this chapter.
- Give yourself ample time to perform the complete warm-up. Your muscles need to be warmed up before you stretch.
- Cool down properly after any and all intensive activities.
- Perform PNF stretching every other day, and perform AIS/static stretching on the days you do not perform PNF stretches. If you are really committed to increasing your flexibility, you can try AIS/static stretching every day in addition to PNF stretching every other day.
- When increasing flexibility, it is also important to strengthen the muscles responsible for holding the stretched limbs in their extended positions. Strengthening methods are discussed in Chapter 8.

Overall, flexibility will increase gradually. However, by following the guidelines presented, you can achieve maximal upper-body flexibility within 1 month and maximal lower-body flexibility within 2 months. Those who are older or more inflexible than the average person will take longer than this. Remember, do not try to increase flexibility too quickly by forcing yourself to overstretch. The stretches should go no farther than your comfortable end point.

OVERSTRETCHING

If stretching is done properly, you should feel minimal or no soreness the day after you perform the stretches. In fact, the opposite should be true—your body should feel good. If you have a great deal of soreness, then you may have overstretched and should reduce the intensity and duration of some or all of the stretches you are performing.

Overstretching simply increases the time it takes to gain greater flexibility. This is because overstretching actually damages muscles, and they need to repair themselves to have the same extensibility as before they were injured. One of the easiest ways to overstretch is to stretch "cold" or without any

FIELD NOTES

I primarily remained injury-free by stretching for 30 to 40 minutes daily, doing aerobic activity, being conscious of body mechanics, and receiving weekly bodywork. I had some thumb issues from performing neuromuscular therapy, so I trained for Thai massage, which took care of the thumb overuse.

To ensure bodywork practitioners remain injury-free, I recommend they *walk the talk*; be a good role model; model healthy behaviors; develop a regular stretching program; constantly assess their comfort levels while working, and if they're uncomfortable, change their positions.

Jerry Weinert, RN, LMT, NCTMB, Certified Thai massage therapist and instructor, certified neuromuscular therapist, author. Professional bodywork practitioner from 1988 to 2006.

warm-up. A maximal cold stretch is not desirable. Just because a muscle can be moved to its limit without warming up does not mean it is ready for the strain that a workout will place on it.

As the extreme ranges of a stretch are reached, sensations include localized warmth of the stretched muscles, followed by a burning or spasmlike feeling, then sharp pain. The localized warming usually occurs at the attachments of the stretched muscles. If these sensations are felt, then you need to decrease the stretch's intensity.

If you ignore the warming sensation, or perhaps do not feel it, and you continue the stretch until you feel a definite burning sensation in the stretched muscles, then you should discontinue the stretch immediately. If you continue the stretch to the point you feel a sharp pain, it is likely that the stretch has already resulted in tissue damage that may cause immediate pain and soreness that persists for several days.

In some cases, you may follow all of the stretching guidelines but still feel some soreness the next day. If this is the case, then it may be a matter of becoming used to stretching. The soreness will decrease over time as you gain more flexibility.

STRETCHING PROTOCOLS

For the body to work at its best, any physical activity should involve four phases:

1. General warm-up
2. Stretches

3. Activity (exercise or the performance of bodywork)

4. Cooldown

As discussed, warming up before stretching helps prevent injury, and it does more than just loosen stiff muscles. When done properly, it can potentially improve performance. On the other hand, an improper warm-up, or no warm-up at all, greatly increases the risk of injury during activity. Warming up should raise body temperature 1.4°F to 2.8°F. Signs that the body is reaching these temperatures include vasodilation of skin blood vessels, causing the skin to become warm and possibly flushed. Temperatures closer to 2.8°F stimulate the sweat glands, causing sweating. Another noticeable sign is increased heart rate.

The goals of the warm-up are to increase awareness, improve coordination, improve elasticity and contractibility of muscles, and achieve a greater efficiency of the respiratory and cardiovascular systems. It is important to note that active stretches and isometric stretches should not be part of the warm-up because they are likely to cause the stretched muscles to become too tired to properly perform the activity, in this case bodywork, for which you are preparing your body. The general warm-up should consist of joint ROM exercises first and some type of aerobic activity second (Kurz, 2003).

GENERAL WARM-UP

The general warm-up begins with joint ROM exercises, starting at either the toes and working up the body or from the fingers and working down the body. The ROM exercises facilitate joint motion by causing synovial fluid to lubricate the entire joint. The synovial fluid becomes less viscous and more slippery, providing better nutrition to the joint structures. Such lubrication permits the joints to function better when performing bodywork.

Joint ROM Exercises

The ROM exercises involve slow circular movements, both clockwise and counterclockwise, or flexion and extension, until the joint feels like it is moving smoothly. An example protocol follows. The exercises can be done in the order presented, or in the reverse order:

1. Fingers in circular motion (Fig. 7-11)
2. Wrists in circular motion (Fig. 7-12)
3. Elbow flexion (Fig. 7-13A) and extension (Fig. 7-13B)
4. Shoulders in circumduction (Fig. 7-14A and B)
5. Neck lateral flexion (Fig. 7-15)
6. Trunk (waist) rotation (Fig. 7-16A and B)
7. Hips in circular motion (Fig. 7-17A and B)
8. Knee flexion and extension (Fig. 7-18A and B)
9. Ankle dorsiflexion and plantarflexion (Fig. 7-19A and B) and inversion and eversion (Fig. 7-20A and B)
10. Toe flexion and extension (Fig. 7-21A and B)

Aerobic Activity

After you have completed the joint ROM exercises, next is at least 5 minutes of light aerobic activity such as jogging, jumping rope, or any other activity that will cause a similar increase in heart rate. The purpose is to raise your core body temperature and

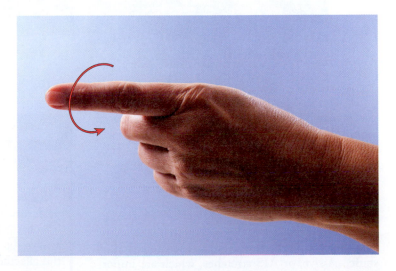

FIGURE 7-11 Finger in circular motion.

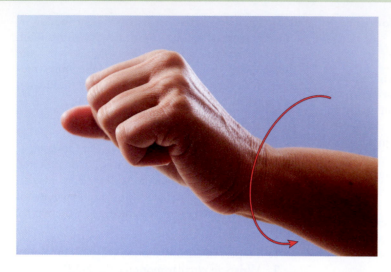

FIGURE 7-12 Wrist in circular motion.

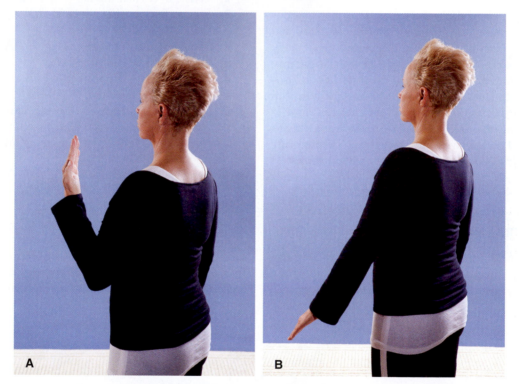

FIGURE 7-13 (A) Elbow flexion. **(B)** Elbow extension.

get increased blood flow to active tissues. Increased blood flow in the muscles warms them, improves muscle performance, and reduces the likelihood of injury.

STRETCHING

Stretching involves two types. The first is dynamic (movement). These stretches are then followed by static, passive, or AIS stretches, which are important to perform after dynamic stretches. Static,

Body Awareness

Do you currently perform a warm-up before doing bodywork? Why or why not? If you do perform a warm-up before doing bodywork, how has it benefited you? If you do not perform a warm-up before doing bodywork, how has this affected your performance of bodywork?

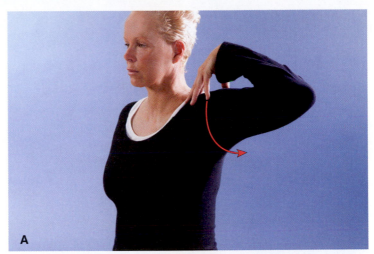

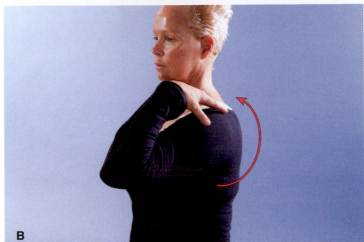

FIGURE 7-14 (A, B) Shoulder in circumduction.

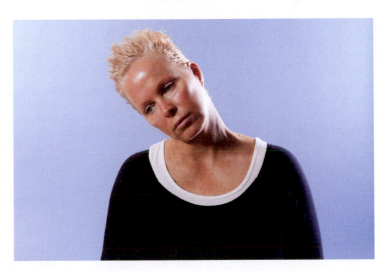

FIGURE 7-15 Neck lateral flexion.

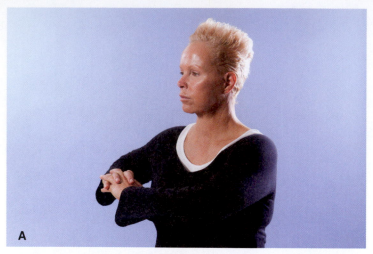

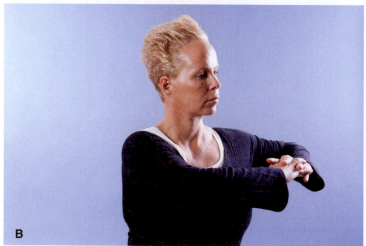

FIGURE 7-16 (A, B) Trunk (waist) rotation.

passive, or AIS stretches can often result in over-stretching, which damages the muscles. Performing dynamic stretches first will help reduce this risk of injury.

Dynamic Stretching

It might be surprising to find dynamic stretching or movement is part of warming up. However, the warm-up is for a workout or bodywork that usually involves a great deal of dynamic activity. Therefore, it makes sense to perform some dynamic stretches to increase dynamic flexibility.

Light dynamic stretching or movements can include thigh raises, which resemble high stepping (Fig. 7-22), and arm swings in all directions (Fig. 7-23). Do this as many times as it takes to reach your maximum ROM in any given direction, but do not work your muscles to the point of fatigue. Remember, this is just a warm-up. The real workout comes later when you are exercising or performing bodywork.

Static, Passive, or AIS Stretches

After you complete the general warm-up and dynamic stretching, your muscles are warmer and more elastic than they were before starting. Slow, relaxed, static, passive, or AIS stretches follow the dynamic stretches. Stretch your back first, then your upper body, followed by your lower body.

An example protocol follows. If you do not have enough time to stretch all these muscles before working out or doing a bodywork session, at

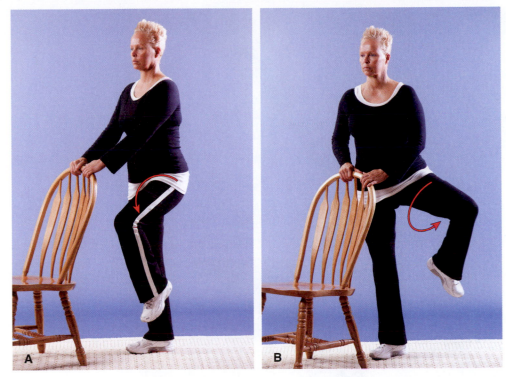

FIGURE 7-17 (A, B) Hip in circular motion.

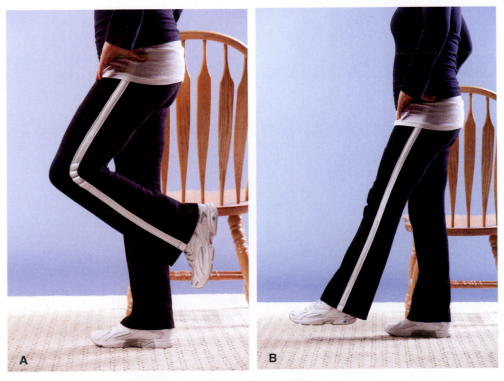

FIGURE 7-18 (A) Knee flexion. **(B)** Knee extension.

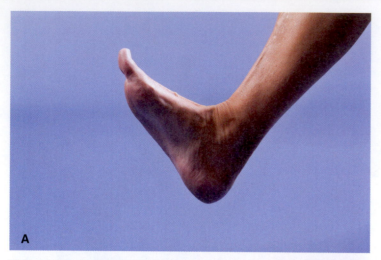

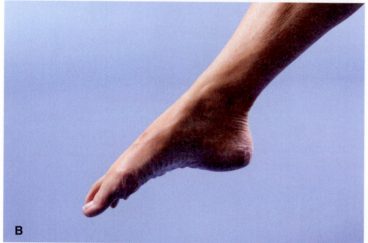

FIGURE 7-19 (A) Ankle dorsiflexion. **(B)** Ankle plantarflexion.

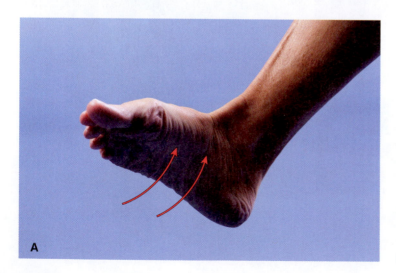

FIGURE 7-20 (A) Ankle inversion.

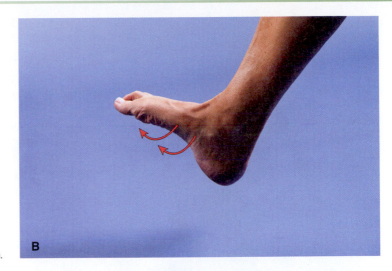

FIGURE 7-20 cont'd (B) Ankle eversion.

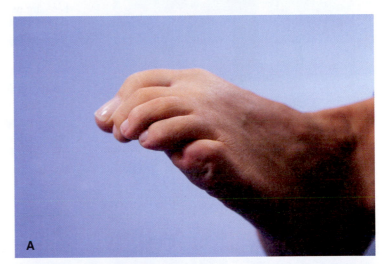

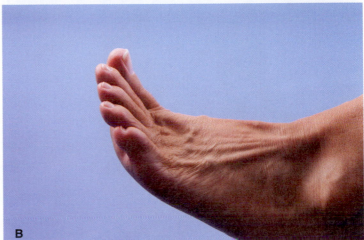

FIGURE 7-21 (A) Toe flexion. **(B)** Toe extension.

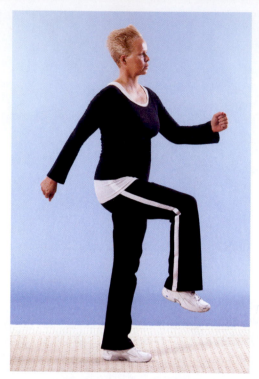

FIGURE 7-22 Thigh raises.

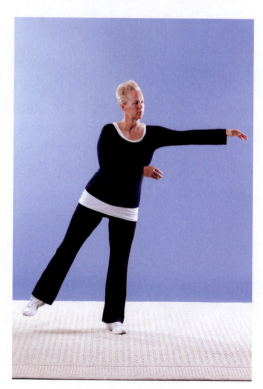

FIGURE 7-23 Arm swings.

least stretch those muscles you will use during the activity.

Stretching reminders:

- Breathe
- Let your muscles relax before stretching them
- Stretch only to the end point
- Maintain a balanced posture
- If doing AIS or static stretches, hold for the time specified for each type of stretch. For AIS stretches, it is 2 to 5 seconds; for static stretches, it is 20 to 60 seconds.

For some of the stretches, you will need a mat, towel, rope, yoga strap, and exercise ball. These are shown in Figure 7-24.

LOW BACK

Lie supine on a mat. Flex one knee and inhale (Fig. 7-25A). Exhale as you drop that knee over the opposite leg and your hip rises off the floor. Keep your shoulders and upper torso on the mat (Fig. 7-25B). You should feel this stretch through your lower back muscles. Take deep breaths and relax into the stretch.

In a sitting position, flex your knees, grasp them with your hands, and inhale (Fig. 7-26A). Exhale as you pull your knees to your chest and roll backward (Fig. 7-26B). Gently roll up and down your spine, keeping your chin down toward your chest and remembering to breathe (Fig. 7-26 C).

ABDOMEN AND BACK

Lie supine on an exercise ball and breathe normally (Fig. 7-27A). Extend your arms over your head to increase the stretch (Fig. 7-27B). To increase the intensity of the stretch, rotate your trunk as you inhale, then tilt your trunk to one side as you exhale (Fig. 7-27C). Repeat on the other side.

LATERAL TORSO

Sit on the floor with an aligned spine. Abduct your legs as far as you can (Fig. 7-28A). Inhale and then exhale as you reach over your head with one arm (Fig. 7-28B). Repeat on the other side. To increase the intensity of the stretch, inhale, then exhale as you gently rotate your trunk to one side (Fig. 7-28C). Repeat on the other side.

MCKENZIE STRETCH (UPWARD FACING DOG)

Lie supine on a mat on the floor. Keeping your hips on the mat, inhale; as you exhale, push your trunk up with one hand. Relax, then repeat on the other side

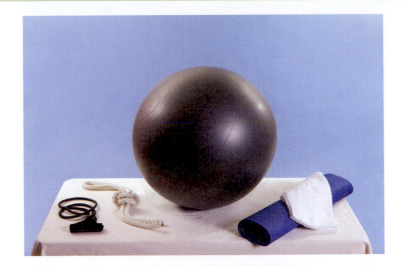

FIGURE 7-24 Mat, towel, dowel, rope, yoga strap, and exercise ball.

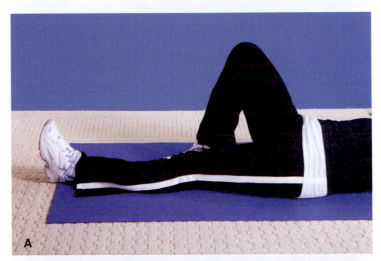

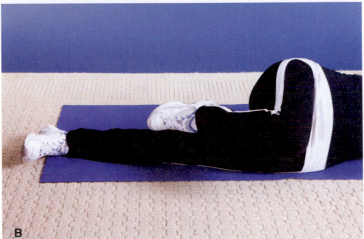

FIGURE 7-25 (A) Flex one knee and inhale. **(B)** Drop that knee over the opposite leg as your hip rises off the floor.

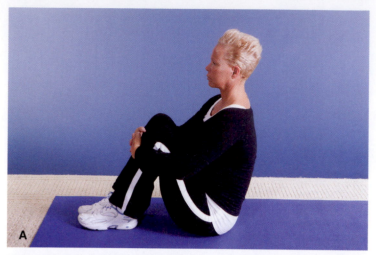

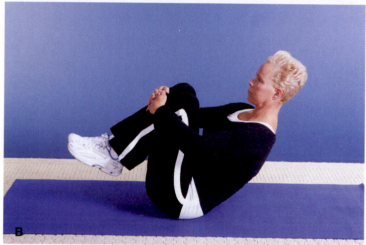

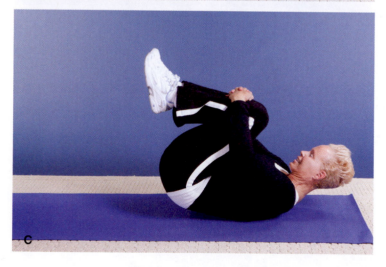

FIGURE 7-26 (A) Flex your knees, grasp them with your hands, and inhale. **(B)** Exhale as you pull your knees to your chest and roll backward. **(C)** Gently roll up and down your spine, keeping your chin down toward your chest.

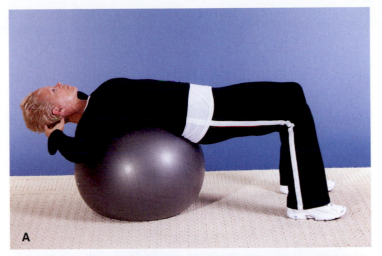

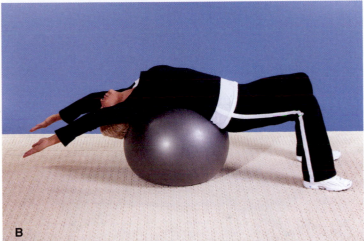

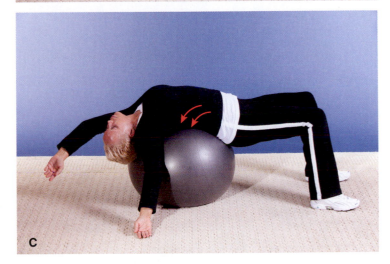

FIGURE 7-27 (A) Lie supine on an exercise ball. **(B)** Extend your arms over your head to increase the stretch. **(C)** Rotate your trunk, then tilt your trunk to one side.

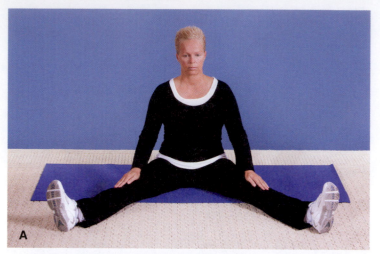

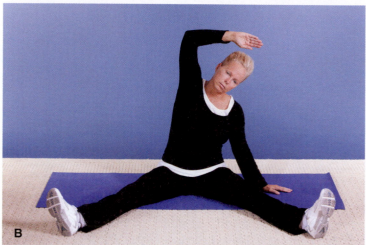

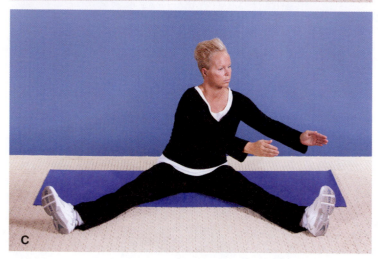

FIGURE 7-28 (A) Abduct your legs as far as you can. **(B)** Reach over your head with one arm. **(C)** Gently rotate your trunk.

of your trunk with your other hand. To increase the intensity of the stretch, rotate your trunk by drawing circles with it (Fig. 7-29).

FORWARD TORSO

Hold on to the back of a chair with your hands shoulder-width apart. Make sure you are far enough away to elongate your trunk. Your focus should be on your upper back, shoulders, and arms during the stretch. Inhale, and then as you exhale, flex at the waist to a 90-degree angle (Fig. 7-30).

NECK

Inhale as you interlace your fingers and place them on the back of your head (Fig. 7-31A). Exhale as you gently pull your head down for a posterior neck stretch (Fig. 7-31B).

Take your hands from the back of your head. Extend your neck backward until your face is toward the ceiling. Inhale, and as you exhale, gently stretch your anterior neck (Fig. 7-31C).

Laterally flex your neck. Inhale as you place your hand from the same side on top of your head and exhale while you gently pull your head down to stretch your lateral neck. Bring your head to center, then laterally flex your neck to the other side and repeat.

FOREARM SUPINATION

With your elbow at a 90-degree angle, tuck it against your side with your palm facing in toward your midline (Fig. 7-32A). With your other hand, inhale as you grasp the radial side of the back of the hand. Exhale as you pull the hand into supination to

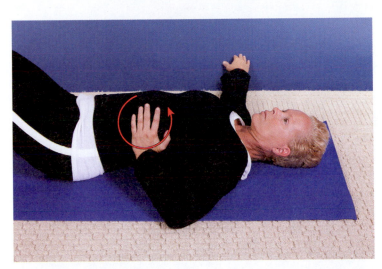

FIGURE 7-29 Rotate your torso by drawing circles with it.

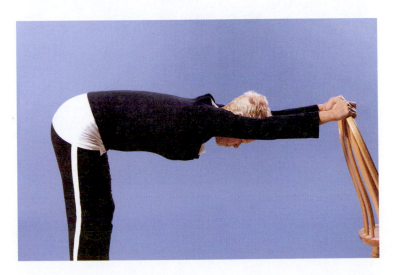

FIGURE 7-30 Hold on to the back of a chair and flex at the waist.

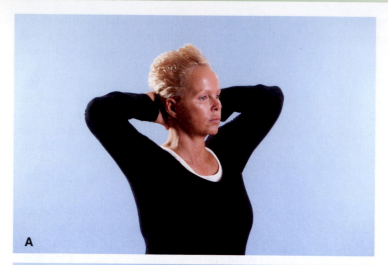

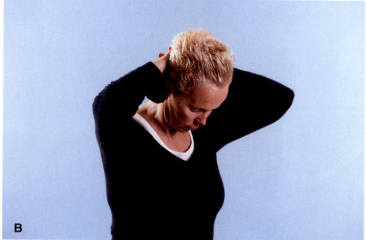

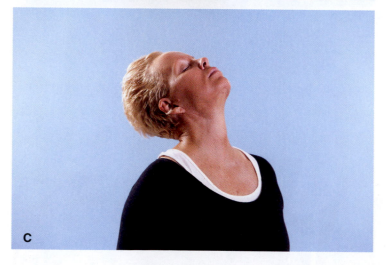

FIGURE 7-31 **(A)** Inhale as you interlace your fingers and place them on the back of your head. **(B)** Gently pull your head down for a posterior neck stretch. **(C)** Gently stretch your anterior neck.

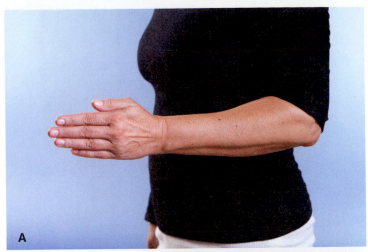

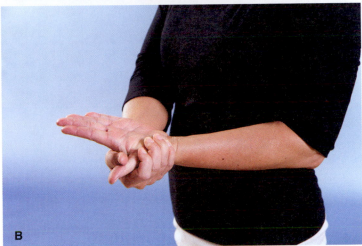

FIGURE 7-32 (A) With your elbow at a 90-degree angle, tuck it against your side with your palm facing in. **(B)** Pull the hand into supination to stretch your forearm.

stretch your forearm muscles (Fig. 7-32B). Repeat on your other arm.

FOREARM PRONATION

With your elbow at a 90-degree angle, tuck it against your side with your palm facing in toward your midline (Fig. 7-33A). With your other hand, grasp the ulnar side of the back of the hand and inhale. Exhale as you pull the hand into pronation to stretch your forearm muscles (Fig. 7-33B).

WRIST FLEXORS AND EXTENSORS

With your elbow at a 90-degree angle, pronate your forearm (Fig. 7-34A). Using your other hand, inhale as you hold it against all your fingers, including your thumb. Exhale as you use your other hand to push (extend) your fingers backward to stretch the wrist flexors (Fig. 7-34B). Repeat on the other arm. To

increase the intensity, supinate the forearm and repeat the stretch.

With your elbow at a 90-degree angle, pronate your forearm. Using your other hand, inhale as you hold all your fingers, including your thumb, and exhale as you (flex) push them downward to stretch the wrist extensors. Repeat on the other arm. To increase the intensity, curl your fingers of the forearm to be stretched into a soft fist and repeat the stretch (Fig. 7-34C).

FINGERS

Place your fingertips together in a tentlike position (Fig. 7-35A). Inhale, and as you exhale, gently push your hands together until you feel a stretch in your fingers (Fig. 7-35B).

Interlace your fingers in front of you (Fig. 7-35C). Pronate your forearms so that your palms are facing

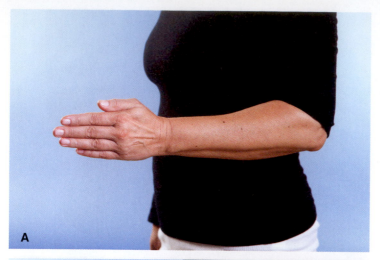

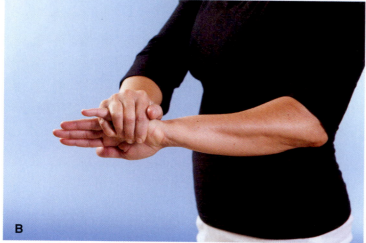

FIGURE 7-33 (A) With your elbow at a 90-degree angle, tuck it against your side with your palm facing in toward your midline. **(B)** Pull the hand into pronation to stretch your forearm muscles.

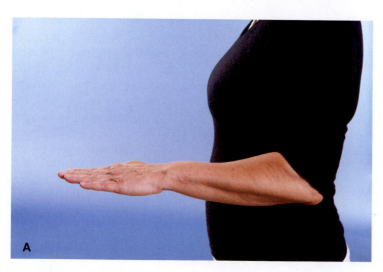

FIGURE 7-34 (A) With your elbow at a 90-degree angle, pronate your forearm.

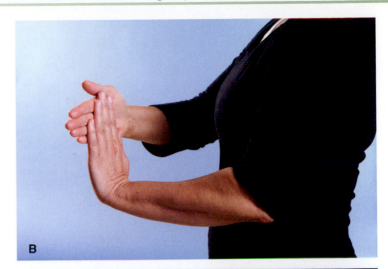

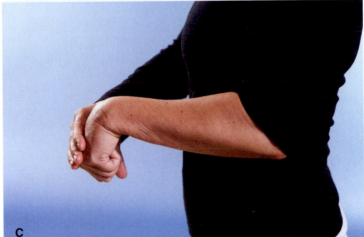

FIGURE 7-34 cont'd (B) Push (extend) your fingers backward to stretch the wrist flexors. **(C)** Stretch the wrist extensors with the fingers curled into a soft fist.

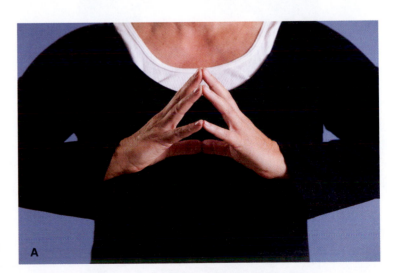

FIGURE 7-35 (A) Fingertips in a tentlike position.

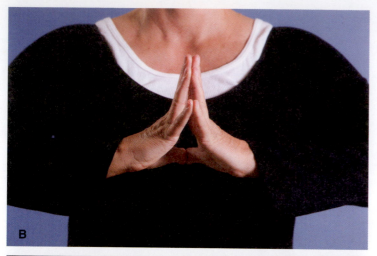

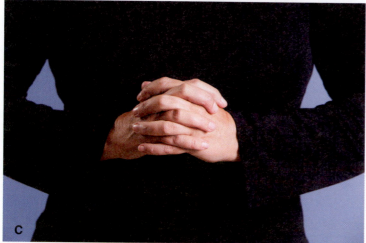

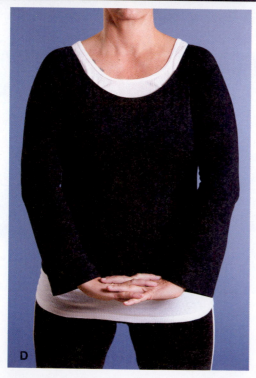

FIGURE 7-35 cont'd (B) Push the hands together to stretch the fingers. **(C)** Interlace your fingers. **(D)** Pronate your forearms so that your palms are facing down. Push your interlaced fingers downward to stretch them.

down. Inhale, and as you exhale, extend your elbows and push your fingers down into a gentle stretch (Fig. 7-35D).

TRICEPS BRACHII

Flex your elbow and raise it until your upper arm is shoulder height and your hand is at your posterior neck (Fig. 7-36A). Place your other hand on the tip of your elbow and inhale. As you exhale, pull your elbow upward with your other hand; your hand should move from behind your neck down your back (Fig. 7-36B).

Add a slight lateral flexion of the trunk to the opposite side to stretch serratus anterior (Fig. 7-36C). Repeat on the other arm.

ANTERIOR DELTOID

Stand with your forearms pronated and by your sides (Fig. 7-37A). Inhale, and as you exhale, slowly slide your arms backward until you feel a stretch in your anterior deltoids (Fig. 7-37B). Stop and hold that position for a few seconds while breathing normally.

PECTORALS AND ANTERIOR DELTOID

Clasp your hands together behind your back (Fig. 7-38A). Inhale, and as you exhale, gently rotate your shoulders back (Fig. 7-38B), and extend your arms until you feel a stretch through the chest and shoulder region. See how far you can raise your arms comfortably (Fig. 7-38C).

PECTORALS

This is the same stretch for medially rotated shoulders, sunken chest, kyphosis, and winged scapulae, discussed in Chapter 3.

Stand in a doorway with arms flexed at the elbows and parallel with the floor (Fig. 7-39A). Slowly lean into the doorway until you feel a stretch in the pectorals, then relax. Modifications: Try varying the position of your arms, as this will stretch the different pectoral fibers (Fig. 7-39B, C, and D).

SHOULDERS

Hold a rope with both hands, overhanded and shoulder-width apart. Inhale, and as you exhale, slowly raise it over your head (Fig. 7-40A).

As your shoulder flexibility improves, you will be able to perform this movement with the rope vertical behind your back. Turn one hand under and keep the other hand over (Fig. 7-40B). Bring your hands as close together as you can (Fig. 7-40C). Repeat this movement by reversing your hand position.

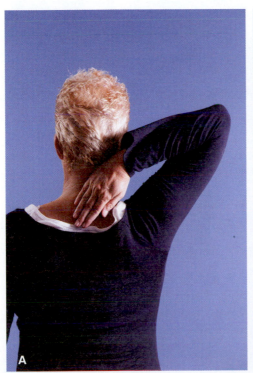
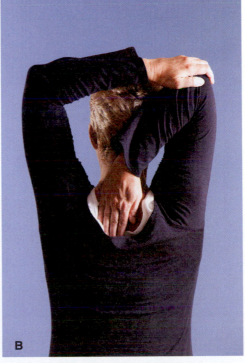

FIGURE 7-36 (A) Flex your elbow and raise it until your upper arm is shoulder height and your hand is on your posterior neck. **(B)** Push your elbow upward with your other hand.

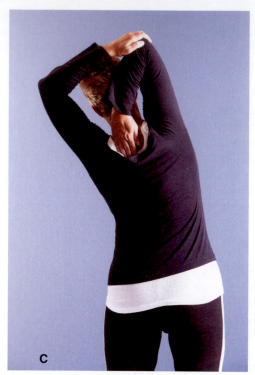

FIGURE 7-36 cont'd (C) Slight lateral flexion of the trunk to stretch serratus anterior.

WALL CLOCK (SHOULDERS)

For this stretch, you will need a wall that is clear of any items that can interfere with your arm movements. Stand in a lunge position next to a wall, approximately 1 foot away. Raise the arm closest to the wall, with your palm facing the wall. This is the 12 o'clock position (Fig. 7-41A). Hold this position while you breathe normally. To increase the intensity of the stretch, crawl your fingers up the wall and hold. Release the stretch. Inhale, and as you exhale, move your hand to the 1 o'clock position (Fig. 7-41B), crawling your fingers up to increase the intensity of the stretch. Hold in this position while you breathe normally. Repeat the stretches with your hand at the 2 and 3 o'clock positions (Fig. 7-41C and D).

Repeat with your other arm by turning around and placing your arm in what will now be the 12 o'clock position. Repeat the stretch with your arm in the 11 o'clock position, then the 10 and 9 o'clock positions.

To benefit the most from this stretch, keep your body facing forward and do not rotate into the wall.

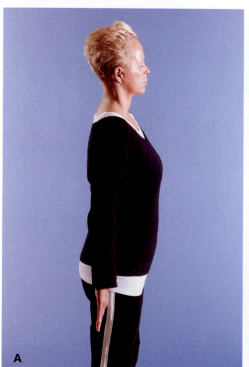
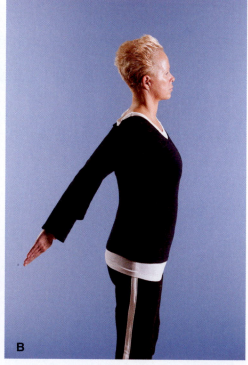

FIGURE 7-37 (A) Stand with your forearms pronated and by your sides. **(B)** Slowly slide your arms backward until you feel a stretch in your anterior deltoids.

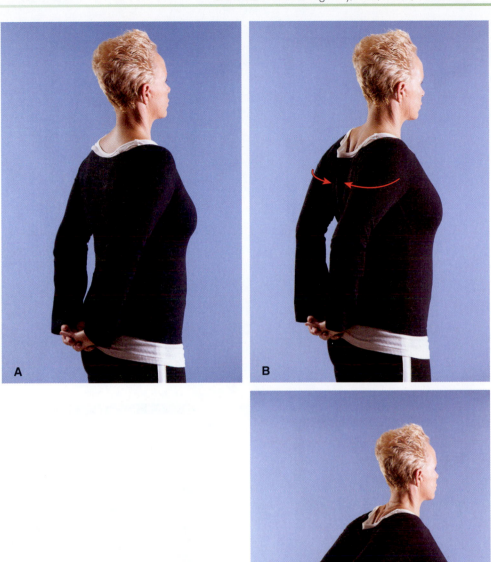

FIGURE 7-38 **(A)** Clasp your hands together behind your back. **(B)** Gently rotate your shoulders back. **(C)** Extend your arms until you feel a stretch through the chest and shoulder region. See how far you can raise your arms comfortably.

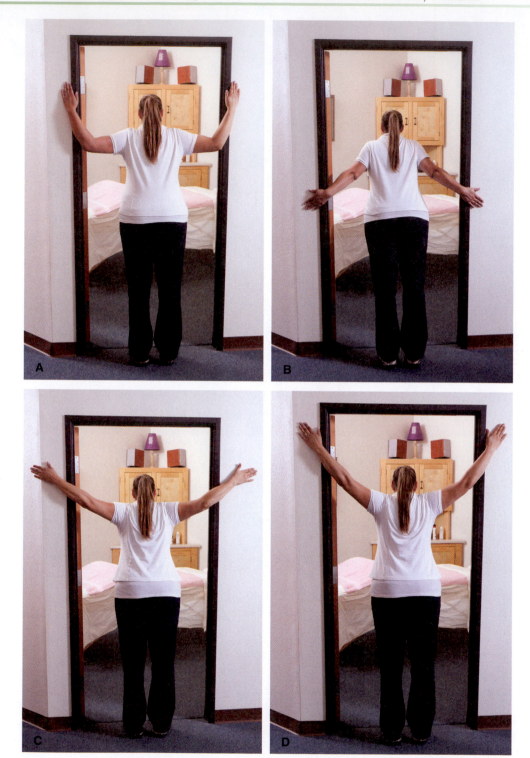

FIGURE 7-39 (A) Stand in a doorway with arms flexed at the elbows and parallel with the floor, and slowly lean into the doorway. **(B, C, D)** Varied positions of the arms.

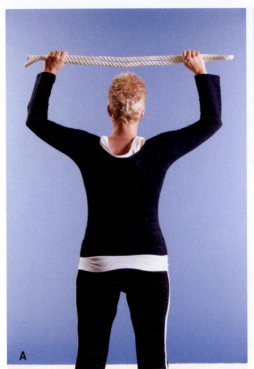

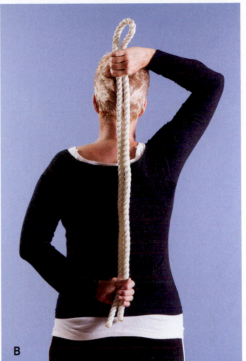

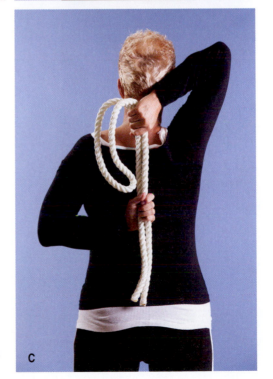

FIGURE 7-40 (A) Hold a towel or dowel in both hands, overhanded and shoulder-width apart. **(B)** Hold the towel or dowel behind your back and turn one hand under and keep the other hand over. **(C)** Bring your hands as close together as you can.

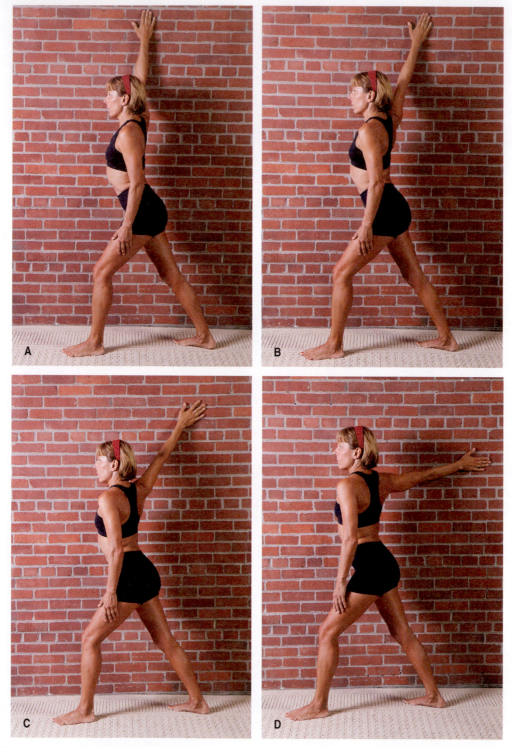

FIGURE 7-41 **(A)** Arm extended in the 12 o'clock position. **(B)** Arm extended in the 1 o'clock position. **(C)** Arm extended in the 2 o'clock position. **(D)** Arm extended in the 3 o'clock position.

ILIOPSOAS

Lie supine on the edge of a bench or at the end of a massage table with one leg hanging freely over the end. Hug the knee of your other leg to your chest to keep your lower back close to the bench or table (Fig. 7-42A). Wait a few seconds to allow iliopsoas of the hanging leg to relax. Inhale, and as you exhale, use one hand to gently push on the thigh of the hanging leg (Fig. 7-42B). To increase the intensity of the stretch, rotate the thigh of the hanging leg by drawing small circles with the knee (Fig. 7-42C).

PIRIFORMIS AND GLUTEALS

These stretches work the hips and lower back but also affect the abdominal muscles, including the obliques.

Lie supine on a mat on the floor. Flex your knees, then cross your left leg over your right leg just above the knee and place your right foot flat on the floor. (Fig. 7-43A). Inhale, and as you exhale, hold the back of your right leg and pull it toward your chest; try to keep both shoulders on the mat. The lower portion of your right leg should be parallel to the floor and your left leg should be perpendicular to the right leg (Fig. 7-43B). Switch legs and repeat.

GLUTEALS

These stretches are mainly for the gluteal muscles but can also affect your inguinal region and hip adductor muscles. Warning: Be very careful not to apply any stress to your knee joints when performing this stretch. Otherwise, serious injury, such as tearing the cartilage, may occur.

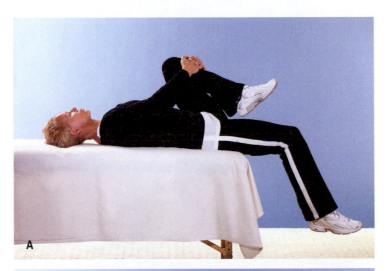

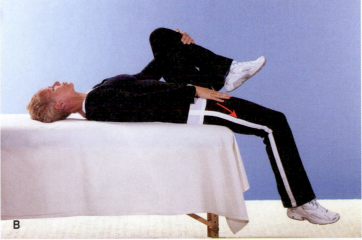

FIGURE 7-42 (A) Lie supine at the end of a massage table with one leg hanging freely over the end. Hug the knee of your other leg to your chest to keep your lower back close to the table. **(B)** Use one hand to gently push on the thigh of the hanging leg.

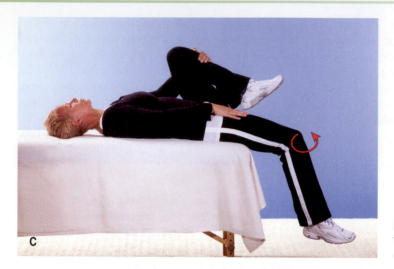

FIGURE 7-42 cont'd (C) Rotate the thigh of the hanging leg by drawing small circles with the knee.

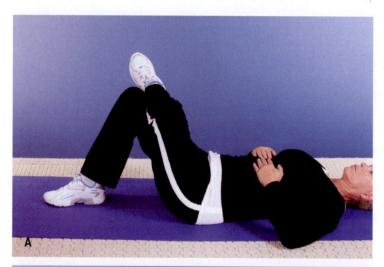

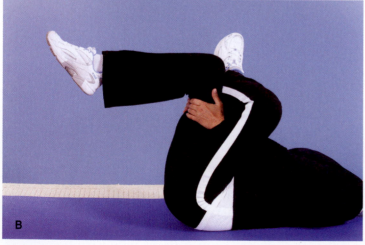

FIGURE 7-43 (A) Cross your left leg over your right leg just above the knee and place your right foot flat on the floor. **(B)** Hold the back of your right leg and pull it toward your chest; try to keep both shoulders on the mat.

Lie supine on a mat on the floor with both knees flexed and your feet flat on the floor (Fig. 7-44A). Grasp your right foot in your left hand, wrapping your hand under your foot so that your fingertips are on its lateral edge (Fig. 7-44B). Hold your leg, with your knee flexed, about 1 to 3 feet above the right side of your chest (Fig. 7-44C). Inhale, and as you exhale, slowly pull your foot over to the side and up toward your head as if you were trying to place your foot about 12 inches to the outside of your left shoulder (Fig. 7-44D). You should feel a good stretch in your gluteals. If you feel any stress at all on your knee, stop at once. You may be pulling up on your foot too much and not enough to the side. Use your free hand to support your knee. Switch legs and repeat.

To perform this as an isometric stretch, when you feel the stretch in your gluteal muscles, continue to pull your foot to the outside of your shoulder while at the same time resisting with your leg so that it pushes against your hand (Fig. 7-44E). No actual leg motion should take place, just the resistance. Stop immediately if you feel any undue stress on your knee.

HIP ADDUCTOR MUSCLES

Lie supine on a mat. Flex your hips and abduct your thighs (Fig. 7-45A). After your muscles have relaxed, inhale and place your hands on your medial thighs. As you exhale, use minimal force to increase the stretch (Fig. 7-45B). You should not feel tension on the medial sides of your knees or in your inguinal region. To increase the intensity of the stretch, rotate your thighs, circling your feet in both directions (Fig. 7-45C).

HIP ABDUCTOR MUSCLES

Lie on a bench or massage table in a side-lying position with the knee of your bottom leg flexed. Be close enough to the edge so your top leg can hang off

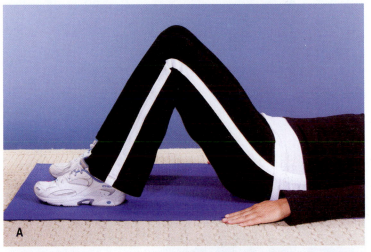

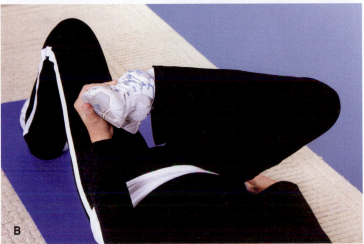

FIGURE 7-44 (A) Lie supine on a mat on the floor with both knees flexed and your feet flat on the floor. **(B)** Grasp your right foot in your left hand, wrapping your hand under your foot so that your fingertips are on its lateral edge.

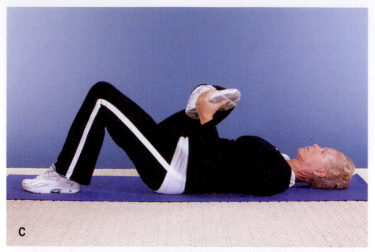

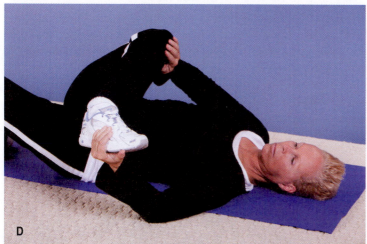

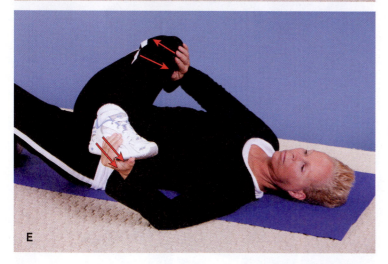

FIGURE 7-44 cont'd (C) Hold your leg, with your knee flexed in the air about 1 to 3 feet above the right side of your chest. **(D)** Pull your foot over to the side and up toward your head as if you were trying to place your foot about 12 inches to the outside of your left shoulder. **(E)** Resist with your leg so that it pushes against your hand.

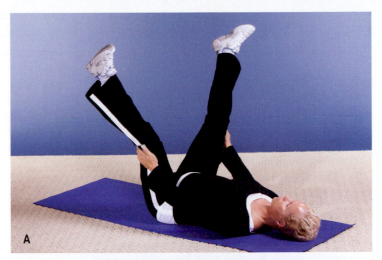

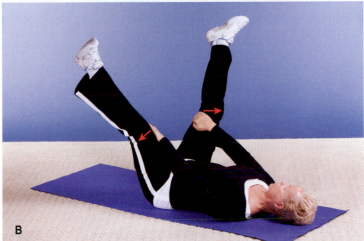

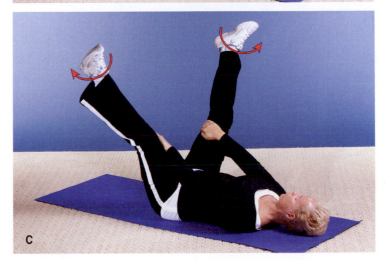

FIGURE 7-45 (A) Lie supine on a mat. Flex your hips and abduct your thighs. **(B)** Place your hands on your medial thighs and use minimal force to increase the stretch. **(C)** Rotate your thighs, circling your feet in both directions.

it (Fig. 7-46A). Inhale, and as you exhale, move your top leg backward, allowing it to relax and lower over the edge of the bench or massage table (Fig. 7-46B). To increase the intensity of the stretch, rotate your stretched thigh by drawing small circles with your foot (Fig. 7-46C). Turn on your other side and repeat the stretch.

QUADRICEPS

Lie on a mat on the floor in a side-lying position. Support your head with the hand of the same side you are lying on and flex both knees (Fig. 7-47A). With your other hand, inhale as you grasp the ankle of the top leg and exhale as you pull back (extending the thigh) to stretch your quadriceps muscles (Fig. 7-47B). Be sure to maintain alignment between your hip and knee joint. Turn on your other side and repeat the stretch.

HAMSTRINGS

Lie supine on a mat on the floor. Flex one knee while keeping your foot flat on the floor (Fig. 7-48A). Inhale as you raise the other leg straight up. Hold the back of this leg just distal to your knee and gently pull the leg toward your chest. Keep the stretched leg extended, but not locked at the knee joint. Exhale as you pull this leg toward your chest (Fig. 7-48B). Repeat on the other leg.

CALF STRETCH

Stand with one foot in front of the other, approximately 2 feet apart (Fig. 7-49A). Inhale as you flex the knee of the forward leg and exhale as you slowly lunge forward, keeping your back leg extended (knee slightly flexed) (Fig. 7-49B). Keep your spine aligned and your toes pointed straight ahead or turned slightly medially, and make sure the knee of

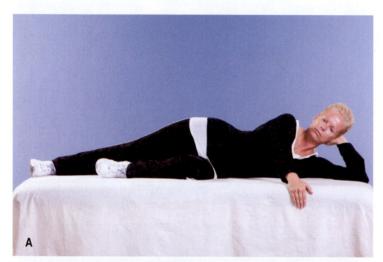

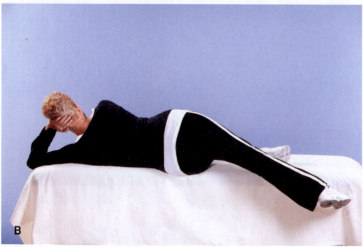

FIGURE 7-46 (A) Lie on a massage table in a side-lying position. **(B)** Cross your upper leg over your lower leg, allowing the upper leg to relax over the end of the massage table.

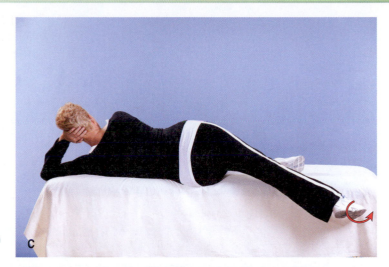

FIGURE 7-46 cont'd (C) Rotate your stretched thigh by drawing small circles with your foot.

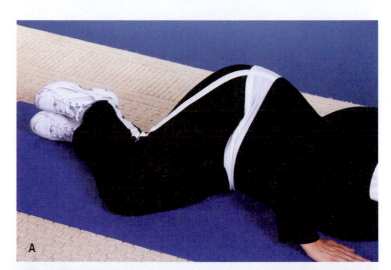

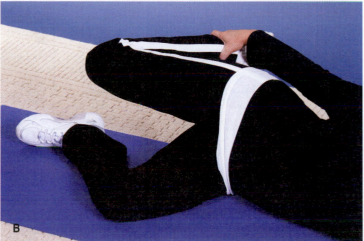

FIGURE 7-47 (A) Lie on a mat on the floor in a side-lying position. Support your head with your arm. **(B)** Flex the knee of your top leg and exhale as you pull back on your ankle.

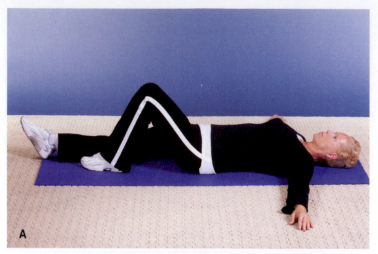

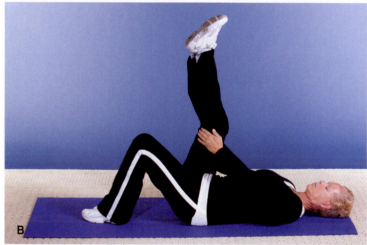

FIGURE 7-48 (A) Lie supine on a mat on the floor. Flex one knee while keeping your foot flat on the floor. **(B)** Raise the other leg straight up, hold the back of it just below your knee, and pull the leg toward your chest.

your front leg does not go past your toes. Repeat the stretch on your other leg.

TIBIALIS ANTERIOR

Stand with one foot in front of the other, approximately 2 feet apart (Fig. 7-50A). Inhale as you extend one leg backward with your ankle in plantarflexion and your toes on the floor (Fig. 7-50B). Exhale as you flex the knee of your forward leg and increase the extension of your back leg to stretch tibialis anterior (Fig. 7-50C). Keep your vertebral column aligned. Repeat the stretch on your other leg.

GASTROCNEMIUS AND SOLEUS

Sit on a mat on the floor with one knee flexed and the foot flat on the floor, and the other knee flexed and the lower leg flat on the floor (Fig. 7-51A). Inhale, and as you exhale, rise up, or push with

Focus on *Wellness*

Ideally, you should complete a general warm-up and then do warm-ups with dynamic movement. After that, you should move into AIS or static stretching, depending on how much time you have. AIS is a great method if your time is limited before a treatment session, and it is great to use in between treatment sessions or incorporated into a treatment where you think both you and the client need to stretch. If you are going to do a workout that is not a bodywork treatment, you could do your general warm-up, followed with some dynamic movement, complete your workout, and then follow with static stretching.

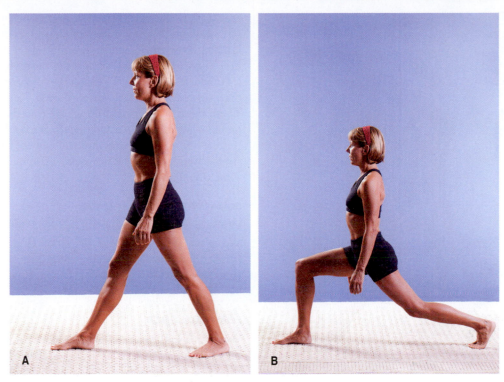

FIGURE 7-49 (A) Stand with one foot in front of the other, approximately 2 feet apart. **(B)** Flex the knee of the forward leg and slowly lunge forward, keeping your back leg extended (knee slightly flexed).

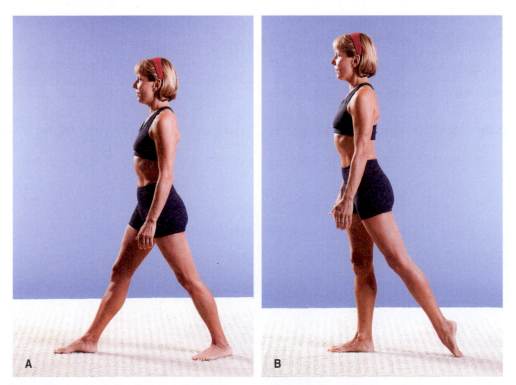

FIGURE 7-50 (A) Stand with one foot in front of the other, approximately 2 feet apart. **(B)** Extend one leg backward with your ankle in plantarflexion and your toes on the floor.

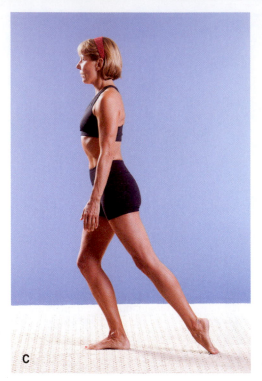

FIGURE 7-50 cont'd (C) Flex the knee of your forward leg and increase the extension of your back leg to stretch.

fingers or soft fists against the floor, and lean forward to stretch gastrocnemius and soleus (Fig. 7-51B). Switch leg positions and repeat to stretch gastrocnemius and soleus in your other leg.

Stretches for Those Performing Bodywork on a Futon

Bodywork modalities that are performed on a client lying a futon, such as shiatsu and Thai massage, require practitioners to have lower centers of gravity because

they work in kneeling, half-kneeling, **seiza**, and wide-seiza positions. *Seiza* is a Japanese term for sitting in a kneeling position in which the gluteals rest on the heels (Fig. 7-52A). Wide seiza is this position with the legs abducted (Fig. 7-52B). Because of these positions, practitioners need to have strong core and leg muscles. These muscles also need to be flexible so that practitioners can perform their treatments in a fluid manner.

The following are stretches you can use to further stretch your legs and core muscles. Also included are some overall stretches.

SQUAT WITH LATERAL LUNGE

While keeping your spine aligned, sink into a squat and place your hands on the floor (Fig. 7-53A). Inhale, and as you exhale, lunge to one side (Fig. 7-53B). Come back to the center. Inhale, and as you exhale, lunge to the other side.

FORWARD LUNGE

While in a squat, turn to face one side. Bring one leg forward and extend the other leg backward, keeping the knee slightly flexed. Place both hands on the floor next to the medial side of the foot of the forward leg. Inhale while keeping your spine aligned, and exhale as you lunge forward (Fig. 7-54). Turn to the other side and repeat.

ADDUCTOR STRETCH

While prone, raise your upper body and support it with your hands on the floor. Abduct your legs, flex your knees, and place the soles of your feet together (Fig. 7-55A). Inhale, and as you exhale, press your abdomen and feet to the floor and extend your arms straight out in front of you (Fig. 7-55B). Depending on your flexibility, you may be able to keep only your

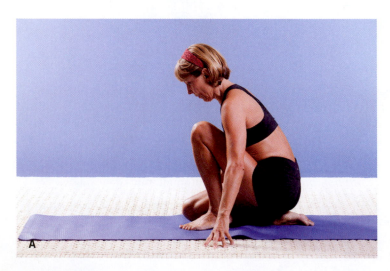

FIGURE 7-51 (A) Sit on a mat on the floor with one knee flexed and the foot flat on the floor, and the other knee flexed and the lower leg flat on the floor.

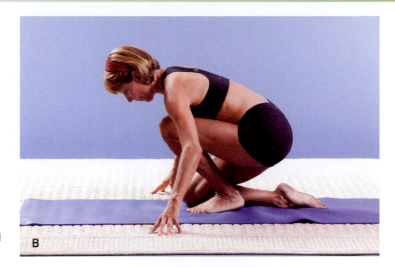

FIGURE 7-51 cont'd (B) Rise up and lean forward to stretch gastrocnemius and soleus.

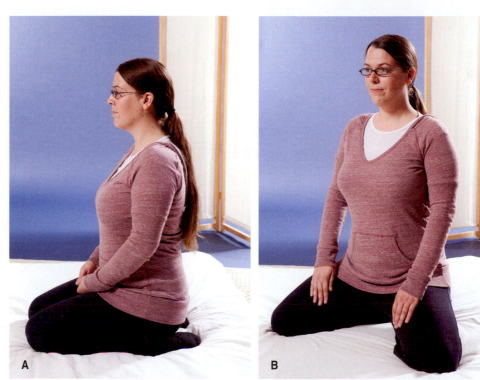

FIGURE 7-52 (A) Seiza. **(B)** Wide seiza.

abdomen pressed to the floor or your feet to the floor but not both. Do the best you can and do not force the stretch. Over time, you may be able to press both your abdomen and feet to the floor.

MAKKA-HO

In the 1970s, a Japanese man named Makka designed a series of stretches based on the Five Element organ channel (meridian) pairs. These are known as *Makka-Ho*, which means Makka's method, or Makka's exercises. Each of the Five Elements—metal, earth, water, fire, and wood—has stretches designed to address their channels.

Performing Makka-Ho has several benefits. They:

- Serve as a reminder for channel locations
- Provide an overall stretch because every area of the body is addressed
- Can bring to the practitioner awareness of imbalances in her own body. If tension, tightness, or pain is felt while performing the Makka-Ho for a particular set of channels, there may be blockages or deficiencies in those channels.

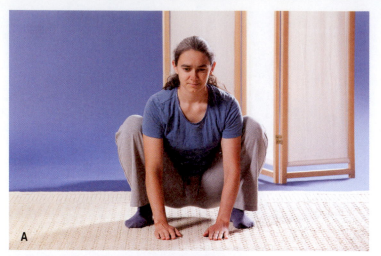

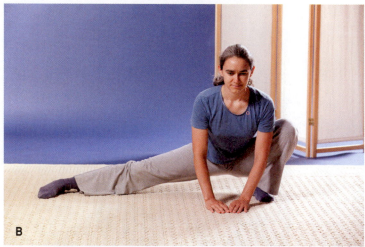

FIGURE 7-53 (A) Sink into a squat and place your hands on the floor. **(B)** Lunge to one side.

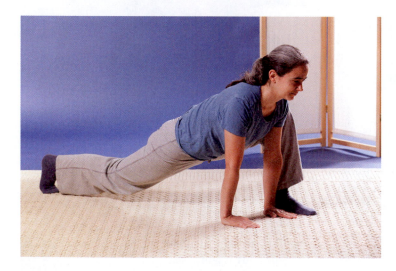

FIGURE 7-54 Bring one leg forward and extend the other leg backward, keeping the knee slightly flexed. Place both hands on the floor next to the medial side of the foot of the forward leg.

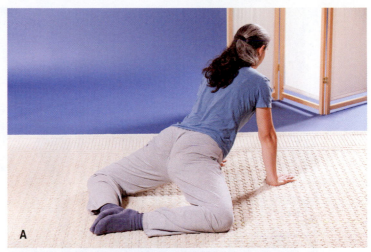

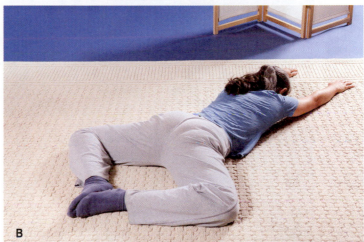

FIGURE 7-55 (A) Abduct your legs, flex your knees, and place the soles of your feet together. **(B)** Press your abdomen and feet to the floor and extend your arms straight out in front of you.

As with all exercises and stretches, it is important to relax while doing them and to remember to keep breathing.

METAL MAKKA-HO (LUNG AND LARGE INTESTINE CHANNELS)

Stand with your feet shoulder-width apart. Behind your back, form an interlocking circle with the thumb and middle finger of both hands. Extend your index fingers down (Fig. 7-56A and B). As you inhale, lean back slightly. Hold for several seconds while breathing normally. Inhale and exhale as you lean forward as far as is comfortable for you, raising your arms as far as is comfortable and keeping your index fingers extended (Fig. 7-56C). Hold for several seconds, release, and stand upright. Interlock your other thumb and middle fingers behind your back and repeat the Makka-Ho.

EARTH MAKKA-HO (STOMACH AND SPLEEN CHANNELS)

Although these stretches are beneficial, there is a potential risk of injury. For some practitioners, the stretches can simply put too much stress on their knee and hip joints. Great care should be used when performing any of these stretches. Note that the second and third methods of performing Earth Makka-Ho are similar to the traditional hurdler's stretch, discussed in the "Stretches to Avoid" section. The stretches in this section are considered risky if they are done incorrectly or without proper training.

Earth Makka-Ho can be done several ways. Stand with your feet flat on the floor and shoulder-width apart. Flex one knee so that the sole of the foot is facing your hamstrings. While balancing on the other foot, grasp the raised foot with the hand on the same side and pull it as close to your hamstrings as you can.

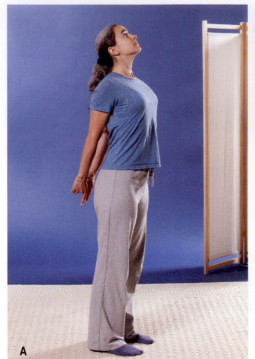

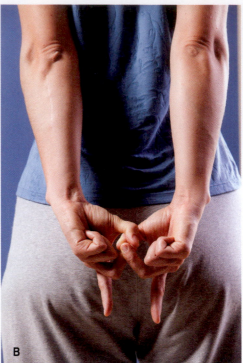

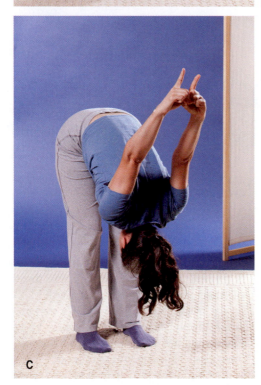

FIGURE 7-56 (A) Behind your back, form an interlocking circle with the thumb and middle finger of both hands. **(B)** Point your index fingers. **(C)** Flex your trunk so that your back is parallel to the floor.

Extend the arm on the other side over your head (Fig. 7-57A). Hold this position for several seconds as you feel your body settle into a stable balance. Release, then repeat with the foot on the other side.

Another method is to sit on the floor with your gluteals resting on your heels. Move your feet out so they are just lateral to your gluteal muscles. Lie back until your back is flat on the floor. Raise both arms over your head and lay them flat on the floor (Fig. 7-57B). Hold for several seconds, then release.

A third way is a modified version of the previous method. Lie back with one foot just lateral to your gluteal muscles and your other leg extended. Raise both arms over your head and lay them flat on the floor above your head (Fig. 7-57C). Hold for several seconds, then release. Repeat with the leg that was

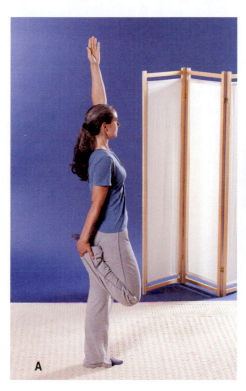

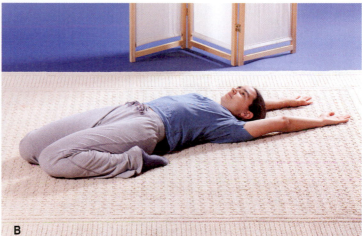

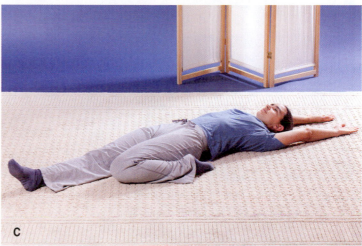

FIGURE 7-57 (A) Flex one knee so that the sole of the foot is facing the hamstrings. While balancing on the other foot, grasp the elevated foot with the hand on the same side and pull it as close to your hamstrings as you can. Extend the arm on the other side of your head. **(B)** Sit on the floor in seiza. Move your feet outward so they are just lateral to your gluteals. Lie down with your back flat on the floor. Raise both arms over your head and lay them flat on the floor. **(C)** Lie with one foot just lateral to your gluteals and the other leg stretched out straight on the floor. Raise both arms over your head and lay them flat on the floor.

extended now with the foot just lateral to the gluteals and the leg that was flexed now extended.

WATER MAKKA-HO (KIDNEY AND URINARY BLADDER CHANNELS)

Sit on the floor with your legs extended in front. Extend your arms and raise them straight over your head (Fig. 7-58A). While keeping your spine aligned and arms extended, flex your trunk and bring your hands toward your feet (Fig. 7-58B). See if you can touch the bottom of your feet with your fingers. Hold for several seconds, then release.

FIRE MAKKA-HO (HEART AND SMALL INTESTINE CHANNELS)

Sit on the floor with your knees flexed and the soles of your feet placed together. Interlace your fingers and use them to grasp your feet. Pull your feet as close into your body as is comfortable, and let your knees relax as much as possible. Inhale, and, keeping your spine aligned, exhale as you flex your trunk and lean forward as far as you can. Keep your elbows in front of your legs (Fig. 7-59). Breathe normally as you hold this position for several seconds, then release.

LESSER FIRE MAKKA-HO (TRIPLE HEATER AND HEART PROTECTOR CHANNELS)

Sit on the floor with your knees flexed and legs crossed. Tuck your inside foot close to your body. Cross your arms and lay your arms flat on the floor in front of you. Inhale, and as you exhale, flex your trunk to lean forward as far as possible, elongating your arms on the floor as you do so (Fig. 7-60). Breathe normally as you hold this position for several seconds, then release. Repeat with your legs and arms crossed the other way.

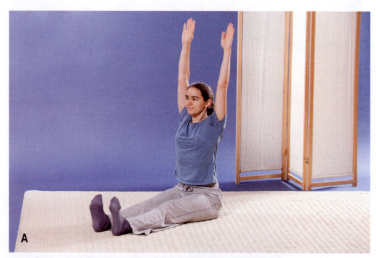

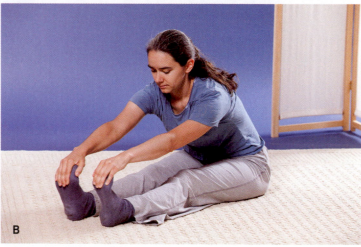

FIGURE 7-58 (A) Sit on the floor with your legs stretched out straight in front of you. Raise both your arms straight over your head. **(B)** While keeping your spine aligned and arms extended flex your trunk and bring your hands toward your feet.

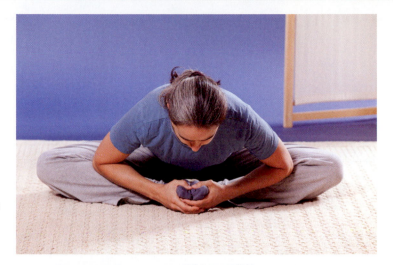

FIGURE 7-59 Sit on the floor with your knees flexed and the soles of your feet placed against each other. Interlace your fingers and grasp your feet with them. Flex your trunk and lean forward as far as you can while exhaling, keeping your elbows in front of your legs.

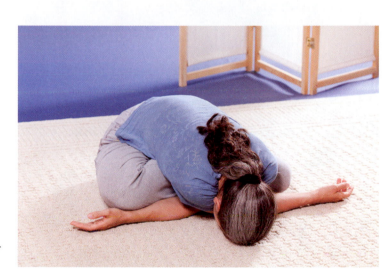

FIGURE 7-60 Sit on the floor with your legs crossed. Tuck your inside foot close to your body. Cross your arms and place your hands in front of your knees.

WOOD MAKKA-HO (LIVER AND GALL BLADDER CHANNELS)

Sit on the floor with your legs extended and abducted at about a 45-degree angle from your body. Raise one arm over your head and keep it extended. While keeping your spine aligned, laterally flex to the opposite side and extend the arm on this side toward your foot (Fig. 7-61A). Hold for several seconds, then release and sit back up straight. Raise your other arm and laterally flex to your other side and repeat. After releasing, sit back up straight. While keeping your spine aligned, flex your trunk and extend your arms out in front of you as far as you can (Fig. 7-61B). Hold for several seconds, then release.

Myth: If I don't feel anything when I stretch, I should just stretch harder.

FACT: Stretching hard may result in injury. If you're not feeling anything when you stretch, consider changing the angle at which you are stretching. Try to identify and isolate the area being stretched. It could also mean that that particular muscle is already flexible and doesn't need to be stretched.

ACTIVITY

The last part of the warm-up is spent executing movements that are similar to the movements you will perform during the exercise activity or bodywork,

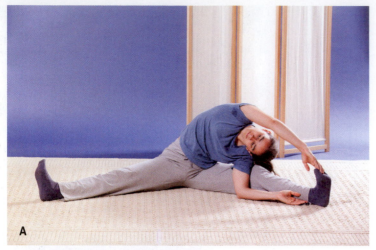

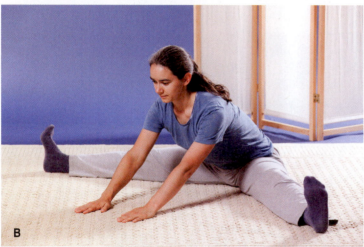

FIGURE 7-61 (A) Sit on the floor with your legs extended and abducted about a 45-degree angle from your body. Raise one arm over your head and keep it extended. Laterally flex to the opposite side and extend the arm on this side toward your foot. **(B)** Flex your trunk and as you lean forward, stretch your arms straight out in front of you as far as you can.

but at a reduced intensity. For example, massage therapists may spend some time doing the motions involved in gliding strokes while lunging. Shiatsu practitioners may spend some time in wide seiza as they rise to their knees, then sit back on their heels. Such activities are beneficial because they improve coordination, balance, strength, and response time, and they may reduce the risk of injury. Once you have done these movements, you are ready to perform your treatments for the day.

COOLING DOWN

After completing the workout or after a long treatment day, the best way to reduce muscle fatigue (caused by the production of lactic acid from maximal or near-maximal muscle exertion) and soreness is to perform a light cooldown. This cooldown is similar to the second half of the warm-up. Recall that the warm-up consists of dynamic movement followed by AIS or static stretching.

Dynamic movement, followed by stretching, can reduce cramping, tightening, and soreness in fatigued muscles and gives an overall feeling of well-being. Doing dynamic movement and stretching as a light cooldown immediately following exertion is a better way of clearing lactic acid from the blood than complete rest. Furthermore, if you experience soreness the next day, a light warm-up or cooldown is a good way to reduce lingering muscle tightness and pain. Another option is to receive a bodywork treatment.

STRETCHES TO AVOID

Although certain stretches may be beneficial in some aspect, the potential risk of injury from performing the stretch must be taken into consideration. Some stretches can simply put too much stress on the joints. They may involve rotations that strain tendons or ligaments, or put pressure on vertebral disks, or require twists or turns that may cause injury to seemingly unrelated parts of the body.

The stretches discussed here have a very high risk of injury for those who perform them. This does not mean that you should never do these stretches. However, use great care when attempting any of them.

In general, any standing stretch in which the trunk needs to be flexed, such as toe touching, requires a lot of training to do correctly. For example, unless the individual is properly trained, the hamstrings contract reflexively to stabilize the pelvis, thereby transferring stress to the lumbar ligaments. Refer to the hamstring example in the "Rules for Successful Stretching" section.

Standing lateral stretches for the adductors and abductors do not work well either. In a standing position, both these sets of muscles usually contract reflexively to stabilize the hip. They cannot stretch because they cannot relax. Standing and seated stretches in which the torso is flexed can place pressure on the sciatic nerve. Done repeatedly, this pressure may damage the nerve.

The knee should never be placed in a weight-bearing position on the ground for any stretch. It is an invitation for ligament or cartilage damage. The common hurdler stretch and the kneeling quadriceps and hamstring stretches, discussed in the next section, are the most risky.

Unless you are an advanced athlete or are being coached by a qualified instructor such as a certified yoga instructor, physical therapist, or fitness trainer, you should avoid these types of stretches. However, when performed correctly, as in using a properly aligned spine instead of flexing the trunk, and with the aid of an instructor, some of these stretches can be quite beneficial.

THE YOGA PLOW

This stretch involves lying supine and sweeping the legs up and over, trying to touch the knees to the ears (Fig. 7-62). This position places excessive stress on the lower back and on the vertebral disks. It also compresses the lungs and heart and can make it difficult to breathe.

This stretch is a prime example of an exercise that is quite easy to do incorrectly. However, with proper instruction and attention to body position and alignment, this stretch can be performed successfully with a minimal amount of risk and can actually improve spinal health and mobility.

THE TRADITIONAL BACKBEND

This stretch involves maximally arching the back with the soles of the feet and the palms of the hands on the floor and the neck extended backward

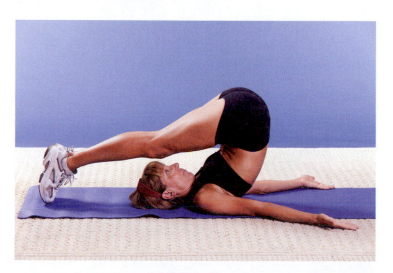

FIGURE 7-62 The yoga plow.

(Fig. 7-63). This position compresses the vertebral disks and can pinch nerves in the back.

THE TRADITIONAL HURDLER'S STRETCH

This stretches the quadriceps muscles in one thigh. It involves sitting on the ground with one leg extended in front and the other knee flexed with the leg behind the individual. The individual leans back to stretch the quadriceps of the flexed leg (Fig. 7-64A). This stretch can also be done by leaning forward to stretch the hamstrings. A modified version involves abducting the thigh and flexed knee, then leaning forward to stretch the hamstrings of the extended leg (Fig. 7-64B).

This stretch can be harmful because it stretches the medial ligaments of the knee and compresses the

menisci. It can also result in the patella slipping off its track due to twisting and compression.

STRAIGHT-LEGGED TOE TOUCHES

This stretch involves standing with the legs either together or hip-width apart while flexing and attempting to touch the toes or the floor (Fig. 7-65). If the individual cannot support much of her weight with her hands when performing this exercise, her knees are likely to hyperextend. Also, the hamstrings cannot stretch in this position because they reflexively contract to stabilize the pelvis.

This position can also place a great deal of pressure on the vertebrae of the lower lumbar spine. Furthermore, if the legs are hip-width apart, it places more stress on the knees, which can result in structural problems.

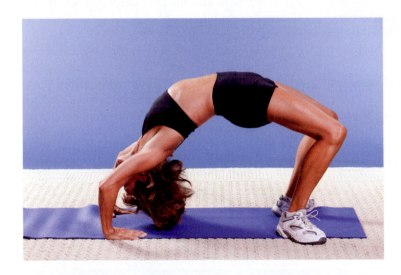

FIGURE 7-63 The traditional backbend.

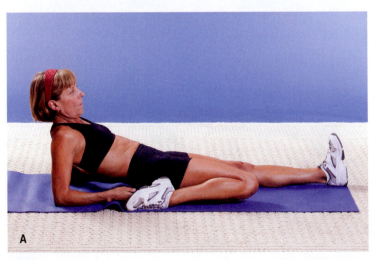

FIGURE 7-64 (A) Traditional hurdler's stretch.

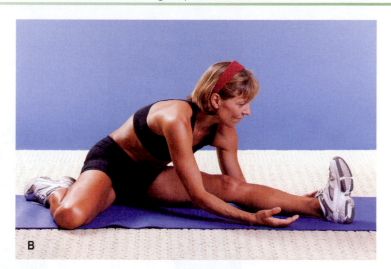

FIGURE 7-64 cont'd (B) Modified traditional hurdler's stretch.

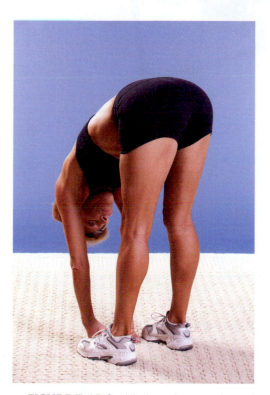

FIGURE 7-65 Straight-legged toe touches.

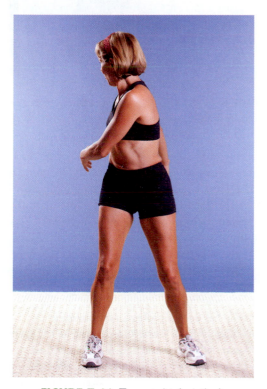

FIGURE 7-66 Torso twist (rotation).

SUDDEN TORSO TWISTS (ROTATIONS)

Performing sudden, intense rotations of the torso, especially with weights, while in an upright position (Fig. 7-66) can tear tissue by exceeding the momentum-absorbing capacity of the stretched tissues and can sprain the ligaments of the knee and low back.

INVERTED STRETCHES

These are stretches in which the individual hangs upside down. This can be accomplished by using inversion boots (Fig. 7-67A) or an inversion table (Fig. 7-67B). Using inversion boots may increase blood pressure and may even rupture blood vessels,

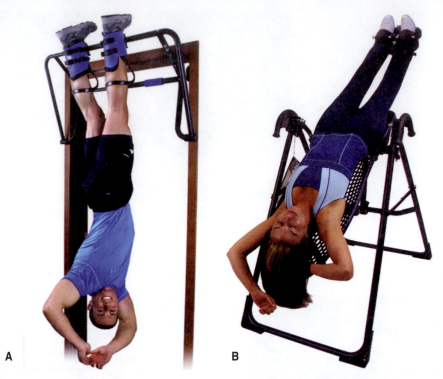

A   B

FIGURE 7-67 (A) Inversion boots. **(B)** Inversion table. (A Teeter Hang Ups EZ-Up Inversion System. Photo courtesy of Teeter, www.teeter-inversion.com.)

especially in the eyes. Inverted positions are discouraged for anyone with spinal issues and for those who do not have clearance from their physicians. The preferred method for this type of stretch is with the use of an inversion table, which poses the least amount of stress on the joints.

Wellness Profile Check In

Looking at the Wellness Profile you completed at the end of Chapter 1, are there any challenge areas you could remedy through a plan for stretching? If

Case Profile

Marvin has been a professional bodywork practitioner for 8 years. Prior to that, he had spent 15 years doing construction work. His bodywork program included classes in wellness, which he thought were a waste of time. After all, he had been doing physical work his entire life, and he didn't need some instructor telling him how to stay fit. He knew how to use his body to do work, and doing some silly stretches certainly weren't going to help his career longevity.

Over the last year, however, Marvin has started to hear noises in and around his right shoulder joint as he moves. He prides himself on being able to perform deep-tissue treatments but has noticed that lately he

is losing some strength in his right arm and hand. He has started to become concerned that soon he may not be able to deliver the treatments he is known for and that he might start losing clientele.

■ *What do you think are the cause of the noises in Marvin's right shoulder?*

■ *What structures may be involved?*

■ *How do you think this is related to his ability to do bodywork?*

■ *What specific recommendations would you give Marvin?*

so, what are they? How would you like these areas improved? What methods or activities will you use to improve these areas? Write down a plan for improvement that includes the methods you will use, a timeline for implementing these methods, and ways you will assess your improvement along the way.

Consult with your physician to see if you have any contraindications for the stretches presented in this chapter and to find out what levels of activity are best for you to start with.

SUMMARY

It is essential that practitioners keep their bodies in the best shape possible. Optimal physical fitness requires flexibility, aerobic activity, and strength training. Flexibility training is used to help correct muscle imbalances, increase joint ROM, relieve abnormal joint stress, maintain normal functional length of muscles, and improve neuromuscular efficiency. Chronically shortened muscles can lead to injury.

Many factors affect flexibility such as the structure and shape of the joint, the joint ligaments and tendons that cross the joint, adhesions from past injuries or surgeries, too much muscle around a joint, shortened muscles, imbalanced muscles, paralysis, neurological disease, joint immobilization, aging, and periods of rapid growth. Benefits of stretching include decreased risk of injury, increased range of motion, increased flexibility, increased mobility, and increased coordination.

The sliding filament mechanism describes how muscles shorten. Each sarcomere has a habitual resting length. Regular stretching will cause the myofibrils to grow longer by growing new sarcomere segments. These new sarcomere segments increase the muscle's ROM and increase the power the muscle can generate. Therefore, stretching increases the muscle's pliability and its strength.

The neuromuscular system has safeguards against severe muscular injury in the form of proprioceptors that can sense changes in muscle tension and muscle length. If a muscle is stretched far enough during a particular movement, the muscle is stimulated to contract, relieving the stretching. The tendon reflex protects tendons and associated muscles from damage by causing muscles to relax when muscle contractions place excessive tension on tendons. Joint kinesthetic receptors respond to pressure and acceleration and deceleration of joints. Articular ligaments contain receptors similar to tendon organs that adjust reflex inhibition of the adjacent muscles when excessive strain is placed on the joint.

Dynamic stretches involve swinging the arms or legs in a controlled manner. Static stretching consists of low force and long duration, holding for 20 or more seconds. Passive or relaxed stretches are similar to static stretches. A position is assumed and held with some other part of the body, with the assistance of a partner or a piece of equipment. Movements should be slow, steady, and gentle to lengthen the soft tissues effectively. Ballistic stretches use the momentum of a moving body or a limb in an attempt to force it beyond its normal end point. AIS involves contracting muscles opposite the target muscles, using the principle that when the agonist contracts, the antagonist relaxes. *PNF* is an umbrella term for several types of contract-relax stretches.

The rules of successful stretching include relaxation, warmth, minimum force, breathing, duration, and patience. When stretching for the purpose of increasing overall flexibility, the stretching routine should train the stretch receptors to become accustomed to greater muscle length and reduce the resistance of connective tissues to muscle elongation.

For the body to work at its best, any physical activity should involve a general warm-up, stretching, activity, and cooldown. The general warm-up includes joint ROM exercises and aerobic activity. When stretching, dynamic stretches should be done first, followed by static, passive, or AIS stretches. The best way to reduce muscle fatigue and soreness after a workout or long treatment day is to perform a light cooldown.

Review Questions

MULTIPLE CHOICE

1. The term for a functional unit made up of the myofascial systems, articular system, and nervous system is
   a. flexibility reserve.
   b. kinetic chain.
   c. flexibility deficit.
   d. neuromuscular efficiency.

2. A cause of inflexibility is
   a. muscle imbalance.
   b. aging.
   c. joint immobilization.
   d. All of the above

3. Within muscle fibers are tiny, threadlike structures called
   a. myofibrils.
   b. epimysium.
   c. collagen fibers.
   d. fascicles.

4. If a muscle is stretched too long, to the point of pain, or if it cannot tolerate the stretch, what type of contraction will occur?
   a. Minimal
   b. Isotonic
   c. Rebound
   d. Elongated

5. Which of the following is the most commonly performed type of stretch?
   a. Static
   b. Ballistic
   c. Dynamic
   d. PNF

6. Which of the following is a contraindication for performing stretches?
   a. Lack of pain the next day
   b. Neuropathy
   c. Strong bones
   d. Hypertension controlled by medication

7. Doing which of the following will increase the success of stretching?
   a. Holding the breath
   b. Using as much force as possible
   c. Relaxing the muscles
   d. Cooling the muscles first

FILL-IN-THE-BLANK

1. A benefit of stretching is that it _____ range of motion.

2. Perimysium surrounds groups of 10 to 100 or more muscles into bundles called _____.

3. The event involved in muscle contraction is called the _____ _____ mechanism.

4. The muscle that is to be stretched is referred to as the _____ muscle.

5. Patterns of biological activity, such as the sleep-wake cycle, that occur in a 24-hour period are called _____ _____.

6. The fastest and most effective way currently known to increase passive flexibility is by performing _____ stretches.

7. The four phases of physical activity are _____,_____ _____, and _____.

SHORT ANSWER

1. Give at least three examples of how inflexibility can lead to injury.

2. Explain how correct stretching lengthens muscle on a microscopic level.

3. Briefly describe dynamic, static, passive, ballistic, AIS stretches, and PNF.

4. Briefly explain the six rules of successful stretching.

5. Describe how to prevent overstretching.

6. Give two examples of joint ROM exercises and two examples of aerobic activity that can be done during a general warm-up.

7. Explain how to do a light cooldown.

Activities

1. Contact at least three professional practitioners. Ask them what stretching routines they do, how they benefit from the stretches, what impact stretching has had on their career longevity, and how they started doing the stretching routines.

2. Consult a personal trainer or yoga instructor for recommendations on how to design a stretching program for yourself using the stretches presented in this chapter.

3. When you start your stretching program, keep a journal for at least 2 weeks. Write down how you feel before you begin the stretches, how it feels as you do the stretches, how you feel after the stretches, and what benefits you are gaining from doing the stretches. At the end of 2 weeks, review your journal to see what progress you have made.

REFERENCES

American College of Sports Medicine. ACSM's *Resource Manual for Guidelines for Exercise Testing and Prescription*, 6th ed. Baltimore, MD: Lippincott Williams & Wilkins, 2009.

Andersen, J. C. Stretching before and after exercise: Effect on muscle soreness and injury risk. *Journal of Athletic Training*, 40;2005: 218–220.

Johnson, April. Indications, Contraindications, and Instructions on PNF Stretches (2007). Retrieved November 2010 from www.associatedcontent.com/article/340274/indications_contraindications_and_instructions.html

Kurz, Thomas. *Stretching Scientifically: A Guide to Flexibility Training*, 4th ed. Island Pond, VT: Stadion Publishing Company, 2003.

Mattes, Aaron L. *Active Isolated Stretching: The Mattes Method*. Sarasota, FL: Aaron L. Mattes, 2006.

Mayo Clinic. Stretching: Focus on Flexibility (2009). Retrieved November 2010 from www.mayoclinic.com/health/stretching/HQ01447.

McAtee, Robert, and Jeff Charland. *Facilitated Stretching*, 3rd ed. Champaign, IL: Human Kinetics, 2007.

Muscolino, Joseph E. *Kinesiology: The Skeletal System and Muscle Function*, 2nd ed. St. Louis, MO: Elsevier Mosby, 2011.

National Strength and Conditioning Association. *Essentials of Strength Training and Conditioning*, 3rd ed. Champaign, IL: Human Kinetics, 2008.

Run the Planet. Factors Limiting Flexibility (2010). Retrieved November 2010 from www.runtheplanet.com/trainingracing/stretching/chap2-limitingfactors.asp.

Tortora, Gerard J., and Bryan Derrickson. *Principles of Anatomy and Physiology*, 12th ed. Hoboken, NJ: John Wiley & Sons, 2009.

Voss, Dorothy E., Marjorie K. Ionta, and Beverly J. Myers. *Proprioceptive Neuromuscular Facilitation*. Baltimore, MD: Lippincott Williams & Wilkins, 1985.

Strengthening: Why, How, When, and Where?

Key Terms

Aerobic
All-or-none response
Cross-training
Fast-twitch muscle fibers
Heart rate
Overtraining
Rating of perceived
  exertion (RPE)
Recruitment
Slow-twitch muscle fibers
Target heart rate (THR)
Weight bearing

Learning Objectives

After studying this chapter, the reader will have the information to:

1. Explain the importance of strength training for health and career longevity in the bodywork profession.
2. Describe an integrated approach to exercise, explain what cross-training is, and know how to prevent overtraining.
3. Explain what aerobic exercise is and list the benefits of doing it.
4. Describe important factors for starting aerobic exercise.
5. Explain how to calculate target heart rate, and how to determine heart rate during exercise.
6. Explain the physiological basis of body strength.
7. Describe the differences between cardiac, smooth, and skeletal muscle tissue.
8. List guidelines to follow when starting a strengthening program.
9. Evaluate how various pieces of equipment and tools can be used during a strengthening program.
10. Integrate a strengthening protocol into daily life.

"Take care of your body. It's the only place you have to live."
—Jim Rohn

INTRODUCTION

According to the Surgeon General's Report, physical inactivity is just about as big a risk factor for coronary heart disease as smoking, hypertension, and high serum cholesterol (surgeongeneral.gov, 2009). In addition to cardiovascular concerns, lack of adequate muscular strength and a decrease in bone density due to aging are definite health concerns of the general population. For bodywork practitioners, whose primary methods of providing treatments are through the use of their bodies, building and maintaining musculoskeletal strength is of utmost importance. Being fit and strong gives practitioners the stamina they need to perform treatments, reduces their risk of injury, and gives them overall health and well-being. All of this adds up to career success and career longevity and provides more quality of life outside of work.

Recall from Chapter 7 the importance of balanced physical fitness and how it can affect career longevity. There are three key components to this balance, and all are equally important:

- Flexibility
- Aerobic activity
- Strength training

AN INTEGRATED APPROACH TO EXERCISE

The act of exercise is not in itself training. While it is certainly an integral part of it, training, including all of the key components discussed in previous chapters, is part of the process of a wellness lifestyle that will lead to career longevity. There are several ways that you can integrate exercise into your lifestyle and several methods that will enhance your workout efforts:

- Heavy resistance training. This involves using dumbbells, barbells, elastic tubing, and so forth, to provide "heavy" external resistance to your musculoskeletal system. Exercises performed with dumbbells and barbells and workout equipment such as exercise bands or exercise tubing that simulates traditional dumbbell and barbell movements constitute weight training.
- Light resistance training. Running, swimming, cycling, rowing, stair climbing, calisthenics, and aerobic dance are all examples of light resistance training. This form of exercise uses your body weight as the sole source of resistance.
- Psychological techniques. Self-hypnosis, mental imagery training, meditation, and other methods of focusing can help improve your strength output, especially the amount needed for the physically demanding job of bodywork. Intense concentration is not necessary *all* the time. This can lead to mental burnout as easily as physical burnout. For example, an Olympic runner does not concentrate on form and speed every time she trains. Sometimes, she just runs for the joy of it. Likewise in exercise, there is no need to visualize every motion of every strength-training movement. To maintain the power of intense concentration, it should be done at selected times, not during every workout.
- Therapeutic modalities. Whirlpool baths, massage and other bodywork modalities, ultrasound, and music are some examples of modalities that can enhance your exercise efforts, both indirectly and directly.
- Medical support. Periodic checkups, preventive care, chiropractic adjustments, and even certain medications prescribed by health-care providers may be necessary when medical problems arise during an exercise program.
- Biomechanics (skills training). Performing techniques or skills optimally almost always results in greater force (meaning increased strength) being applied, whether you are applying it to a piece of equipment, a client, an opponent in sports, or against gravity. Skillful performance involves using prime movers, stabilizers, and synergistic muscles in an efficient and effective manner.

- Healthy diet. Eating healthy helps ensure increased muscle strength both immediately and over time. Practitioners who are engaging in exercise programs are encouraged to see nutritional specialists to design healthy, balanced diets. More about this is presented in Chapter 9.
- Nutritional supplements. The average American diet is often lacking in some of the nutrients needed to build and maintain strength. Practitioners who are engaging in exercise programs are encouraged to see nutritional counselors to determine what may be lacking in their diets. More about this is presented in Chapter 9.

CROSS-TRAINING

Cross-training means using several modes of training to develop a specific component of fitness. It is an effective approach for maximizing fitness levels while minimizing the risk of being injured. By combining modes of exercise, the same muscle groups and bones are not stressed over and over. The repetition of a given activity over an extended period of time can lead to minor or even major musculoskeletal issues. In other words, cross-training reduces the likelihood of being injured by decreasing the likelihood of overtraining or overstressing a given bone or muscle.

Cross-training can also make exercising more fun. Doing different types of exercises means less chance of boredom with a given routine. Having variety in an exercise program also increases the chances of sticking with it.

Myth: If I stay consistent with my program, no matter what, I will eventually have success.

FACT: Many times people stick faithfully to a program that is not producing results, hoping to suddenly see results. As obvious as it may seem, if you continue to do the same thing, you will continue to get the same results. If you are not consistently seeing results on a monthly basis, you need to reassess your exercise regimen.

AEROBIC ACTIVITY

Under all circumstances, the body strives to meet the energy requirements placed on it in the most efficient manner possible. When muscles need oxygen, the cardiovascular system must be able to efficiently deliver it to them. When there is an increase in

Voice of Experience

In the bodywork profession, business rarely remains at the same steady level throughout the entire year. There are busy times and slow times, particularly if you work in a spa or resort setting. You need to be able to handle the busy seasons without wrecking yourself. We treat people with all manner of aching muscles; bad backs, necks, and shoulders; carpal tunnel syndrome, lateral and medial humeral epicondylosis thoracic outlet syndrome; and other orthopedic conditions. If bodywork practitioners don't practice a self-care plan, they are likely to wind up with some of the same conditions as those of their clients. I've known plenty of practitioners who stopped doing bodywork because their bodies couldn't take it.

If you are going to have a lengthy, injury-free career, you have to approach it like you are training for an athletic event—the athletic event being your workday. In fact, as a bodywork practitioner, you are working as an *industrial athlete*, similar to any profession involving physical labor. In order to last, you need to build strength, stamina, endurance, and flexibility. As a sports massage therapist and trainer, a number of my clients are also practitioners who are seeking to get strong and in shape and stay that way so that they will be up to the physical demands of their profession. We focus on building functional strength using weights, resistance bands, and plyometric exercises; increasing stamina and endurance conditioning through running, rowing, biking, and swimming; and increasing flexibility through the use of self-stretching and assisted-stretching routines.

Self-care is an extremely important part of what we do. For your own self-care, develop and maintain an exercise routine that addresses building strength, increasing endurance, and improving flexibility. In addition to all the other important benefits of exercise, you will begin to find those busy, heavily booked days and weeks a much less daunting prospect.

Eric Mackey, BA, CSCS, NCTMB, LMT. Certified personal trainer, CrossFit certified trainer, co-owner of Wildcat CrossFit, Tucson, AZ, and owner of Sonoran Athletic Therapies. Licensed massage therapist since 2004.

and lungs can be strengthened while they effectively distribute nutrients and oxygen to tissues and take away wastes. Performing aerobic exercise regularly has many other health benefits as well. The following illustrates the links among fitness, wellness, and career longevity:

- It burns body fat. Engaging in aerobic exercise can burn up to 1,000 calories an hour, depending on the type and intensity of the activity. Practitioners who want to reduce their level of body fat can use this positive, user-friendly option over trying to starve the weight off (a risky and unhealthy way to lose pounds and inches). Being more lean and fit increases a practitioner's mobility, strength, and stamina, and makes it easier to perform bodywork techniques. Adhering to sound nutritional principles and practices (discussed in Chapter 9) increase the body's ability to burn fat while performing aerobic exercise. These principles and practices are also a much better way to maintain health.

- It increases life span. Research indicates that for every hour spent exercising aerobically, life is extended 2 hours. That is an extremely good return on investment. Aerobic exercise also can improve quality and the quantity of life. For practitioners, this means being able to perform treatments, and perform them well, for a great many years with a reduced chance of injury.

- It increases energy levels. The old adage "Add life to your years, as well as years to life, by exercise" has considerable merit. A properly designed aerobic exercise program gives practitioners more energy to do the activities they enjoy, including performing bodywork.

- It aids in relieving depression. In her book *Mental Skills for Physical People*, Dr. Dorothy V. Harris concluded that "exercise is nature's best tranquilizer." For example, researchers have found that individuals suffering from moderate to light depression typically experience a dramatic improvement in their condition when they engage in aerobic exercise for 20 to 30 minutes at least every other day.

- It enhances self-image. Research has shown that people who exercise regularly feel better about themselves than do sedentary people. This can add to practitioners' self-confidence, increasing their chances of career success.

- It relieves stress and anxiety. Exercise dissipates the stress hormones (adrenaline and corticosteroids,

wastes (such as carbon dioxide and other metabolic by-products) from increased muscular activity, the respiratory and cardiovascular systems must be up to the task. This is the functional basis of **aerobic** fitness. *Aerobic* means "with oxygen."

Aerobic fitness, activity, or exercise is generally meant to be performed at a moderate level of intensity for extended periods of time. This way the heart

the most common of which is cortisol) and other chemicals that build up during periods of high stress. Exercise also generates a period of substantial emotional and physical relaxation that sets in approximately an hour and a half after an intense workout. Therefore, exercise is a great way to prepare for a long workday or to unwind afterward. It can help put practitioners in a better mood and mind-set for dealing with the day-to-day issues involved in maintaining a bodywork practice. It can also help them focus on the larger, more complicated matters that arise, such as how to expand their practice or choose what marketing methods to use.

- It slows the aging process. Aerobic exercise strengthens the body and counterbalances the decrease in cardiovascular efficiency and loss of muscle strength that typically occurs with aging. Aerobic exercise helps maintain and sustain the ability to perform work and to be independent. This is essential for a long and successful career in bodywork.

- It improves quality of sleep. Researchers have found that exercisers go to sleep more quickly, sleep more soundly, and are more refreshed than individuals who do not exercise. Sleep is essential for the body and mind to recuperate from the stresses of life and work. Having enough sleep helps practitioners perform bodywork treatments effectively, which enhances career success.

- It improves mental sharpness. Numerous studies have shown that individuals who exercise regularly have better memories, better reaction times, and a better level of concentration than those who do not exercise. Mental sharpness is essential for building rapport with clients, performing client-centered treatments, maintaining a successful bodywork practice, and making wise decisions for career longevity (Dinas, Koutedakis, and Flouris, 2010; Mayo Clinic, 2010; nami.org, 2010; U.S. Department of Health & Human Services, 2008).

Body Awareness

Do you or have you participated in aerobic exercise? What type and for how long? How did you feel while you were doing it? Did you find it beneficial? Why or why not?

IS AEROBIC EXERCISE REALLY NECESSARY?

Some practitioners may be skeptical about the need for and the benefits of aerobic training. Perhaps they are interested in only one particular aspect of exercise, such as well-defined muscles. Others may be naturally thin and so think their level of fitness is just fine. Or they may be young with bodies that function perfectly and think their bodies will always remain this way. Yet others may think it takes too much time, effort, and money, and as long as they can perform their bodywork treatments, there is no need to change anything.

There are many myths and misconceptions about the hows and whys of aerobic training. It is important to be able to separate myths from facts regarding aerobic fitness. This list includes the most common myths about aerobic fitness:

Myth: Aerobic fitness is not important for everyone.

FACT: Everyone needs to be able to efficiently take oxygen into their lungs and blood and have their heart pump it to their working muscles, where it is used to metabolize carbohydrates and fats to produce energy.

Myth: All time spent exercising aerobically would be better used in strength training.

FACT: Aerobic fitness is among the most preventative medicines available. How strong the individual is, how well sculpted her body is, and how good she feels about herself does not make much difference if she becomes seriously ill. While muscular fitness is certainly important, aerobic fitness is just as essential as the other components of fitness—flexibility and strength training.

Myth: Aerobic training improves only the cardiovascular and respiratory systems, not the muscular system.

FACT: The muscles are the primary target of aerobic training, which increases the muscles' ability to use fat as a source of energy. It also increases the size and number of mitochondria (the organelle inside cells that produces energy the cells use) within each muscle fiber and increases the levels of muscle enzymes required for the aerobic transformation of glucose (a simple carbohydrate) into energy. Aerobic training improves the condition and efficiency of the breathing muscles and the heart (undoubtedly the most important muscle in the body). Therefore, in aerobic fitness, muscles do matter.

Myth: The best aerobic exercise is running.

FACT: The best aerobic exercise for an individual is one that he enjoys, one that is safe for him, and one that he will perform regularly. It is best that practitioners choose an aerobic activity that they like—using a stair-climber or a treadmill, swimming, cycling, and so forth—and make it a regular part of their workout regimen.

Myth: Aerobic exercise is expensive.

FACT: The costs for aerobic training can range from inexpensive to costly, depending on the chosen activity. Many aerobic activities such as walking and running require little or no equipment. However, if you choose to run, then you will need good running shoes. They usually range from $50 to $150. A fitness club membership may be necessary if you choose to swim or use exercise equipment such as a stair-climber. The costs for those who prefer to cycle depend on the type and quality of bicycle they want to use. It is possible to get just as good an aerobic workout on a low-cost bicycle as on one that costs hundreds of dollars.

Myth: Aerobic training is extremely time-consuming.

FACT: Most exercise scientists recommend exercising aerobically 20 to 30 minutes per workout. Some practitioners may choose to exercise for longer periods of time, but such a time commitment does not appear to be necessary.

Myth: Aerobic fitness is achieved by raising the **heart rate** (the number of times the heart beats per minute).

FACT: Aerobic fitness involves elevating the metabolic rate and oxygen consumption in the muscles; the elevation needs to be maintained long enough for the aerobic enzymes to burn through the supply of glucose in the muscle. Raising the heart rate is only a by-product of this process.

Myth: The harder you exercise, the faster your level of aerobic fitness will improve.

FACT: Exercise scientists suggest that the best way to approach aerobic conditioning is "to make haste slowly." Trying to do too much, too soon will usually result in either injury or discouragement. It takes time for the body to adapt to the physiological changes needed for optimal aerobic fitness. It is recommended to perform aerobic exercise at an intensity level ranging from 55% to 85% of the maximum heart rate. Those who are quite aerobically fit should be at the higher end of the range, and those who are just beginning should be at the lower end of the range. This is discussed in more detail in the "Exercise Intensity" section.

Myth: The joints need to be sacrificed for the heart.

FACT: Not all aerobic activities involve orthopedic trauma, commonly known as high-impact exercises. Three popular aerobic activities are non-impact: cycling, rowing, and independent stair-climbing. In independent stair-climbing machines, each foot has its own stepper (as opposed to machines in which both feet step off one step). Independent steppers replicate the user's normal movement patterns. Compared to cycling and rowing, independent stair-climbing not only eliminates the stress on skeletal joints (because it replicates normal movement patterns, the person can step as high or low as he wants) but it also offers the additional and critical advantage of being a **weight-bearing** activity. Weight-bearing exercise increases the strength of the bones because it requires muscles to work against gravity, and muscles are, of course, attached to bones.

Myth: It may be too late to begin an aerobic training program.

FACT: The benefits of aerobic fitness can be gained regardless of how sedentary a lifestyle an individual has had previously. The initial level of fitness influences the rate of aerobic improvement. In fact, the less active and fit an individual is, the faster she will improve aerobically. Gains in health occur immediately. For example, even a 70-year-old person can expect a substantial improvement of about 10% in aerobic fitness from regular exercise. In short, it is never too late.

CHOOSING AN AEROBIC ACTIVITY

In order for an activity to be considered aerobic, it needs to be rhythmic and continuous for at least 20 minutes. It also needs to involve a large percentage of the body's muscle mass. Examples include walking, jogging, swimming, cycling, rowing, circuit training, and cross-country skiing. Activities such as playing golf and football are not considered aerobic because of their start-stop nature. Singles tennis can be aerobic if it does not have a lot of starts and stops; doubles tennis is not aerobic. Walking a dog may be aerobic if the dog walks continuously, but not if he pauses frequently to check out his surroundings.

Deciding what type of aerobic exercise is best for you may be easier said than done. In reality, not all forms of aerobic exercise offer the same features and benefits to everyone. Some aerobic exercises are safer to perform for certain people than others. For example, for someone with joint issues, swimming is a safer exercise than running. Aerobic activity that one person finds exciting may be boring to someone else. Some activities enhance more than one aspect of fitness at a time. For example, rowing builds muscular strength while building cardiovascular and respiratory strength. Cost may also be an issue. A practitioner may want to join a fitness club and use a variety of aerobic training machines but may have a budget for only a good pair of athletic shoes and so must walk or run instead.

Some activities involve a slightly longer learning curve than others. For example, it may take a while to master the skills involved in rowing or cross-country skiing. The aerobic exercise equipment of choice may require upkeep, such as a particular machine for home use or a bicycle. Some pieces of equipment will withstand greater use, such as a rowing machine, whereas others will need to be replaced periodically, such as running shoes.

For the best exercise results, the key is making an informed decision about what type of aerobic exercise is best for *you*. Such a decision involves taking the time to evaluate the advantages and disadvantages of each exercise option and determining the impact on your interests and needs. In other words, do your homework to find out what is the most interesting and cost-effective aerobic exercise for you to do.

HOW TO GET STARTED

Before beginning any fitness program, you should consult with your physician to see if you have any contraindications for the exercises and to find out what levels of activity are best for you to start with. Here are suggested guidelines when beginning an aerobic program:

- If you choose walking or running, purchase a pair of supportive walking or running shoes and use them *only* for your aerobic exercise. This helps protect your ankle, knee, and hip joints.
- If you are walking or running, purchase a pedometer, which will track the number of steps you take. Set a goal of at least 10,000 steps (2,000 to 2,500 steps equal about 1 mile. This burns about 100 calories for a 150-pound person).
- If you are walking or running, walk on relatively flat areas for the first month or so. Hills require more effort from your heart and joints.
- Avoid walking during the hottest or coldest parts of the day.
  - In hotter weather, staying hydrated can be more challenging, potentially giving rise to heat sickness. Your heart rate will naturally go up 1 beat per minute for each degree above 77°F. Therefore, while you may not be going faster, your body is working harder.
  - In colder weather, muscles may be more prone to injury. Breathing in cold air tends to dehydrate the body, so staying hydrated, even though you are not thirsty, can also be a problem. In areas that get snow, there are also the dangers of slipping on icy surfaces and frostbite, especially on the nose, cheeks, and ears.
- If you are walking or running, do so slowly as you warm up for 5 minutes. Another way to warm up is to perform the dynamic movements presented in Chapter 7.
- Increase your activity for the next 20 minutes. To see how hard you are working, one rule of thumb is if you can sing while performing the aerobic activity, you need to work harder and faster, and if you have difficulty carrying on a conversation, you need to work less hard and slow down.
- Stretch after your aerobic activity. Use the stretches presented in Chapter 7.

What Do You Think?

What aerobic activity appeals to you most? Why? Are you likely to do this activity? Why or why not?

- After your activity, perform the cooldown presented in Chapter 7.
- Do your aerobic activity three to five times weekly, and increase your distance or speed over a few months.
- If you have been ill or are considerably out of shape, perform your aerobic activity for only 10 minutes. Increase by 5 minutes every week so you can follow the suggestions listed above. Monitoring your increase in exercise is important

to avoid injury. Consider journaling or using your Wellness Plan to measure your progress.

You can still gain aerobic benefits if you do not have 20 or 30 minutes available in one time frame. For example, if you can walk for 10 minutes three or four times daily, you reap some of the same benefits as from a sustained 30-minute walk. However, this method is more beneficial for burning fat than significantly increasing aerobic capacity.

Focus on Wellness

Scan the shelves of any sports equipment store, and it would seem that there are more types of athletic shoes than there are sports for which to wear them. However, all that specialization does matter because you need to wear the best shoe, not only for your chosen activity, but also for *you*. This means you should consider your foot size, shape, and how you habitually run, walk, jump, and land. No matter what you need, there is a shoe out there just for you—and you can learn how to find it.

Try shoes on late in the day; if you go in the morning, your foot will be smaller and tighter than it is after a day of walking around. You do not want shoes that fit fine in the store but become too small after you wear them all day. Also, when buying the shoes, wear socks you will wear when you exercise in the shoes. The correct shoe fit takes the sock size and thickness into account.

Before going shoe shopping, it is helpful to know a few terms. A *neutral foot strike* means the heel and ball land evenly, with no rotation of the ankle. People who *overpronate* or *overevert* (they often have flat or fallen arches) tend to roll the ankle too far medially. People who *underpronate* or *underevert* (who often have high arches and stiff feet) do not have enough flexibility in their stride. Ankle and arch support issues permeate all activities so, if possible, have an expert watch your walking and running stride to determine if you over- or underpronate. More about how to determine what type of arch you have is discussed in Chapter 10.

Perhaps the greatest variety of shoes exists for runners. Because good foot motion is so important to prevent injury for runners, it is imperative that you find a shoe that provides exactly what you need. Motion-control running shoes are often the sturdiest, and thus the heaviest, of the running shoes on the market. They provide solid arch

curvature for those with flatter feet and help keep the ankle from rolling too far when the heel strikes. If you overpronate or have fallen arches, look for shoes with strong motion control.

If you have high arches, you should investigate cushioning shoes. These are built on a curved last. A last is a form in the shape of a human foot used in the manufacture of shoes; a curved last curves medially at the insole. The shoes also have padding in the heel or under the ball of the foot. These features encourage a rolling motion through the heel strike to the ball push-off.

If you are a neutral strider, you can find excellent shoes that offer a middle level of cushioning, motion control, and stability that will encourage an efficient running motion without providing too much extra support. Stability shoes are lighter than motion-control runners but are a bit heavier than cushioning runners.

The average runner will often find stability shoes to be the most comfortable, because they do not create a particular stride motion. However, if you run at an elite level, you will probably focus most on the shoe's weight and be drawn to lightweight training shoes. Some of these incorporate motion-control or cushioning aspects, but mostly they tend to sacrifice therapeutic controls to become as light as possible. Severe over- or underpronators should not look into lightweight shoes, but average striders should be quite comfortable in them.

The same concerns exist for walking shoes, but you need to consider the anatomical differences of walking. Because the foot is in contact with the ground longer, and because the motion creates a different type of impact, walkers often feel soreness in the lower back rather than in the knee. While pronation is still a key factor in buying the correct shoe, the types of shoes offered for walking vary greatly from those marketed for running. Walking shoes tend to be stiffer overall than running shoes, with greater cushioning in the ball, even for motion-control shoes. You need to find a shoe that does have some flexibility, because the walking stride requires a rolling action from the heel throw to the toe box. Many advanced walkers seek out a shoe with a heel that is flat relative to the ball, because it promotes that rolling motion and eases lower back strain.

Cross-training shoes take an entirely different motion into consideration. You want a pair of cross-trainers if you take aerobic classes that involve any lateral (sideways) motion in addition to impact, such as step or kickboxing. Running or walking shoes are built for the forward motion of running and do not provide any ankle stability for side-to-side motion; only cross-trainers are designed to prevent injury and support lateral moves. You should also wear cross-trainers when weight lifting, because they provide the most multidirectional support. Most cross-trainers have a wider outsole than running or walking shoes, which contributes to their excellent stability for lateral motion. This type of shoe is a great choice for bodywork practitioners (discussed in more detail in Chapter 10).

The last type of specialized shoe you might seek out is a basketball shoe. These shoes are a combination of a running, walking, and cross-training shoe. Basketball involves running, stopping, jumping, and sliding, so basketball shoes must provide flexibility, support, stability, and lateral control. If you are a competitive basketball player, you will want more shock absorption than a recreational player, who will need more support and stability. Find a shoe with the kind of pronation control you need, and consider other features after that.

Of course, buying the right size of any athletic shoe will provide the key to the best fit. Have your foot measured professionally, and seek out a shoe built on a narrow or wide last if you have a foot that is not average width. Take your shoes for a test drive—if you are a runner, jog around the store, if possible with a shoe specialist watching your stride in your original shoes and then in the shoes you are testing. Make sure that the shoe is comfortable and supportive in movement. After you buy your new shoes, take care of them. Do not wear a running shoe for a kickboxing class or a walking shoe to shoot hoops with your friends.

Buying exercise shoes is something most people do *too* seldom. Wearing worn-out exercise shoes is one of the main causes of exercise injuries. If you have a few pairs of exercise shoes that you trade off wearing, than your shoes will last longer. The average time is 7 months if you exercise 5 to 6 days per week, or 300 to 400 miles of walking or running. If you wear one pair of shoes, they generally lose their effectiveness after about 3 to 4 months if you exercise 5 to 6 days a week. If you exercise only 3 days per week, your shoes may last a bit longer.

Consider keeping the receipt for your exercise shoes: You will have the receipt if you need to return the shoes, and you will have the date to refer to for the age of your shoes. You can write the day on your calendar as well. Find a way to post the date you started wearing your shoes so you will have something to refer to when it is time to get new exercise shoes.

EXERCISE INTENSITY

Perhaps the most important component of fitness is the level of exercise intensity. The best level of intensity is one that is sufficient to overload the cardiovascular system but is not so severe that it overtaxes any of the other body systems. As previously discussed, one way to do this is to have your heart rate be between 55% and 85% of your maximum heart rate. This is called **target heart rate (THR)**. This level means the optimal amount of oxygen can be transported to your muscles during the activity. Again, those who have been relatively sedentary should keep their heart rate at the lower end of the scale, and those who have good aerobic conditioning should keep their heart rate at the higher end of the scale.

During exercise, the heart beats faster to meet the demands of the muscles for more blood and oxygen. The more intense the exercise, the faster the heart beats. Therefore, monitoring heart rate during exercise accurately reflects how efficiently you are exercising.

In order to calculate THR, you must first calculate your maximal heart rate. This is done with the following formula.

For a low estimate:

$$\text{Maximal heart rate (HR)} = 220 - \text{age}$$

or for a high estimate:

$$\text{Maximal heart rate (HR)} = 210 - (0.5 \times \text{age})$$

In the formula, 220 is the maximum rate any human heart can beat. Therefore, your safe maximal heart rate is calculated by subtracting your age from 220 for a low estimated maximal heart rate. If you are a well-trained athlete, then it is safe for you to have a higher maximal heart rate. This is calculated by subtracting half of your age from 210.

For example, Helen is a 35-year-old shiatsu practitioner who is beginning an aerobic fitness program for the first time. Her maximal heart rate should be a low estimate:

Helen's maximal HR = 220 − 35 (Helen's age)
Helen's maximal HR is 185.

Gordon is a 24-year-old craniosacral therapist who is also a triathlete. His maximal heart rate should be a high estimate:

Gordon's maximal HR = 210 − (0.5 × 24)
Gordon's maximal HR = 210 − 12
Gordon's maximal HR = 198

After calculating maximal HR, you can calculate THR using the following formula:

THR range = maximal HR × 0.55 (low end of the range) to 0.85 (high end of the range)

Since Helen is just beginning her aerobic fitness program, she should calculate her THR this way:

THR = maximal HR × 0.55
Helen's THR = 185 × .55
Helen's THR = 101.8 which can be rounded off to 102

Since Gordon is already quite fit aerobically, he should calculate his THR this way:

THR = maximal HR × 0.85
Gordon's THR = 198 × .85
Gordon's THR = 168.3 which can be rounded off to 168

Another way to measure exercise intensity is to use **rating of perceived exertion (RPE)**. *Perceived exertion* refers to the physical strain individuals believe they are experiencing while exercising. Perceived exertion feedback is helpful because it is a practical way for you to realize what your exercise intensity should be. During exercise, your perception of your effort is influenced by a variety of cues, such as feeling muscular discomfort or strain, your heart rate, your breathing rate, and so forth.

Figure 8-1 is the Borg RPE scale. It is named after its developer, Swedish psychologist Gunnar Borg. His numbering system closely correlates to heart rate. When a "0" is added to each category number, the result is a range of numbers comparable to the target heart range. Practitioners using

Body Awareness

According to the American Heart Association (AHA), the following table shows estimated target heart rates (HR) for different ages. Look for the age category, and then read across to find your target heart rate.

Age (in years)	Target Heart Rate Zone 50–85% (beats per minute)	Average Maximum Heart Rate 100% (beats per minute)
20	100-170	200
25	98-166	195
30	95-162	190
35	93-157	185
40	90-153	180
45	88-149	175
50	85-145	170
55	83-140	165
60	80-136	160
65	78-132	155
70	75-128	150

(American Heart Association, 2010)

Remember, your maximum heart rate is 220 minus your age. This table depicts averages, so use them as general guidelines.

Note: A few high blood pressure medications lower the maximum heart rate and thus the target zone rate. If you are taking such medicine, contact your physician to find out if you need to use a lower target heart rate.

RPE to monitor their exercise intensity decide which verbal description of the *perceived exertion during exercise* matches what they are experiencing, and they can see if the rating matches their THR.

BORG RPE SCALE	
Rating	Perceived Exertion During Exercise
6	Very, very light
7	Very, very light
8	Very, very light
9	Very light
10	Very light
11	Fairly light
12	Fairly light
13	Somewhat hard
14	Somewhat hard
15	Hard
16	Hard
17	Very hard
18	Very hard
19	Very, very hard
20	Very, very hard

FIGURE 8-1 Borg RPE scale.

Checking Target Heart Rate During Exercise

To ensure that you are staying at your target heart rate during exercise, you can purchase a heart rate monitor (Fig. 8-2). An alternative is to take your pulse periodically while exercising to check your heart rate.

The pulse can be taken at areas of the body where arteries are superficial enough that the surge of blood coming out of the heart can be palpated. Figure 8-3A shows the pulse points of the body. When taking the pulse, the thumb should not be used because there is a pulse at its tip. Instead, place the index and middle finger over the area until you feel the pulse (see Fig. 8-3B for the pulse being taken over the common carotid artery). Once the pulse is felt, it should be timed for 10, 20, 30, or 60 seconds. If it is timed for 10 seconds, the number of pulses felt should be multiplied by 6 to calculate the number of beats in 60 seconds. If the pulse is timed for 20 seconds, the number of pulses should be multiplied by 3; if the pulse is timed for 30 seconds, the number of pulses should be multiplied by 2.

Tips for counting the number of pulses include:

- When you start timing the pulses, the first one felt should be counted as "0," the second one as "1," the third one as "2," and so forth. Otherwise, the pulse count will be one more than actually occurred.
- When exercising, do not take your pulse at the radial artery (wrist). Exercise causes such a surge of blood through the upper extremities that both hands and all the fingers will be pulsing, so it is

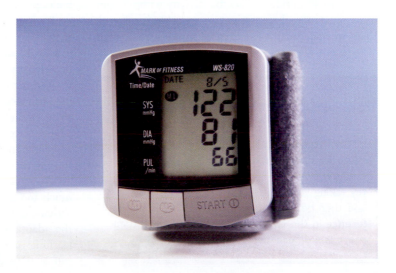

FIGURE 8-2 Heart rate monitor.

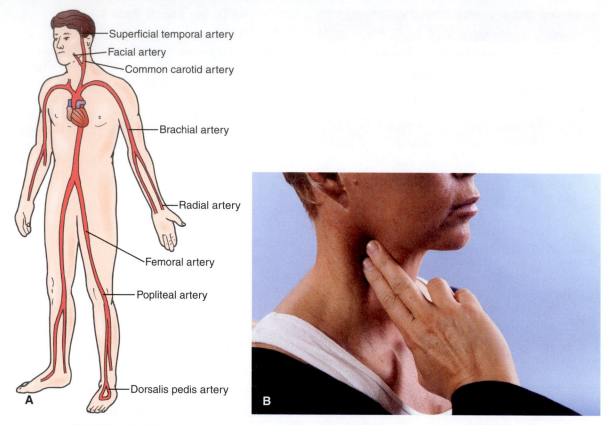

FIGURE 8-3 (A) Pulse points of the body. **(B)** Taking the pulse over the common carotid artery.

impossible to feel the pulse at the wrist. It is better to take the pulse at the common carotid artery because it has quite a strong pulse due to its proximity to the heart.

Injury Prevention

Twenty to 45 minutes of aerobic activity within target heart rate range, three to five times weekly, is optimal. Keep in mind that most exercise injuries occur with an increase of intensity or duration. For example, if an individual is accustomed to walking a mile in 20 minutes but feels good and chooses to walk that mile in 15 minutes, he might be at a higher risk for injury. There is an even greater risk if he chooses to walk faster and twice as long, say 40 minutes. Gradual buildup is the best way to proceed. For example, if you walk a mile in 20 minutes, the next time you walk, try to decrease your time by 2 minutes, thus walking your mile in 18 minutes. If this proves to be too much, try decreasing your time in 1-minute increments.

Another caution is for resuming exercise after having been sick or discontinuing for some other reason. When resuming aerobic activity, it is better to start at a much lower intensity and duration to rebuild stamina and endurance over a few weeks. This greatly decreases the chance of injury after being sedentary for a while.

Overtraining can lead to overuse, or doing too much too fast. When the body is faced with a new activity, it does its best to adapt to the challenge, but the adaptation takes time, whether it is exercise or learning new bodywork techniques. Overtraining can lead to chronic injuries. It takes time for the

Body Awareness

Have you ever calculated your target heart rate? If not, try it right now. Have you ever taken your pulse? If not, try it right now. Also, try taking your pulse first thing in the morning and then before you go to bed. What is the difference in the two readings? Why do you think there is a difference?

bones, tendons, and muscles to adapt to the stress of workouts. How much you exercise really comes down to being able to listen to your body and make adaptations in your workouts as needed. This will help you remain injury-free to ensure your career longevity. This is discussed in more detail in the section "over training."

It is important to watch for warning signs during aerobic activity. These include:

- Angina, which is a feeling of squeezing, burning, pressure, heaviness, or tightness under the breastbone that may spread to your left arm or shoulder, back, throat, or jaw. Angina goes away when you stop exerting yourself. However, if the sensations continue after you stop exercising, you may have a more serious heart issue.
- Feeling light-headed, dizzy, or confused.
- Feeling extremely tired after physical activity.
- Unusual or extreme shortness of breath.
- Fast or uneven heartbeat.
- Any of the above accompanied by nausea and sweating.

If you experience these signs during or after physical activity, you need to see your physician immediately. If you cannot get in to see your physician immediately, call either 911 or have someone take you to the nearest emergency room.

STRENGTH CONDITIONING

As discussed in previous chapters, bodywork practitioners use the lower extremities and core muscles in the performance of techniques. It is extremely important that these muscles and muscle groups are strong in order to withstand long treatment days and all ADL. Strength conditioning for the entire body is another way to help remain injury-free, reduce fatigue, increase stamina, and help use body weight instead of muscular strength during treatments.

In this section, the focus is on muscles of the lower extremity and core muscles. Also included are some strengthening exercises for the upper body for muscular balance. Presented are ways to strength condition using no equipment and exercises using equipment such as weights, exercise balls, and elastic tubing. As always, you should consult with your physician before starting any exercise program.

WHAT IS STRENGTH?

Strength is defined as the ability to exert musculoskeletal force against an external object such as a barbell, the ground, or an opponent (as in sports or combat). Strength comes from four main sources:

1. The construction and physiology of the body
2. The body's internal systems working together to create energy and promote repair, remodeling, and growth in response to training
3. Skills, attitudes, belief systems, and tolerance to pain that can interconnect to ensure the body functions at peak efficiency
4. Factors external to the body such as weather, gravity, and equipment that can be used to produce greater force output

PHYSIOLOGICAL BASIS OF STRENGTH

The human body is an efficient machine. All body movements—walking, running, and even circulating blood—depend upon the actions of muscles. Over 600 muscles work together with the support of the skeletal system to create motion. An additional 30 or so muscles are required to ensure the passage of food through the digestive system, to circulate blood, and to operate specific internal organs such as the contraction of the bladder to expel urine.

Types of Muscle Tissue

Because of their underlying cellular structure, muscles differ in appearance when observed under the microscope. Two appearances are recognized: striated (striped) muscle tissue and smooth (not striped) muscle tissue. Based on functional and structural differences, muscle tissue is divided into three types (cardiac, smooth, and skeletal):

- Cardiac muscle tissue. The majority of the heart wall is made of cardiac muscle tissue. It contracts to pump blood out of the heart into blood vessels that carry it throughout the body. Cardiac muscle is involuntary (meaning it cannot be voluntarily

What Do You Think?

What do you think strength is? Why do you think this? What do you think are your body strengths?

controlled), and its cells appear striated like skeletal muscle fibers because they have the same type of sarcomeres (Fig. 8-4A). However, they are connected to each other in such a way that nerve impulses spread easily from one cardiac muscle fiber to another. This ensures synchronized contraction of the heart. Additionally, cardiac muscle contracts 10 to 15 times longer than skeletal muscle, and it does not fatigue easily; it needs only a brief period of rest in between contractions. Even during periods of intense exercise, the skeletal muscles will fatigue but cardiac muscle will not. In fact, the heart beats about 100,000 times every day, which adds up to about 35 million beats a year. This means about 2.5 billion beats in the average lifetime. It is capable of contracting continuously, without interruption, for over 100 years.

- Smooth muscle tissue. The digestive, respiratory, and genitourinary tracts all contain smooth muscle. It is also found in the walls of blood vessels and large lymphatic vessels, in gland ducts, and within the eye (the iris and ciliary body), and it is the muscle that pulls hairs upright. Smooth muscle functions to move substances along their respective tracts and ducts, change diameter of blood vessels, change the diameter of pupils and the shape of lens,

and pull hairs upright. Like cardiac muscle tissue, smooth muscle tissue cells are elongated but have pointed ends. They have thin and thick filaments, but they are not arranged in sarcomeres like skeletal muscle tissue, giving the cells a smooth appearance (Fig. 8-4B). Smooth muscle is involuntary and contracts more slowly than striated muscle; therefore, it does not fatigue easily.

- Skeletal muscle tissue. Skeletal muscle is attached to bones. It also controls the movements of the eye and moves food during the first part of swallowing in the upper third portion of the esophagus. Skeletal muscle tissue is voluntary and is made up of long muscle fibers that are striated (Fig. 8-4C). Skeletal muscle tissue cannot sustain prolonged contractions and is easily fatigued. The focus in this chapter is on the skeletal muscles (Tortora and Derrickson, 2009).

Types of Contractions

Recall from Chapter 7 the basic skeletal muscle cellular anatomy and physiology. The functional unit is the sarcomere, and associated proprioceptors are the Golgi tendon organ and the muscle spindle. The sliding filament mechanism describes how a myofibril contracts and thin filaments slide over thick filaments. Chemical bonds and receptor sites on the thin and

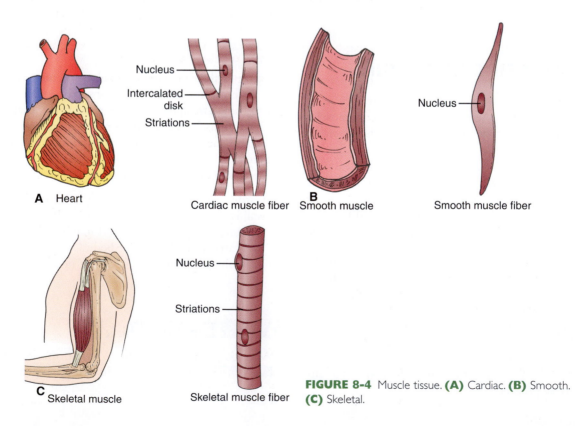

FIGURE 8-4 Muscle tissue. **(A)** Cardiac. **(B)** Smooth. **(C)** Skeletal.

thick filaments form the connection between them and maintain the contraction until fatigue interferes. The strength of contraction in a muscle depends, in large part, upon the number of muscle fibers involved: the more muscle fibers, the stronger the contraction.

When a nerve carries an impulse of sufficient magnitude down to the muscle cells it innervates, the myofibrils will do only one thing—contract. Each myofibril does not do this by degrees but rather contracts totally. This is called the **all-or-none response**. In other words, a muscle fiber is either completely relaxed or fully contracted; it is never partially contracted.

However, not all of the muscle cells in a muscle are activated during any given movement. If more muscle cells are needed to contract, such as when lifting a heavy object like a massage table or futon, then they will be stimulated. This is called **recruitment**. If few muscle cells need to contract to perform an action such as lifting a bottle of massage lotion, fewer of them will be recruited. Muscle recruitment is very rarely at 100%; it usually occurs only during absolute maximal exertions such as occurs during extreme exercise or during fight-or-flight responses.

Recall from Chapters 2 and 7 that proprioceptors are part of regulatory mechanisms that allow muscles to adjust automatically to different loads and length requirements. These sensors provide constant information to the nervous system regarding body movement and positions, speed of joint movements, and length and tension of muscles.

Recall from Chapter 3 that the term *contraction* does not always refer to the shortening of a muscle. Technically, it refers to the development of tension within a muscle. There are two major types of contractions. A contraction in which the muscle develops tension but does not shorten is called *isometric*. A contraction in which the muscle shortens but maintains constant tension is called *isotonic*. For example, a practitioner is trying to lift the limb of a client who has a larger body size but strains against the weight. The practitioner's arm muscles develop tension but do not shorten because the amount of resistance generated by the weight of the client's limb is greater than the tension generated by the practitioner's muscles. The practitioner's muscles are contracting isometrically.

However, if the client has a smaller body size, then his limb would not be as heavy. The load on the practitioner's muscles is lightened, and they can now shorten as they contract. They are contracting isotonically. Recall from Chapter 3 that when muscles shorten by overcoming resistance to a load, the isotonic contraction is considered concentric. When the muscles lengthen while contracting, such as occurs while lowering the client's limb, they maintain a constant tension during the lengthening movement. This type of isotonic contraction is considered eccentric (Tortora and Derrickson, 2009).

Energy for Muscle Contraction

The energy for muscle contraction is derived from the chemical reaction between food components and oxygen. The body's preferred source of energy is glucose, which is a type of sugar and a simple carbohydrate. All carbohydrates taken into the body are converted to glucose. Glucose can also be made from proteins and fat, either those ingested or those already in the body. The body stores a limited supply of glucose (in a form called *glycogen*), which can also be converted into proteins and lipids. This happens to a small amount of glucose daily. Usually excess glucose is changed into lipids and stored that way until the body needs it.

When the body uses glucose for energy, it is eventually broken down to just carbon dioxide and water. During this chemical breakdown, energy is released and used by muscle proteins to power contractions. This chemical reaction requires a ready supply of oxygen, which is delivered by the blood. During intense exercise, the blood supply is often insufficient to carry enough oxygen to the muscles.

The muscles solve this problem by breaking glucose down anaerobically (without oxygen), which still releases an ample amount of energy. However, one of the by-products of anaerobic metabolism of glucose is lactic acid. Some of the lactic acid can be converted into a molecule called *pyruvic acid* and can enter the mitochondria to be completely broken down for energy. However, lactic acid still accumulates. This accumulation limits the intensity at which muscles can be exercised and ultimately prevents continuation of the exercise at the same intensity. The result is fatigue.

The lactic acid eventually enters the bloodstream, typically within 45 minutes to an hour. It is circulated to the liver where it is reassembled into glucose and returned to the bloodstream, or reassembled into glycogen and stored in the liver and the skeletal muscles.

Skeletal muscles call upon this storehouse of glycogen during high-intensity, short-duration activities, such as weight lifting. This is different from the caloric draw during a low-intensity, long-duration activity, such as long-distance running, which uses a mixture of glucose from glycogen and fatty acids from lipid stores (Tortora and Derrickson, 2009).

Slow-Twitch and Fast-Twitch Muscle Fibers

Skeletal muscle tissue is composed of two general types of muscle fibers: **fast-twitch** and **slow-twitch**. The percentage of each varies from person to person and from one muscle to another in the same person.

Fast-twitch fibers are selectively recruited when heavy workloads are demanded of the muscles and strength and power are needed, such as in high-intensity, short-duration work. They contract quickly, yielding short bursts of energy, and are recruited in high numbers during brief, intense exercises such as sprinting, weight lifting, or performing the massage techniques percussion and vibration. But these fast-twitch muscle fibers exhaust quickly and are quite susceptible to injury. Pain and cramps settle in rapidly as they become vulnerable to lactic acid buildup.

Slow-twitch muscle fibers produce a steadier, low-intensity, repetitive contraction, characteristic of endurance activities. They are capable of sustaining workloads of low intensity and long duration, such as occurs during most bodywork techniques and long-distance running. Slow-twitch fibers are highly resistant to fatigue and injury, but their force output is very low.

Individuals involved in high-intensity activities, such as weight lifting, wrestling, and sprinting, tend to have a greater percentage of fast-twitch muscle fibers. Individuals who participate in low-intensity activities, such as long-distance running, tend to have a higher percentage of slow-twitch fibers (Tortora and Derrickson, 2009; University of California, San Diego, 2000).

GETTING STARTED

The body works in harmony; every system is vital to growth and development. The neuromuscular system, which includes the nervous system, joint tissues, and muscles, works together to produce movement. The brain oversees everything, the central and peripheral nervous systems deliver nerve impulses to the muscles, the muscles produce the force necessary for movement, and the connective tissues (particularly the tendons) help regulate it.

Teach the brain to ask for more and it will. Allow the rest of the nervous system to deliver more and it will. Demand the muscles to produce more and they will. Finally, ask the tendons and ligaments to allow more and they will.

Before starting any strengthening program, the following are guidelines to follow:

- Get a physical from your physician, especially if you are overweight or have not exercised in a while. In addition, if you are over 35, you should have an exercise stress test. An exercise stress test is a screening tool to test how exercise affects your heart. This typically involves walking on a treadmill or pedaling on an exercise bicycle while the electrical activity of your heart is measured with an electrocardiogram (ECG), and blood pressure readings are taken. The stress test measures your heart's reaction to your body's increased need for oxygen as you exercise. It provides an overall look at the health of your heart.

- A fitness assessment, which can be conducted by a qualified fitness professional, is the next step. This establishes a baseline of your current fitness and helps determine what sort of exercise you can safely perform. The assessment often includes simple measurements of your blood pressure and heart rate, strength, flexibility, body composition (how much body fat and lean muscle mass you have), cardiovascular endurance, exercise history, and goals and interests. A variety of assessment protocols (e.g., having you exercise on various machines) are used, and these are often repeated at regular intervals to gauge your progress. The information gathered from this assessment will determine your fitness level. Typically, if you measure fair or poor, the fitness professional will direct you to see your physician before beginning any exercise program.

Beginning an exercise routine can be vigorous and demanding, and you must be in good health to get good results.

The following are guidelines:

1. *Stick to one program, at least in the beginning.* Do not be influenced by what you read or by what your friends say. The result can be confusing information. Besides, there is no one method that works best for everyone, because everyone is different.

2. *Keep a record, like a journal.* Plan your exercise activities at the beginning of each week and write them down for each day. After each workout, write down information like the number of sets and repetitions (discussed in the "Exercise Sets and Repetition" section) and the weight used (if any) for each exercise. This eliminates guesswork and shows your progress. It can also help you identify areas

you need to work on. Figure 8-5 is an example of an exercise journal.

3. *Set goals that you can reach.* If your goals are too high, you might become discouraged or, worse, injured. On the other hand, if you set goals that are too low, you will see little progress or it will be slow, which may make you think about giving up.

4. *Set long-term goals.* Set a goal that takes perhaps a year to achieve. Then set several short-term goals that, as you reach them, show you the progress you are making. Each short-term-goal triumph can encourage you to reach the next goal. Before you know it, you will have reached your long-term goal.

5. *Put a time limit on your goals.* Do not just say, "Someday . . . ," but promise yourself that by a certain date, you will achieve a specific goal. If you have not met your goal by that date, you will then have an opportunity to determine what is working and what is not working for you so you can reschedule the achievement of that specific goal.

Here are suggestions when starting to work out:

1. *Be sure to warm up.* Recall from Chapter 7 the importance of warming up. Use the suggested warm-up in that chapter as a guide.

2. *Take it easy.* If you go to a gym, do not watch how others are working out. Sometimes this can make people think they need to be doing what others are doing, such as lifting the same weights. It can be discouraging to feel like a beginner, but if you try to do what they are doing, you increase the risk of being injured. Work at *your* optimal speed and intensity, and do not compare yourself to others.

3. *Pay attention to previous injuries.* If you are hurting, do not "work through the pain." Switch to an exercise that works the same area but is not

EXERCISE JOURNAL

DATE: ___/___/_____   WEEK: _____   DAY: _____

CARDIOVASCULAR	LEVEL/ PROGRAM		INTENSITY		DURATION/ MINUTES
CHECK ONE	CIRCLE ONE		CIRCLE ONE		CHECK ONE
☐ TREADMILL	1	2 3	BEATS/10 SEC		☐ 0–15
☐ STAIRCLIMBER	4	5 6	15 16	17	☐ 16–30
☐ STATIONARY BIKE	7	8 9	18 19	20	☐ 31–45
☐ STATIONARY ROWER	10	11 12	21 22	23	☐ 46–60
☐ AEROBIC/STEP CLASS	13	14 15	24 25	26	☐ 61–75
☐ ELLIPTICAL TRAINER			27 28	29	☐ 76–90
☐ OTHER _____	OTHER _____				

WEIGHT TRAINING										
REST BETWEEN SETS SEC: _____	SET #1		SET #2		SET #3		SET #4		SET #5	
EXERCISES	REPS	WT	REPS	WT	REPS	WT	REPS	WT	REPS	WT

FIGURE 8-5 Example of an exercise journal.

painful for you (this is where cross-training can be useful). A light, pain-free workout of an affected area gets the blood moving, helps move out metabolic wastes, and speeds healing.

4. *Do not worry about your body weight when starting.* You may actually *gain* weight at first, since muscle weighs more than fat. It takes a 3,500 calorie deficit to burn 1 pound of fat. Over time, you will lose weight and inches as you burn fat and build muscle.

5. *Do not worry about your diet when you are first starting.* It is not a good idea to change everything at the same time. If you try too many changes in lifestyle at once, it can be stressful

Focus on Wellness

The key to success in anything is to *rehearse success rather than rehearse failure.* Most of us have extremely demanding schedules but need to make time for taking care of ourselves. The strategies and skills listed here will help you learn to keep your thoughts positive and constructive, release needless tension, and redirect your attention when you become discouraged.

A simple way to practice accentuating the positive is to keep your workouts upbeat and work on positive thoughts the same way you work with your clients. Avoid thoughts like, "Things keep piling up around me, so I'll have to skip working out today," or "I'll never get things done properly, so it's better if I don't take the time to exercise." If the time you devote to exercise is the only time you have all day that is just for you, then it is important to keep your commitment to your health.

Here are some mental skills that can help you reframe negative thoughts about making those important changes in wellness necessary for a long and successful career in bodywork:

Negative Thought	Reframed Thoughts
I can't.	I can do it. I have done it many times before.
I'm tired. I can't go on.	It's almost over; I know I can finish. The hard part is over.
I'm getting worse instead of better.	I need to set daily goals and evaluate my progress on a regular basis.
I'm really nervous and anxious.	I'll be less nervous and anxious as soon as I get started.
I'm afraid I'll make a fool of myself.	I can accomplish a lot if I face the challenge. Everyone has to start somewhere.
I don't want to fail.	What is absolutely the worst that could happen to me? I could lose or not finish. If so, I'll work harder the next time.
I don't think I'm prepared.	I've been practicing and exercising, so I'm ready to do well.
I'm defeated again. I'll never be a winner.	I can learn from defeat. I need to talk with a personal trainer to get some help in the areas I need to improve.
It's not fair. I work just as hard as everyone else, but I don't do as well.	I may have to work harder than others to accomplish some things. I'm willing to work as hard as I have to because I want to succeed.
I never seem to be able to do this.	I'm going to think things through and mentally prepare myself to do this.

Accomplishment, in anything, occurs when you *focus* on a goal, ignoring outside distractions. As a bodywork practitioner, you narrow the band of attention to the task at hand such as perfecting a bodywork technique or creating an effective treatment plan for a client. You can apply this to your exercise program as well.

and you might be more likely to give up. Once you start getting encouraging results, the other things will fall into place. Be patient, stay focused, and, most importantly, never give up.

6. *Watch for the development of muscle tone.* This can be one of the first positive and exciting effects of your new exercise program.

EQUIPMENT CONSIDERATIONS

When deciding on a strength-training program, consider the use of resistance devices in your workout. These tools and pieces of equipment can be used to train more efficiently:

- Body weight. Body weight is a source of resistance in many exercises such as those to strengthen the core, wall squats, and push-ups (presented under "Strengthening Protocols"). If body weight is sufficient, it will provide enough load to the muscles to strengthen them.
- Exercise bands and exercise tubing (Fig. 8-6). When used appropriately, these tools increase the intensity of the workout. They can be purchased at many department stores, sporting goods stores, and through the Internet. They are cost-effective and easy to use.
- Dumbbells (Fig. 8-7). There are several advantages to using dumbbells during a workout. Some

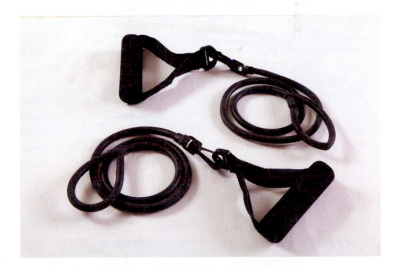

FIGURE 8-6 Exercise tubing.

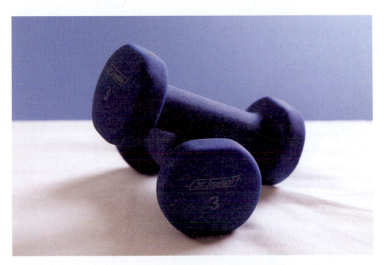

FIGURE 8-7 Dumbbells.

dumbbells are adjustable, meaning the weight they provide can be changed. These are usually less expensive and take up less space than traditional dumbbells. Using dumbbells requires constant adjustment and readjustment of their positions. Therefore, synergistic and stabilizer muscles contract more prominently, which improves overall strength and protects against potential injury. Dumbbells also allow joints to go through full ranges of motion.

- Exercise balls (see Fig. 7-24). These were originally used in physical therapy but have crossed over to the fitness and bodywork fields with great success. With the exception of free weights, there is possibly no other training tool that can be used for so many different functions. An exercise ball allows abdominal training through a full range of motion that cannot be accomplished from exercises done on the floor. All weight-training exercises done on weight-training benches can also be performed on exercise balls with the added benefit of core muscle contraction and greater proprioceptive awareness. When choosing the ball, be aware that its diameter should be relative to the user's height and weight. Proper sizing reduces the chance of injury to the low back and the knees. Information about the proper ball to choose can be found on the ball's packaging. Also, exercise balls come in either burst or antiburst varieties. If using an exercise ball while using weights, an antiburst ball is highly recommended. The ball needs to be filled with air according to the instructions on the package. A ball stand can also be purchased, which may be necessary to use during certain exercises to keep from rolling off and being injured.

EXERCISE SETS AND REPETITIONS

How many sets? A set is a fixed number of repetitions (reps), or repeated movements of an exercise. There should be a rest period in between each set. If the goal is muscle building, rest 30 to 60 seconds between sets. However, to make the exercise aerobic, do not rest between sets. Instead, move from one activity to another, just like in circuit training, which combines strength and aerobic training. This is also a time saver. The best strength gains come from three to five sets per exercise. Use Table 8.1 as a guide for reps and sets.

TABLE 8.1 Training Sets and Reps

Training Goals	Repetition Guidelines	Working Sets
Endurance	12 or more	2 to 3
Hypertrophy	6 to 12	3 to 6
Strength	6 or fewer	2 to 6
Power	1 to 2	3 to 5

How much weight? If weights are used, the rule of thumb is to use as much as is comfortable for 12 reps. The last rep should be fairly challenging. Use the first few sessions primarily as testing sessions to see how much weight is comfortable. Also, when using weights, the primary focus should be on the eccentric contraction. This is where muscle tone will be developed.

When to increase weights? Once it is comfortable to do more than 12 reps, increase the weight.

How often should you lift weights? A general recommendation is to start with two to three workouts per week, spending 30 to 45 minutes each session, with a rest day following each workout. The best results generally occur when you alternate a hard workout day and an easy workout day. This allows for cellular changes to occur on the rest days so that your muscle fibers can recover from the stress of the workout and rebuild themselves stronger.

Why are rest days important? Left to its own resources, the body will recover fully from most exercise sessions, but the body is in no hurry to do so. The key is to speed up this process. As the difficulty of the exercise regimen increases, it is even more important to pay attention to recuperation. As a general rule, allow 24 to 48 hours of rest in between working muscle groups. For example, do not work hip and leg muscles two days in a row. Instead, work hip and leg muscles one day and shoulder and arm muscles the next day. Also, be sure to have a rest day or two in which you do not do your usual workout. It is important to give the body time to recover. An option for the rest day is to choose a low-impact exercise like walking, cycling, swimming, or playing tag with children.

Myth: Heavy weights with low repetitions make muscles bigger, and lighter weights with high repetitions make muscles defined.

FACT: High repetitions (15 or more) are best for muscular endurance but are not conducive to gaining muscular mass. The lighter loads used in high repetition workouts recruit relatively few muscle fibers. When heavier weights with lower reps are used in resistance training, more muscle fibers are recruited. The more muscle fibers recruited for an exercise, the greater the extent of remodeling in the entire muscle.

OVERTRAINING

Overtraining is defined as excessive training that can lead to injuries, insomnia, depression, and chronic muscle soreness. It also slows down workout recovery, which can lead to delays in reaching exercise goals. It can also impact practitioners' abilities to perform treatments, thereby affecting their income and career longevity.

Symptoms of overtraining include:

- Decreased performance
- Delayed-onset muscle soreness (see Chapter 6)
- Elevated heart rate
- Loss of body weight
- Chronic fatigue
- Boredom with the exercise routine
- Increased susceptibility to infection

Ways to prevent overtraining include:

- Varying training methods
- Following sound nutritional and supplementation practices (this is discussed in more detail in Chapter 9)
- Using proper body mechanics when working out
- Getting optimum amounts of rest and sleep

Body Awareness

Are you currently participating in a strengthening program? If so, how do you feel while you are performing the exercises? What benefits do you think you are getting from it? If you are not in a strengthening program, why not? What would make you more likely to participate in one?

- Engaging in modalities that promote restoration such as meditation, whirlpool baths, massage, and bodywork
- Avoiding stressors that can interfere with training efforts
- Keeping a journal of daily activities, including exercise, to see how much effort is being expended each day

WEIGHT TRAINING AND FLEXIBILITY

Recall from Chapter 7 that resistance training contributes to increased joint flexibility. In fact, no matter what your level of flexibility, the primary concern is adequate strength throughout your joints' full ranges of motion. Therefore, when building strength, it is key to perform resistance exercises through each joint's full range of motion (ROM) and to work antagonistic pairs of muscles equally.

When weight training is performed correctly, it results in increased joint flexibility. When performed incorrectly, it can actually *decrease* joint flexibility. Whether it is successful depends on how you do the exercise, how much weight you use, and whether you use full ROM of your joints. It is also important to remember that weight training for beginners is different from more experienced individuals who use more weight.

If relatively light loads are used so that full ROM can be performed, flexibility will increase. For example, in exercises such as a lateral arm raise, if a full ROM is achieved so that the arm ends up directly overhead, shoulder flexibility will increase. This is also true for front arm raises, lateral prone raises, back raises, and so forth. Exercises such as reverse trunk twists are excellent for increasing rotational flexibility of the spine and for strengthening the internal and external abdominal obliques.

As repetitions and sets are increased, and as greater resistance is used, weight training will result in a loss of flexibility. There are two reasons for this:

1. When very heavy weights are used, the limbs are rarely fully extended because of the loss in mechanical advantage of the muscles.
2. The use of heavy weights brings about residual tone in muscles, which, when sufficiently strong, keeps the muscles in a shortened state after the workout.

When performing a greater number of repetitions or sets, invariably as that last repetition or set is begun, ROM decreases. This typically occurs when fatigue begins to set in or when the muscles begin to tighten from the amount of work being done. The more work the muscles do, the greater the likelihood flexibility in the affected joints will decrease.

Because of this, all heavy or intense weight-training programs should be supplemented with stretching, preferably after the workout. This is especially important when the spine is involved in weight-bearing exercise. The spine may become compacted as when holding weights on the shoulders or overhead. Active stretching at this time can be done to regain the normal ROM in the involved joints. Following the protocol outlined in Chapter 7 is recommended.

STRENGTHENING PROTOCOLS

Recall from Chapter 7 that prior to exercise or activity, it is important to:

- Warm up using dynamic movements
- Use light weights and more repetitions to further warm up your muscles and get them ready for movement (refer to Chapter 7, "Activity" under "General Warm-up"): In the last part of your warm-up, perform movements that are less-intense versions of the movements that you will be performing during your workout activity. This is beneficial because it improves coordination, balance, strength, and response time, and may reduce the risk of injury.

Other key points to remember:

- Remember to breathe. Exhale on the most difficult part of the movement and inhale on the easiest part of the movement.
- Maintain a balanced posture throughout movements. This is crucial to injury prevention.
- Keep moving. This will decrease recovery time.
- Take 5 to 10 minutes to cool down using dynamic movement and static stretching.

SAFETY AND INJURY PREVENTION

The following are guidelines for safety and injury prevention while working out:

- If you are lifting weights, try not to train alone. Even at home, have someone there to help if you need it (this person is usually called a *spotter*). Most weight-training injuries occur when the lifter is training alone. Having a spotter provides safety if for some reason you are not able to

properly use the weights or if something goes wrong with the equipment.
- Use proper positions (called *form*) for all exercises. Use all the body mechanics information in this text to make sure you do so.
- Do not jerk or twist when lifting. These movements increase stress on your body and can lead to injury.
- If it hurts, do not do it. Decrease your intensity, reps, sets, or weight. Cross-train as necessary to make sure you do not overtrain or become injured.
- Be especially careful doing the following exercises:
  - Full squats: This puts a great deal of stress on the lower back and the ligaments and tendons in the knees.
  - Any exercise involving your knee being moved forward over your toes.
- Always maintain proper joint alignment.

The strengthening protocols in this chapter are basic guidelines to follow. It is recommended you seek the advice of a health and fitness professional such as a certified fitness trainer before beginning any strength-training regimen. Here are Internet resources for finding a health and fitness professional in your area:

American Council on Exercise (ACE): www.acefitness.org

American College of Sports Medicine (ACSM): www.acsm.org

American Fitness Professionals and Associates (AFPA): www.afpafitness.com

MUSCLE GROUPS

When devising an exercise plan, consider working the larger group of muscles before the smaller ones. Why? If the smaller muscle groups fatigue first, the larger muscle groups cannot be worked adequately. A typical order of exercises would be:

1. Abdominals. Exercising the abdominal muscles is a great way to warm up your whole body.
2. Hips and legs. Since the legs automatically bring the muscles of the lower back into play, be sure you are thoroughly warmed up before working your legs, especially your thighs. The thighs have the largest muscle groups in the body.
3. Chest
4. Back. Since most musculoskeletal injuries involve the back, make sure you are thoroughly warmed up before working these muscles.

5. Shoulders

6. Arms and forearms

7. Hands and fingers

> **Myth:** With the proper exercises, I will be able to control the shape of each one of my muscles.
>
> **FACT:** Your genes determine your individual muscle shapes. Exercise will make them big or strong. However, you can shape your body and shape a body region comprised of several muscles.

Before presenting strengthening protocols, it is necessary to review core strength. Recall from previous chapters that the body's core is important for bodywork practitioners. It is the source of balanced posture and strength necessary to perform treatments.

THE CORE

The body's core includes the trunk, pelvis, hips, abdominal muscles, and the small muscles along the spinal column. Specifically, the muscles of the core are transverse abdominis, external abdominis oblique, multifidus, and the erector spinae group (Fig. 8-8A). Other muscles involved with core stabilization are gluteus medius, rectus abdominis, and internal abdominis oblique (Fig. 8-8B).

The thoracolumbar fascia (TLF; Fig. 8-8C) provides tensile support to the lumbar spine when deep muscles of the trunk contract. Transverse abdominis and internal abdominis oblique both attach to the TLF. This fascia wraps around the torso, connecting the deep trunk muscles. The basis of core training is to increase the recruitment efficiency of the smaller, deeper "stabilizing" muscles around the hip and pelvis.

The body's core muscles are the foundation for all other movement. The muscles of the trunk stabilize the spine and provide a solid foundation for movement in the extremities. When these muscles contract, they stabilize the spine, pelvis, and shoulders, creating a solid base of support. The biggest benefit of core strengthening is functional fitness—fitness that is essential to both daily living and regular activities. For example, strengthening all the abdominal muscles is a useful preventative approach for low back pain.

Core-strengthening protocols should not involve recruiting deep stabilizing muscles in isolation. Instead they should focus on the core muscles working efficiently and in coordination to maintain alignment of the spine and pelvis while the limbs are moving. The current thinking in physiotherapy and fitness training is to focus on core stability training, which specifically targets the smaller and deeper lumbar spine and trunk muscles. The aim of core stability training is to effectively recruit the trunk musculature and then learn to control the position of the lumbar spine during dynamic movements.

Testing for Core Strength

The following core muscle strength and stability test is a way to monitor the development of the abdominal and lower back muscles. If core strength is poor, then the trunk will move unnecessarily during motion and waste energy. Good core strength indicates that the individual can move with great efficiency. To perform the test, you will need a flat surface, a mat, and a watch or clock.

1. Position the watch or clock on the ground where you can easily see it.

2. Assume the basic press-up position, which is similar to the position for performing push-ups except that your knees and elbows are on the floor (Fig. 8-9A).

3. Hold this position for 60 seconds.

4. Lift your right arm off the floor (Fig. 8-9B). Hold this position for 15 seconds.

5. Return your right arm to the floor and lift your left arm off the floor (Fig. 8-9C). Hold this position for 15 seconds.

6. Return your left arm to the floor and lift your right leg off the floor (Fig. 8-9D). Hold this position for 15 seconds.

7. Return your right leg to the floor and lift your left leg off the floor (Fig. 8-9E). Hold this position for 15 seconds.

8. Lift your right leg and left arm off the floor (Fig. 8-9F). Hold this position for 15 seconds. Return your right leg and left arm to the floor.

9. Lift your left leg and right arm off the floor (Fig. 8-9G). Hold this position for 15 seconds.

10. Return to the basic press-up position (see Fig. 8-9A). Hold this position for 30 seconds and then relax.

For increased strength, you can start and end with the basic press-up position but with your knees off the floor—your body weight is resting on your toes and forearms (Fig. 8-9H).

Cautions:

● For those with low back issues, begin with both knees on the floor, pushing up with the upper body; be sure to engage the core. Once this becomes easy, leave one knee on the floor and push up with the other leg.

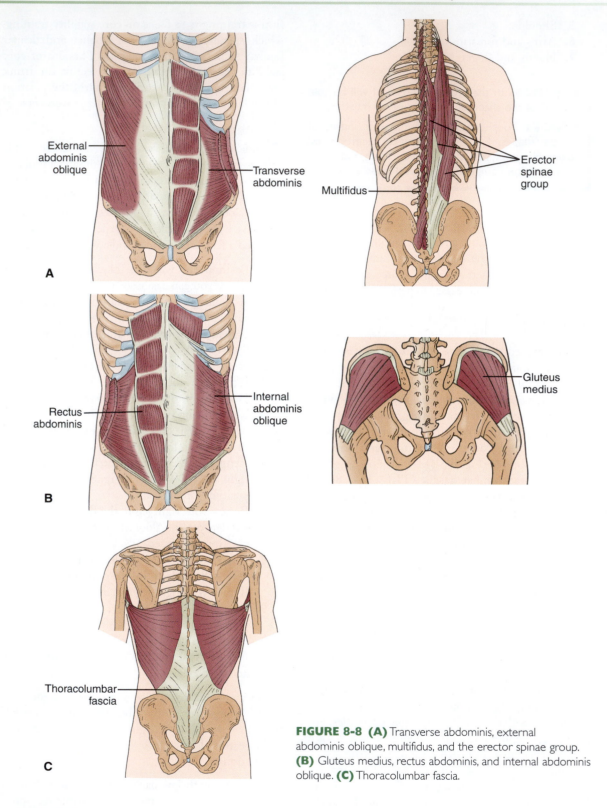

FIGURE 8-8 (A) Transverse abdominis, external abdominis oblique, multifidus, and the erector spinae group. **(B)** Gluteus medius, rectus abdominis, and internal abdominis oblique. **(C)** Thoracolumbar fascia.

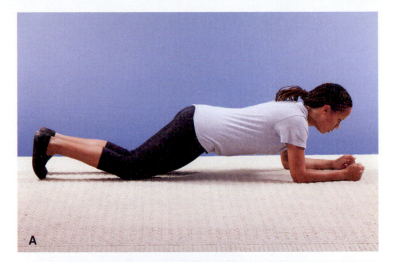

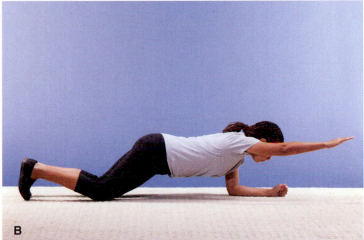

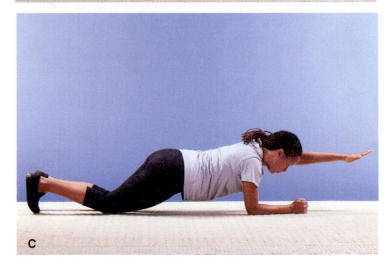

FIGURE 8-9 (A) Basic press-up position.
(B) Lift your right arm off the floor.
(C) Return your right arm to the floor
and lift your left arm off the floor.

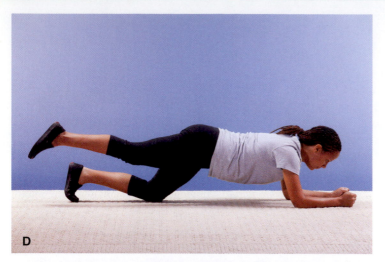

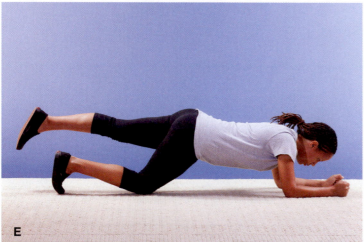

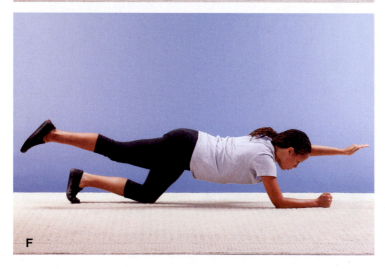

FIGURE 8-9 cont'd (D) Return your left arm to the floor and lift your right leg off the floor. **(E)** Return your right leg to the floor and lift your left leg off the floor. **(F)** Lift your right leg and left arm off the floor.

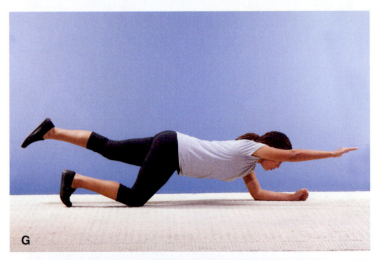

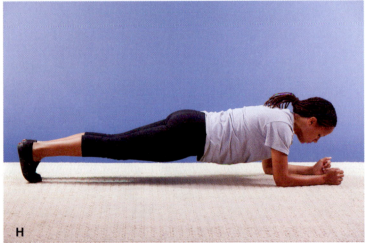

FIGURE 8-9 cont'd (G) Lift your left leg and right arm off the floor. **(H)** Basic press-up position with the knees off the floor and the weight resting on the toes and forearms.

- Remember to inhale on the downward phase of the movement (eccentric contractions) and exhale on the upward phase (concentric contractions).
- Breathe normally while you are holding the position.

If you were able to complete this test, then you have good core strength. If you are unable to complete the test, then repeat the routine three or four times a week until you can. Compare the results each time you do the test with the results of previous tests. Over time, with appropriate training between each test, you should see improvement.

Exercises for Core Strength and Stability

Core-stability training begins with learning to co-contract transverse abdominis and multifidus effectively. This is key to supporting the lumbar region of the body. To co-contract transverse abdominis and multifidus, perform the following

"abdominal hollowing" protocol with your spine aligned:

1. Lie supine on a mat with your knees flexed and your feet flat on the mat. Your lumbar spine should be neither arched nor flattened against the mat but aligned normally with a small gap between the floor and your back. This is the optimal neutral lumbar position (Fig. 8-10A).
2. Inhale deeply and relax all your abdominal muscles. Exhale and, as you do so, draw your lower abdomen inward as if to pull your navel toward the floor (Fig. 8-10B). Tip: Pilates instructors describe this as "zipping up," as if you are fastening up a tight pair of jeans.
3. Hold the contraction for 10 seconds while staying relaxed. Breathe normally as you hold the tension in your lower abdomen. Release your abdominal muscles (Fig. 8-10C)
4. Repeat 5 to 10 times.

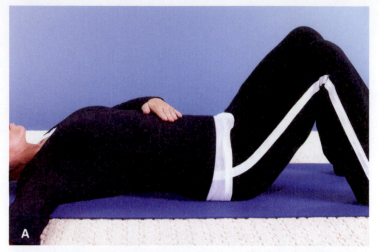

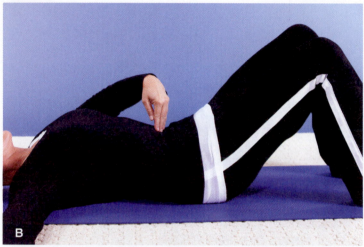

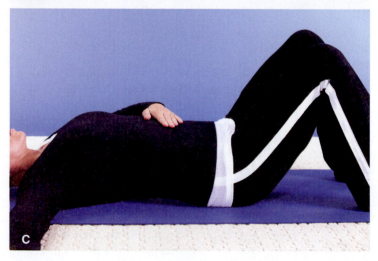

FIGURE 8-10 (A) Lie supine on a mat with your knees flexed and your feet flat on the mat with your back in the optimal neutral lumbar position. **(B)** Draw your lower abdomen inward as if to pull your navel toward the floor. **(C)** Release your abdominal muscles.

Once you have mastered the abdominal hollowing lying on your back, practice it while lying prone, while on your hands and knees, while sitting, and while standing. In each position, make sure you are in the optimal neutral lumbar position before you perform "abdominal hollowing."

Stabilizing Exercises

Prone Superman. Lie prone on an exercise ball with your waist in the center; support your hands with soft fists so you do not compromise your wrists (Fig. 8-11A). Inhale, and as you exhale, contract your abdominal and back muscles to raise your chest, and extend your arms in front of you and your legs behind (Fig. 8-11B). The goal is to look like Superman flying. This will take some practice. If you cannot do this at first, leave your feet on the floor while stretching out your arms. Be sure to keep your head in line with your spine; do not look up. Hold this position for 10 seconds while breathing normally, and then relax.

Tip: If you are unable to keep the exercise ball from rolling as you lift your arms and legs, place the ball on a ball stand to keep it stationary.

Prone Arm/Leg Superman. Start in the same position as Prone Superman. Inhale, and as you exhale, contract your abdominal and back muscles to raise your chest, and extend your right arm forward and your right leg back. Hold this position for 10 seconds while breathing normally, and then relax. Repeat with your left arm and left leg.

For a variation and a more difficult exercise, inhale, and as you exhale, contract your

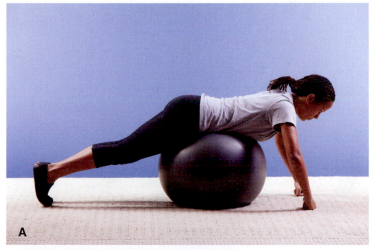

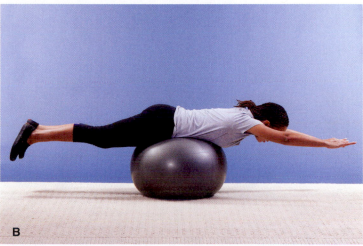

FIGURE 8-11 **(A)** Lie with your waist in the center of an exercise ball. **(B)** Tighten your abdominal and back muscles to raise your chest, and extend your arms in front of you and your legs behind you.

abdominal and back muscles to raise your chest, and extend your right arm forward and your left leg back. Hold this position for 10 seconds while breathing normally, and then relax. Repeat with your left arm and right leg.

Prone Arm Walk. Lie prone on an exercise ball with your chest in the center (Fig. 8-12A). While breathing normally, use your hands to walk forward, rolling the ball toward your feet (Fig. 8-12B). Keep your spine, including your neck, aligned. Roll back to the starting position. Repeat as many times as you like.

Supine Bridging. Lie supine on an exercise ball with the center between your scapulae (Fig. 8-13A). Inhale, and as you exhale, raise your hips until your neck, back, and thighs are parallel (Fig. 8-13B). Slowly extend your left knee and raise your leg until it is parallel to your right thigh (Fig. 8-13C). Breathe normally as

you hold for 10 seconds. Place your hands on your stomach as a reminder to contract your abdominal muscles. Relax. Repeat with other leg.

Tip: If you are unable to keep the exercise ball from rolling as you lift your leg, place the ball on a ball stand to keep it stationary.

Supine Torso Lift. Lie supine on the floor with your knees flexed over an exercise ball (Fig. 8-14A). Inhale, and as you exhale, slowly lift your trunk as high as is comfortable. Keep your arms on the floor to assist with balance (Fig. 8-14B). Breathe normally as you hold for 10 seconds. As your balance improves, place your hands on your abdomen.

The ultimate aim of core-stability training is to ensure the deep trunk muscles are working correctly to control the lumbar spine during dynamic movements,

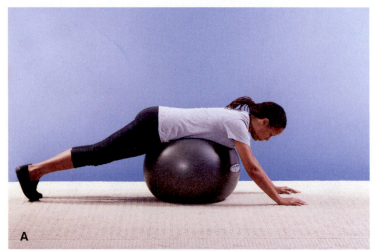

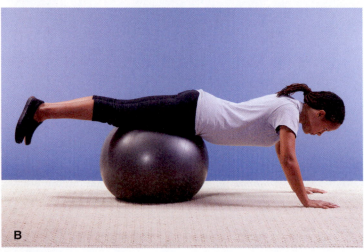

FIGURE 8-12 (A) Lie prone on an exercise ball with your chest in the center. **(B)** Use your hands to walk forward, rolling the ball toward your feet.

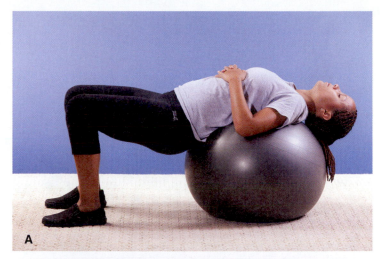

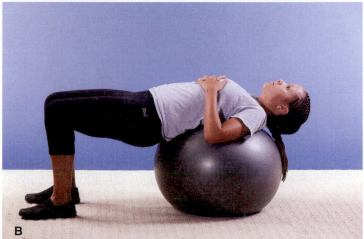

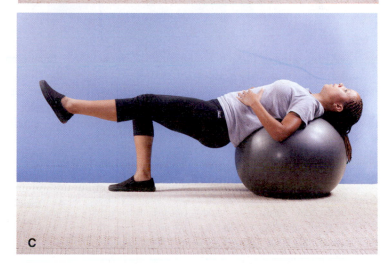

FIGURE 8-13 (A) Lie supine on an exercise ball with the center between your scapulae. **(B)** Raise your hips until your neck, back, and thighs are parallel. **(C)** Slowly extend your left knee and raise your leg until it is parallel to your right thigh.

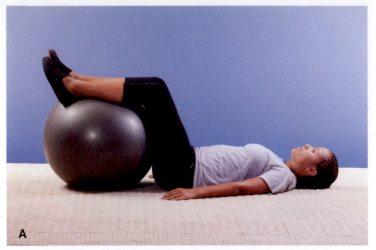

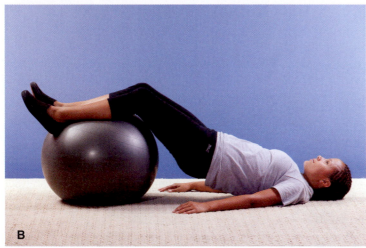

FIGURE 8-14 (A) Lie supine on a mat on the floor with your knees flexed over an exercise ball. **(B)** Slowly lift your trunk as high as is comfortable. Keep your arms on floor to assist with balance.

such as lifting a client's heavy leg during a treatment or running. Therefore, it is important that once you have achieved proficiency in the simple core exercises, you should progress to achieving stability during movements that you will do when performing bodywork. Try these exercises:

The Lunge. This is a classic exercise, which, when performed slowly and with care, can teach you a great deal about body awareness and core stability. Many people wrongly initiate the up movement by pulling their head and shoulders back first. This extends the lumbar spine, losing the neutral position. Others cannot keep their pelvis level while performing the lunge. See stationary lunges in the "Resistance-Training Total-Body Work-out" section for more information and how to do them.

Balancing Disks. These are plastic disks that are filled with air (Fig. 8-15). The air volume can be adjusted to increase or decrease instability. The user either sits with the feet on the disks or stands on the disks. Since the air is shifting within the disk, the user recruits stabilizing muscles whether seated or standing. There is a slightly changing and unstable surface. While it is unlikely bodywork practitioners will be performing treatments while standing on unstable surfaces, using balancing disks can be helpful for increasing overall stability and balance.

Myth: You can burn fat from specific regions of the body by exercising those areas.

FACT: The phenomenon of "spot reduction" has absolutely no basis in fact. When you exercise, you use energy produced by metabolizing fat from

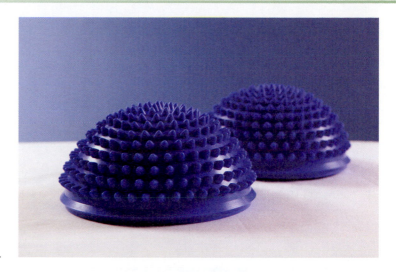

FIGURE 8-15 Balancing disks.

all the regions of your body—not just the specific muscles involved in the exercise. Performing sit-ups, for example, will not trim the fat off your abdominal region any more rapidly than off your gluteal region or thighs. The exercise may firm up the muscles in the area but will not make the fat disappear.

WEIGHT-BEARING TOTAL-BODY WORKOUT

Complete the exercises here for a full-body workout. Depending on time constraints, repetitions, sets, and rest periods in between, sets can be customized for individual needs.

The Plank

The plank, similar to the press-up position presented in the "Testing for Core Strength" section, is an excellent way to build core strength. Lie prone on a mat on the floor with your weight resting on your forearms, knees, and toes (Fig. 8-16A). For extra padding, you can place a towel under your forearms. Raise yourself up so that your knees are off the floor (Fig. 8-16B). Hold for several seconds, then slowly lower yourself back to the starting position (Fig. 8-16C). Repeat several times. Increase the time you hold as your stamina increases.

If you cannot raise yourself off both knees, you can modify the position by leaving one knee down while rising up on the other leg (Fig. 8-16D). Hold for several seconds, then lower yourself back to the starting position. Repeat with the other knee down.

Another modification is to perform the plank in a side-lying position (Fig. 8-17A). Keep your spine aligned as you raise yourself up (Fig. 8-17B) and slowly lower yourself down (Fig. 8-17C). You can also try putting your hand behind your head (Fig. 8-17D) and rotating your trunk to touch your elbow to the floor to increase the intensity of this exercise (Fig. 8-17E).

FIELD NOTES

My situation does not really involve a specific injury. I have scoliosis and experience chronic low back pain from time to time. I had sciatica for about 1 year due to a bulging disk putting pressure on the spinal cord. I also have previous injuries that act up on occasion. I tore my right ACL (anterior cruciate ligament of the knee) out of the bone in my right knee during a skiing accident and broke my right collarbone when I was in college playing intramural softball.

I used VAX-D to address the sciatica issues that proved very effective for me overall. It is a form of decompression stretch on the spine to lengthen the spine and create a vacuum inside the column that draws fluids and health nutrients into the cord, which help it heal. The collarbone is not really an issue anymore, and the knee just has arthritis and gets achy from changes in the weather, especially cooler temperatures. I walk every day and do some mild stretches to keep it limber.

My advice is to understand and be conscious of good vs. bad body mechanics. It is good to engage in regular exercise (even low impact is better than nothing), and stretches. The obvious reminders include rest, low stress, and a healthy diet.

Kathy Lee, BS, LMT. Director of Career Services, Cortiva-Tucson. Massage therapist since 1997.

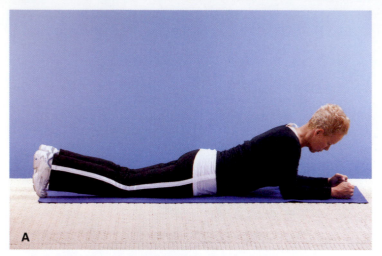

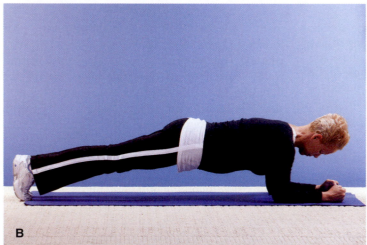

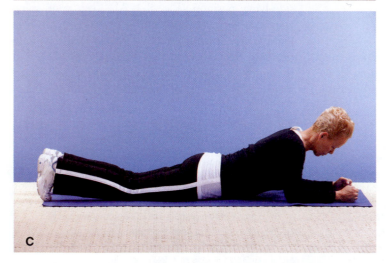

FIGURE 8-16 (A) Plank starting position. **(B)** Raise yourself up so that your knees are off the floor. **(C)** Slowly lower yourself back to the starting position.

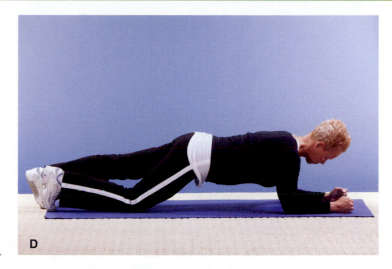

FIGURE 8-16 cont'd (D) Leave one knee down while rising up on the other leg.

Cautions:

- For those with low back issues, begin with the bottom knee flexed (Fig. 8-17F) and push up with the top leg (Fig. 8-17G).
- Remember to inhale on the downward phase of the movement (eccentric) and exhale on the upward phase (concentric).
- Remember to breathe while you are holding the position.

Wall Squat for the Legs

Stand against a wall with your feet at or slightly wider than shoulder-width apart. Position your feet far enough in front of you so that when you descend into the squat, your knees are not going over your

toes. If your knees go over your toes, it can cause undue stress on your knee joints. Figure 8-18A shows the starting position.

Tip: Continue to keep your back against the wall with your spine aligned throughout the exercise.

Inhale and exhale as you slowly lower your body as far as is comfortable for you; do not lower your hips below your knees (Fig. 8-18B and C). This can cause undue stress on your knee joints. Contract your gluteal and hamstring muscles.

While breathing normally, hold this position for as long as is comfortable (until you begin to feel slight discomfort).

Slowly extend your legs and rise up to your original start position (Fig. 8-18D).

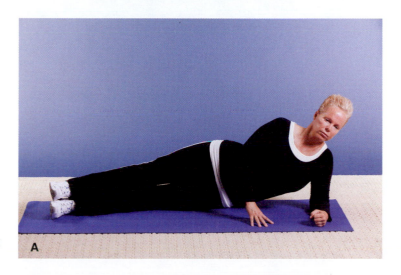

FIGURE 8-17 (A) Plank in side-lying position.

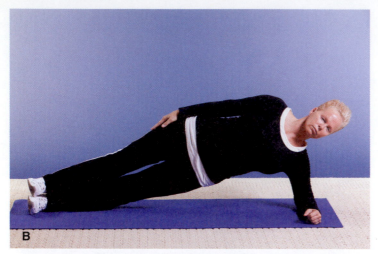

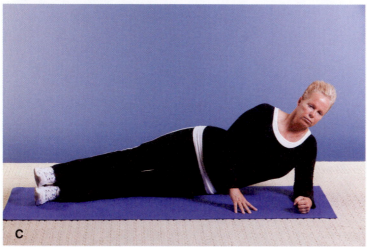

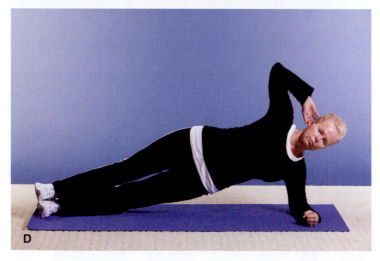

FIGURE 8-17 cont'd (B) Keeping the spine aligned while rising up. **(C)** Return to the starting position. **(D)** Put your hand behind your head.

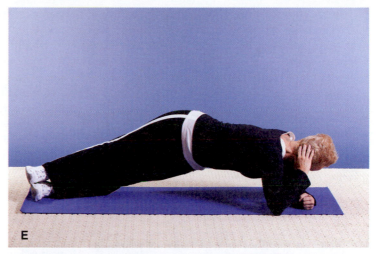

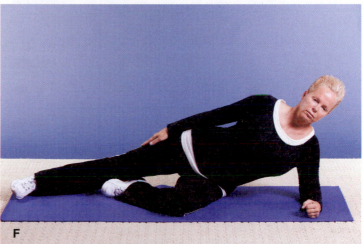

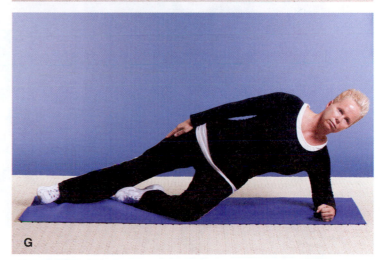

FIGURE 8-17 cont'd (E) Rotate your trunk to touch your elbow to the floor. **(F)** Begin with the bottom leg flexed. **(G)** Push up with the top leg.

Modifications:

To intensify this exercise, try crossing one foot over your opposite knee (Fig. 8-18E). Or have someone sit on your legs once you have lowered yourself as far as is comfortable for you (Fig. 8-18F).

Tips:

- Avoid having your heels come off the floor.
- Keep your knees behind your toes.
- Keep your hips aligned with your knees and feet.
- Keep your shoulders back.

Military-Style Push-ups for the Shoulders and Arms

Lie prone on the floor with your hands positioned under your shoulders (Fig. 8-19A). This is the starting position.

Inhale, and as you exhale, push up with your hands and feet while maintaining an aligned spine (Fig. 8-19B).

Return to the starting position and repeat.

To increase the intensity, you can adjust the angle of your hand positions to work the different fibers of the pectoral muscles (Fig. 8-20A, B, and C).

Modifications:

If this exercise is difficult for you, begin with your knees on the floor (this is also known as *women's push-ups*; Fig. 8-21).

If you have shoulder discomfort, try standing in front of a wall, approximately 1 to 3 feet away, with your elbows tucked into your sides. Place your hands on the wall and perform the push-ups by pushing away from the wall (Fig. 8-22). The farther you are away from the wall, the higher the intensity of the exercise. You can also increase the intensity by adjusting the angle of your hand positions. These will also work the different fibers of your pectoral muscles.

RESISTANCE-TRAINING TOTAL-BODY WORKOUT

The resistance-training total-body workout can be used with weights, exercise tubing, or an exercise ball. In fact, using these tools can help make the

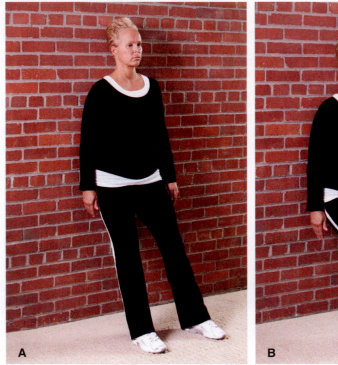 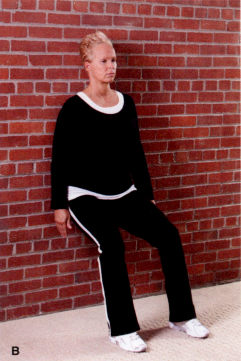

FIGURE 8-18 (A) Stand against a wall with your feet at or slightly wider than shoulder-width apart. Position your feet far enough away from your body so that when you descend into the squat, your knees do not go over your toes. **(B)** Slowly lower your body as far as is comfortable for you, but do not lower your hips below your knees.

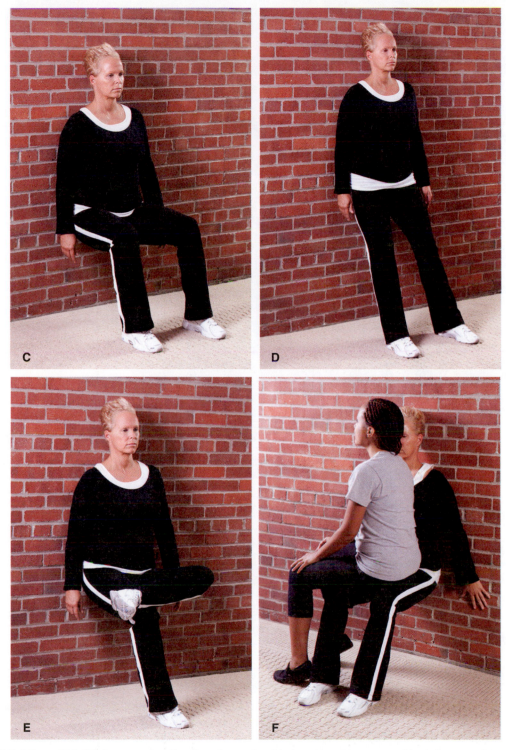

FIGURE 8-18 cont'd **(C)** Lower yourself as far as is comfortable, but do not lower your hips below your knees.
(D) Slowly extend your legs and rise up to your original starting position. **(E)** Cross one foot over your opposite knee.
(F) Have someone sit on your legs once you lowered yourself as far as is comfortable for you.

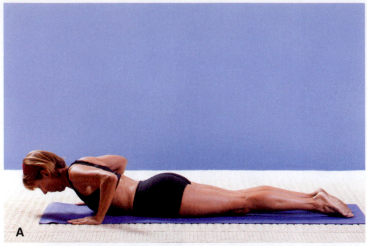

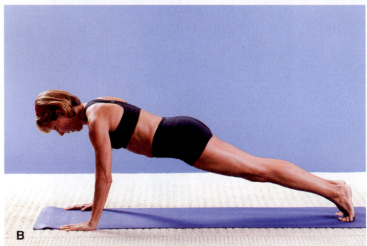

FIGURE 8-19 **(A)** Lie prone on the floor with your hands positioned under your shoulders. **(B)** Push up with your hands and feet while maintaining an aligned spine.

workout exciting. If hand weights are not available, you can use cans of food or water bottles filled with sand. If using the floor modifications suggested, a mat will be needed.

Abdominals

CRUNCH

Lie supine on a mat with your feet on a bench or chair. Make sure your hips and knees are flexed at 90 degrees and rest your arms across your chest (Fig. 8-23A).

Inhale, and as you exhale, flex your head and neck to move your chin to your chest by contracting your abdominal muscles. Keeping your low back aligned, pull your rib cage up and over your pelvis (Fig. 8-23B).

Slowly allow your trunk to uncurl; then allow your neck to extend back to the starting position while maintaining tension in your abdominal muscles.

Modifications:

You can include a rotation on the concentric contraction phase of this exercise, taking your elbow to the opposite knee. This engages internal and external abdominis oblique.

This exercise can also be performed on a bench or exercise ball to help isolate the abdominal muscles.

Cautions:

- Always keep your lower back pressed firmly against the floor mat.
- Do not place pressure on your neck by placing your hands behind your head.
- Work in a slow, controlled manner, concentrating on maintaining contraction of the abdominal muscles.

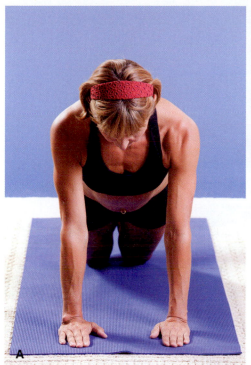

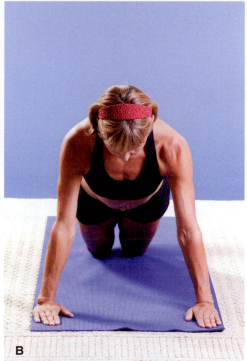

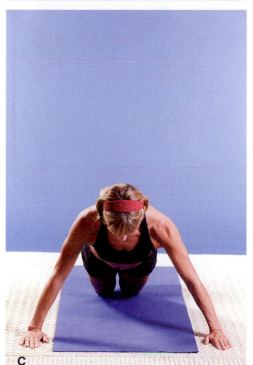

FIGURE 8-20 (A, B, C) Adjust the angle of your hand positions to work the different fibers of the pectoralis muscles.

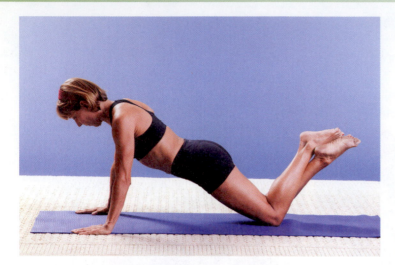

FIGURE 8-21 Begin with your knees on the floor.

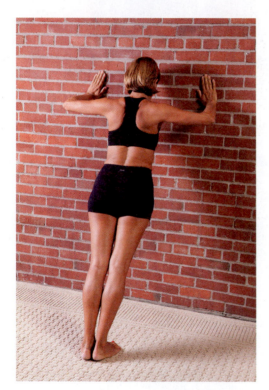

FIGURE 8-22 Perform the push-ups by pushing away from the wall.

Hips and Legs

BASIC SQUAT

This is similar to the wall squat for the legs in the "Weight-Bearing Total-Body Workout" section.

Stand with your feet at or slightly wider than shoulder-width apart. Align your shoulders with your knees and feet. Slightly flex your hips and knees and flex your trunk forward slightly.

Inhale, and as you exhale, slowly lower your body as far as you can comfortably go (but not past a 90-degree angle at your knees), while maintaining an aligned spine. Contract your hip and hamstring muscles. Keep your heels on the floor and your shoulders back.

Slowly extend your legs as you rise up to return to your original starting position while maintaining an aligned spine.

Modifications:

This exercise can be done while standing against a wall, as done in the wall squat for the legs (Fig. 8-24).

To increase the intensity, place weights on your anterior thighs.

To engage vastus medialis more completely, adjust the angle of your feet so that your toes point slightly medially. If you adjust the angle of your feet and you are using weights on your thighs, be sure to lighten the weights.

To engage the vastus lateralis more completely, adjust the angle of your feet so that your toes point slightly laterally. If you adjust the angle of your feet and you are using weights on your thighs, be sure to lighten the weights.

Caution: Do not allow your knees to move over your toes or move past the 90-degree angle. This will cause undue stress and strain to your knees.

STATIONARY LUNGES

Standing with your feet shoulder-width apart, let your arms hang down to your sides while holding weights. Keep your eyes focused straight ahead on a fixed point (Fig. 8-25A).

Take a large step forward. Keeping your spine aligned, firmly plant your forward foot while keeping

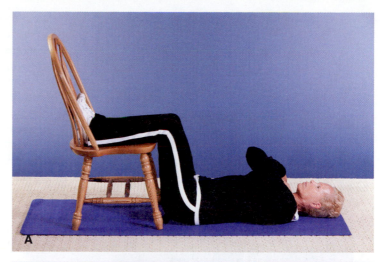

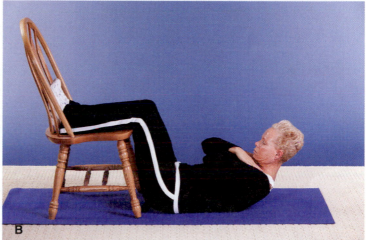

FIGURE 8-23 (A) Lie supine on a mat. Place your feet on a bench or chair with your hips and knees flexed at 90 degrees, and rest your arms across your chest. **(B)** Flex your head and neck to move your chin to your chest by contracting your abdominal muscles. Begin by pulling your rib cage up and over your pelvis.

your back foot in place. Both feet should be pointed forward (Fig. 8-25B).

Inhale, and as you exhale, slowly flex your forward hip and lower your back knee until it comes within 1 to 2 inches from the floor (Fig. 8-25C).

Inhale, and as you exhale, contract the quadriceps muscles of your forward leg to push back up to the starting position (Fig. 8-25D). Remember to keep your spine aligned.

Modifications:

Lunge around a room or lunge side to side. Or, without weights, hold on to the back of a chair or a counter and alternate lunges.

Cautions:

- Do not allow the forward knee to move past your toes. This will cause undue stress and strain to your knee.

- Do not allow your legs to bow medially or laterally during any phase of the exercise.
- Do not allow your equipment to swing at your sides more than 2 inches forward, back, or out to the side.

STANDING CALF RAISES

Facing a wall, stand approximately 1 foot away with your feet hip-width apart and pointed toward the wall. Place your hands on the wall (Fig. 8-26A).

Inhale, and as you exhale, push up onto the balls of your feet (plantarflex your ankles) as far as is comfortable for you (Fig. 8-26B). Make sure to keep your knees extended but not locked. Hold for approximately 10 seconds.

Slowly lower your heels back to the starting position. Repeat.

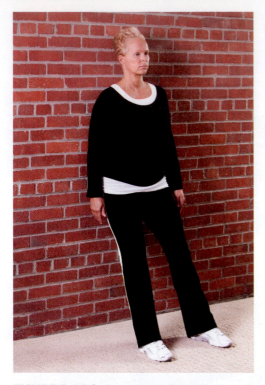

FIGURE 8-24 Basic squat standing against a wall.

Modifications:

To further engage gastrocnemius and soleus, use a door frame that has a step down. This allows for greater range of motion as your heels drop and your ankles dorsiflex.

To isolate and engage soleus, slightly flex your knees.

Change the position of your feet to engage different fibers of your leg muscles. An effective method for increasing your flexibility is to stretch different fibers of the muscles in between strengthening sets (Fig. 8-27 A, B, and C).

Cautions:

● Make sure the surface you are on is stable, with no chance of you slipping and injuring yourself.
● Do not allow your ankles to supinate (invert) or pronate (evert) during the movement.

Chest

PEC FLIES

Lie supine on a mat on the floor. Flex your knees and plant your feet firmly on the floor, keeping them planted throughout the exercise. Place your head, scapulae, and sacrum firmly on the mat. Grasp the weights, exercise tubing, or other equipment (e.g.,

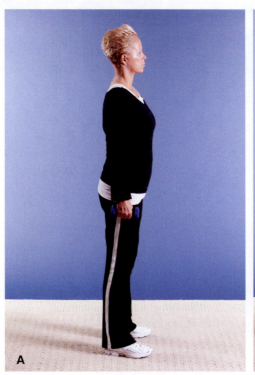

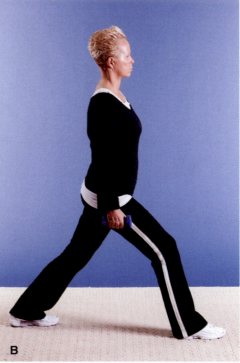

FIGURE 8-25 (A) Stand with your feet shoulder-width apart. Let your arms hang down to your sides while holding weights. Keep your eyes focused straight ahead on a fixed point. **(B)** Firmly plant your forward foot while keeping your back foot in place. Both feet should be pointed forward.

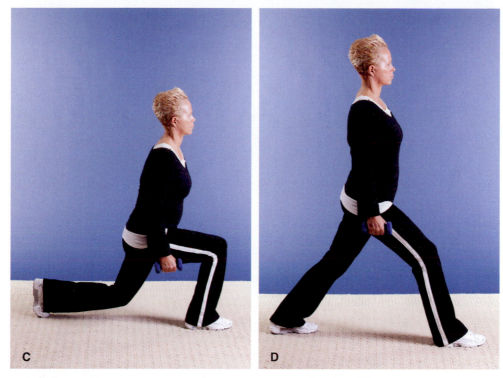

FIGURE 8-25 cont'd (C) Flex your forward hip and lower your back knee until it comes within 1 to 2 inches from the floor. **(D)** Contract the quadriceps muscles of your forward leg to push back up to the starting position.

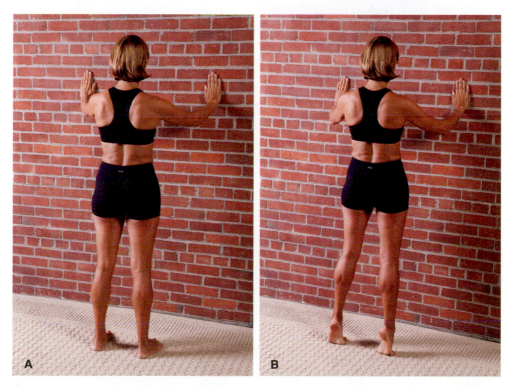

FIGURE 8-26 (A) Stand approximately 1 foot away from a wall with your feet hip-width apart and pointed toward the wall. Place your hands on the wall. **(B)** Push up onto the balls of your feet (plantarflex your ankles) as far as it comfortable for you.

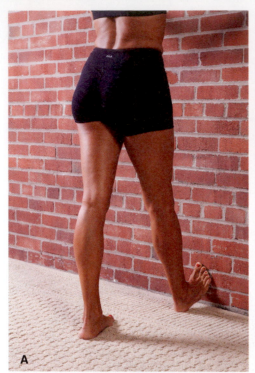

A

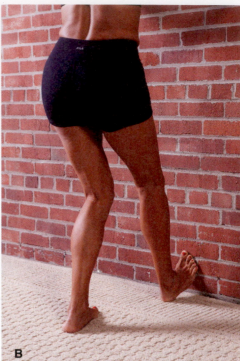

B

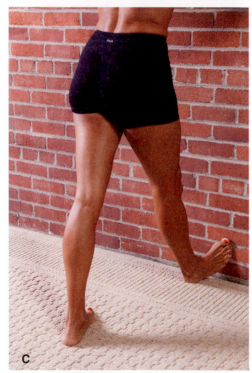

C

FIGURE 8-27 (A, B, C) Increase leg muscle flexibility by changing your foot position to stretch different fibers.

can of food, water bottle filled with sand) with a pronated grip (Fig. 8-28A). Keep them placed firmly on the mat throughout the exercise. Make sure your spine is aligned.

With your shoulders abducted and your elbows flexed at 90 degrees, hold your tool perpendicular to your body (Fig. 8-28B).

Inhale, and as you exhale, slowly extend your elbows keeping your elbows slightly flexed, lifting your tools straight up (Fig. 8-28C).

Slowly bring your tools back down to the starting position (Fig. 8-28D).

Modifications:

This exercise can also be performed lying supine on a mat, a bench, or an exercise ball.

To increase the intensity, try using a position of incline or decline. This also works the different muscle fibers of pectoralis major.

Cautions:

- Do not use a weight that is too heavy or you might risk dropping it on yourself.
- Keep your wrists aligned.
- Do not bounce at the bottom of the movement.

Back
BENT-OVER ROWS

Stand with your feet slightly wider than shoulder-width apart. Flex your knees slightly and flex your trunk until you are slightly above parallel to the floor.

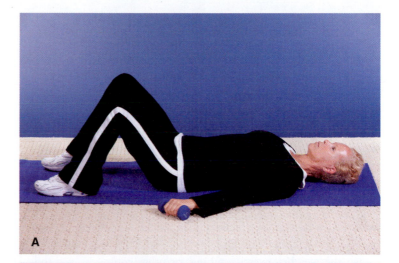

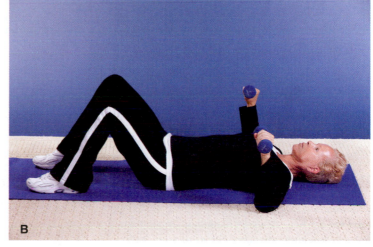

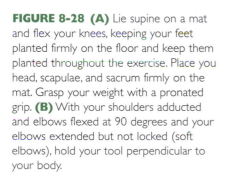

FIGURE 8-28 (A) Lie supine on a mat and flex your knees, keeping your feet planted firmly on the floor and keep them planted throughout the exercise. Place you head, scapulae, and sacrum firmly on the mat. Grasp your weight with a pronated grip. **(B)** With your shoulders adducted and elbows flexed at 90 degrees and your elbows extended but not locked (soft elbows), hold your tool perpendicular to your body.

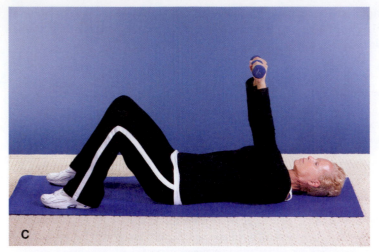

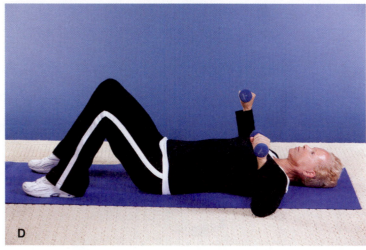

FIGURE 8-28 cont'd (C) Slowly extend your elbows, lifting your weights straight up. **(D)** Slowly bring your weights back down to the starting position.

Grasp the weights, exercise tubing, or other equipment with a pronated grip and your hands slightly wider than shoulder width. Allow your tool to hang with your elbows extended (Fig. 8-29A) but not locked.

Inhale, and as you exhale, retract your scapulae and pull the tools up toward your chest. Continue to contract latissimus dorsi middle trapezius, and rhomboids until your elbows are pointed directly upward (Fig. 8-29B). Continue to contract these muscles, keeping your hands and arms as relaxed as possible.

Inhale, and as you exhale, return to the starting position in a controlled manner.

Tip: To keep your head and neck aligned, focus your eyes a short distance ahead of your feet.

Modifications:

This exercise can also be performed seated on a mat, a bench, or an exercise ball. This position allows you to isolate the muscles of the shoulder girdle and thoracic region.

Cautions:

- Be sure to use slow, controlled movements. Abrupt movements may trigger spasms in your midthoracic region.
- Avoid jerking your trunk when performing the movements.
- Maintain an aligned spine throughout all the movements
- Keep your trunk and knees in the same position throughout the exercise.

Shoulders

MILITARY PRESS

Stand with your feet slightly wider than shoulder width apart with your knees extended but not locked. Grasp the weights, exercise tubing, or other

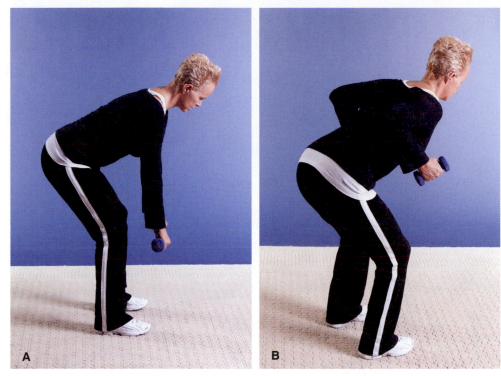

FIGURE 8-29 (A) Stand with your feet slightly wider than shoulder-width apart. Keep your knees slightly flexed. Flex your trunk until you are slightly above parallel to the floor. Grasp the weights or exercise tubing with a pronated grip, and place your hands slightly wider than shoulder width. Allow the tool to hang with your elbows extended but not locked. **(B)** Retract your scapulae and pull the tool up toward your chest.

equipment with a pronated grip and your hands slightly wider than shoulder width. Abduct your shoulders and flex your elbows (Fig. 8-30A).

Inhale, and as you exhale, slowly press your tool overhead until your elbows are fully extended but not locked (Fig. 8-30B). Keep your wrists aligned and your palms facing forward. Do not arch your back while pressing up.

Slowly lower the equipment back to the starting position (Fig. 8-30C).

Modifications:

This exercise can also be performed seated on a mat, a bench, or an exercise ball. Try alternating the movement by holding your tool with one hand and moving it up and over your head. This position allows you to isolate the muscles of the shoulder girdle.

Cautions:

- Do not lift past a 90-degree angle if you have shoulder discomfort.
- Keep your elbows directly under your hands.

Arms

ONE-ARM TRICEPS BRACHII EXTENSIONS

Stand with your feet slightly wider than shoulder-width apart with your knees extended but not locked. Hold the weight or tool in one hand with your shoulder flexed and your elbow extended. The weight is at your upper back. Rest your other arm across your abdomen (Fig. 8-31A).

Inhale, and as you exhale, slowly extend your elbow to raise the tool straight up over your head (Fig. 8-31B).

Inhale, and as you exhale, flex your elbow, bringing the tool down back down to your upper back (Fig. 8-31C). Make sure you do not lean forward.

Repeat with your other arm.

Modifications:

This exercise can also be performed seated on a mat, a bench, or an exercise ball, or while lying supine on a mat, a bench, or an exercise ball.

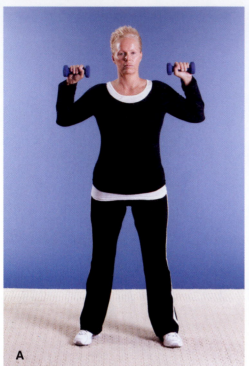

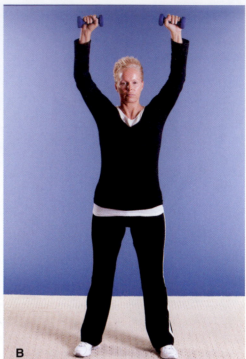

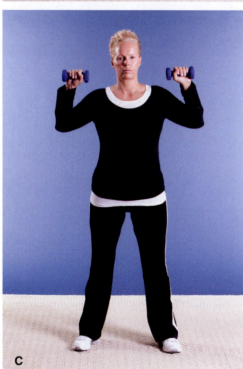

FIGURE 8-30 (A) Stand with your feet slightly wider than shoulder-width apart with your knees extended but not locked. Grasp the weights with a pronated grip and your hands slightly wider than shoulder width. Abduct your shoulders and flex your elbows. **(B)** Slowly press the weights overhead until your elbows are fully extended but not locked. **(C)** Slowly lower the weights back to the starting position.

Hold the tool with both hands while extending (Fig. 8-31D) and flexing your elbows (Fig. 8-31E). Make sure you do not lean forward as you are doing this.

Cautions:

- Do not use a weight that is too heavy or you might risk dropping it on yourself.
- Keep your arm stable during the exercise.
- Make sure to maintain an aligned spine.

BICEPS BRACHII CURLS

Stand with your feet slightly wider than shoulder-width apart with your knees extended but not locked. Supinate your forearms, extend your elbows, and tuck them into your sides while holding the weight or other tool (Fig. 8-32A). Do not lock your elbow in extension, as this will place too much stress on your ligaments and tendons.

Inhale, and as you exhale, contract one of your biceps brachii, flexing your elbow through a comfortable range of motion. Isometrically contract the muscle at the end of the concentric contraction and hold for several seconds (Fig. 8-32B).

Return to the starting position with the elbows aligned under the shoulders and slightly flexed.

Repeat with your other biceps brachii.

Modifications:

Pronate your forearm and perform the curl. This will engage the brachialis.

Rest your arm on a mat, a bench, or an exercise ball and perform the curl. This will isolate the muscle.

Hold the tool over your head with both hands while flexing (Fig. 8-32C) and extending your elbows (Fig. 8-32D). Make sure you do not lean forward as you are doing this.

Cautions:

- Use slow, controlled movements to prevent undue stress on the elbow joint.
- Avoid any twisting or rotating of your shoulders or elbows during execution.
- Do not allow your elbows to come forward in order to lift the weight.

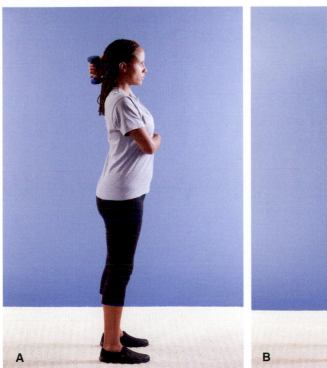
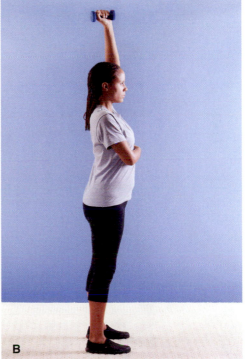

FIGURE 8-31 **(A)** Stand with your feet slightly wider than shoulder-width apart with your knees extended but not locked. Hold the weight in one hand with your shoulder flexed and your elbow extended. Rest your other arm across your abdomen. **(B)** Extend your elbow to raise the tool straight up over your head.

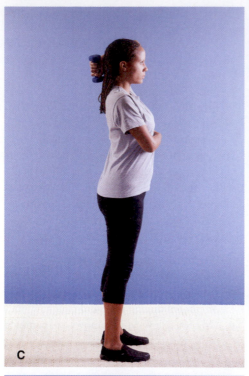

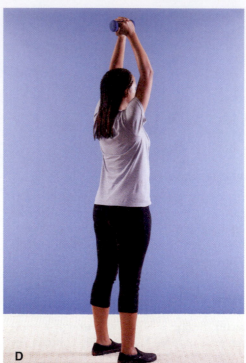

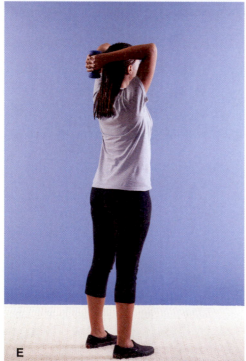

FIGURE 8-31 cont'd (C) Flex your elbow, bringing the tool down behind your head. **(D)** Hold the weight with both hands while extending and **(E)** flexing your elbows.

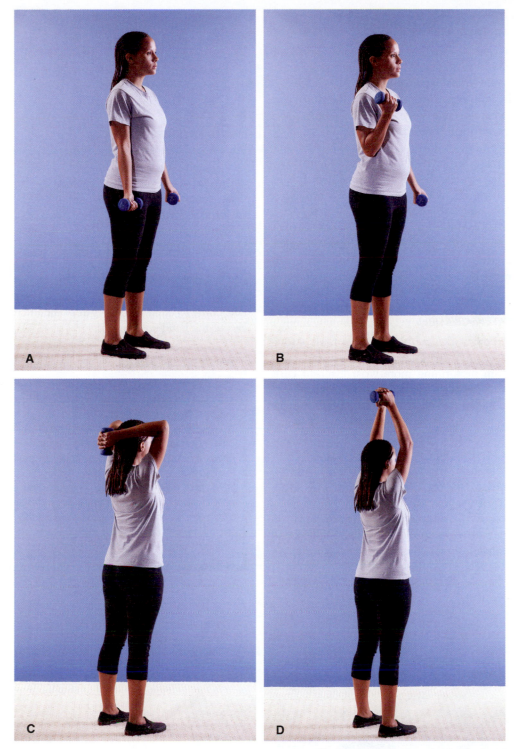

FIGURE 8-32 (A) Stand with your feet slightly wider than shoulder-width apart with your knees extended but not locked. Supinate your forearms and tuck your elbows into your sides while holding the weight. **(B)** Contract your biceps brachii, flexing your elbow through a comfortable range of motion. **(C)** Hold the weight over your head with both hands while flexing and **(D)** extending your elbows.

Forearms

WRIST FLEXOR CURLS

Sit on a chair, bench, or exercise ball. Grasp the weight or other tool with a supinated grip while keeping your wrist aligned (Fig. 8-33A).

Inhale, and as you exhale, slowly flex your wrist through a comfortable range of motion (Fig. 8-33B).

Repeat with your other forearm.

Modification:

To increase the intensity, drop the weight down so that your wrist is slightly hyperextended. Inhale, and as you exhale, slowly flex your wrist through a comfortable range of motion.

Caution: Do not use a weight that is too heavy or you will place undue stress on your wrist and fingers. This exercise is most effective with lighter weights and more reps.

WRIST EXTENSOR CURLS

Typically, bodywork practitioners have fairly strong flexors to begin with. Practitioners may find more benefit from performing more wrist extensor curls than wrist flexor curls.

Sit on a chair, bench, or exercise ball. Grasp the weight or tool with a pronated grip while keeping your wrist aligned (Fig. 8-34A).

Inhale, and as you exhale, slowly extend your wrist through a comfortable range of motion (Fig. 8-34B).

Repeat with your other forearm.

To increase the intensity, drop the weight down so that your wrist is slightly hyperflexed. Inhale, and as you exhale, slowly flex your wrist through a comfortable range of motion.

Caution:

- Do not use a weight that is too heavy or you will place undue stress on your wrist and fingers.
- This exercise is most effective with lighter weights and more reps.

Fingers

FINGER EXTENSION EXERCISE

Place a rubber band around the distal end of all your fingers (Fig. 8-35A).

Inhale, and as you exhale, extend your fingers with slow, controlled movements (Fig. 8-35B). Return back to the starting position.

Modifications:

Instead of extending all your fingers at one time, try one finger at a time. This will increase the intensity of the exercise.

Caution: Begin slowly with this exercise, as it takes time to build the strength in the intrinsic muscles of the hand and fingers.

Myth: Muscles turn to fat when you stop exercising.

FACT: Muscles cannot turn to fat. Muscle and fat (adipose) are two separate and distinct types of tissues. They simply do not have the physical capability to change from one type of tissue into another. However, muscles have the unique property of "use it or lose it." If you do not use a muscle, it will literally waste away or atrophy. This process is perhaps best illustrated when someone has to wear a cast on a broken leg. When the cast is eventually removed, the relatively unused leg muscles are considerably smaller than they were prior to the injury.

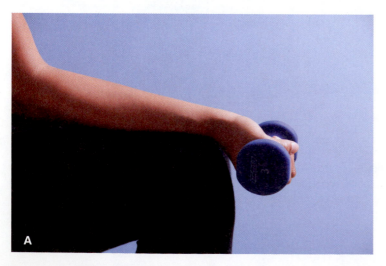

FIGURE 8-33 (A) Sit on a chair, bench, or exercise ball. Grasp the weight with a supinated grip while keeping the wrist in neutral.

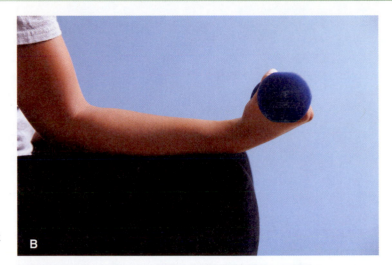

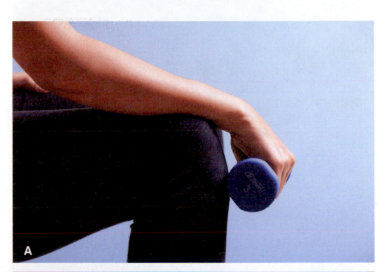

FIGURE 8-33 cont'd (B) Flex your wrist through a comfortable range of motion.

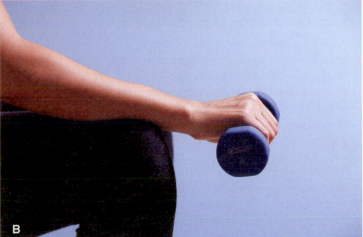

FIGURE 8-34 (A) Sit on a chair, bench, or exercise ball. Grasp the weight with a pronated grip while keeping the wrist in neutral. **(B)** Extend your wrist through a comfortable range of motion.

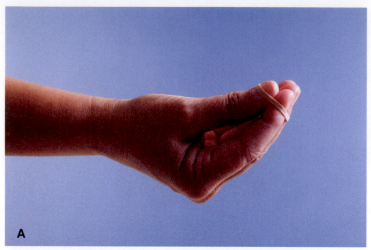

A

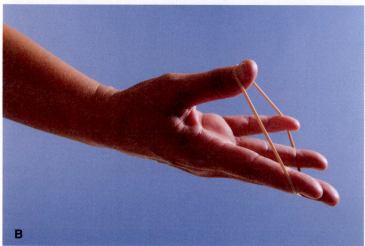

B

FIGURE 8-35 (A) Place a rubber band around the distal end of all your fingers. **(B)** Extend your fingers with slow, controlled movements.

Case Profile

Nadira has been a professional bodywork practitioner for 2 years. Prior to that, she was a receptionist on a part-time basis, while most of her time was spent coaching for a local amateur softball league. She has always thought that she is in great physical condition, so she rarely participates in any physical activities outside of performing her bodywork treatments and coaching her team.

Over the past 6 months, Nadira has been experiencing some tenderness and cramping in the medial aspects of her right elbow, extending down her forearm and into her hand. She knows she mainly uses her hands during treatments and has become concerned that these symptoms may hamper her ability to deliver effective treatment sessions. Additionally, she has been cutting back her softball coaching, especially since her discomfort seems to become worse after practices.

- *What do you think are the cause(s) of the tenderness and cramping in Nadira's elbow?*

- *What body structures may be involved?*

- *How do you think this is related to her ability to do bodywork? Coaching?*

- *What specific recommendations would you give Nadira?*

Wellness Profile Check In

Looking at the Wellness Profile you completed at the end of Chapter 1, are there any challenge areas you could remedy through a plan for strengthening? If so, what are they? How would you like these areas improved? What methods or activities will you use to improve these areas? Write down a plan for improvement that includes the methods you will use, a timeline for implementing these methods, and ways you will assess your improvement along the way.

Consult with your physician to see if you have any contraindications for the exercises presented in this chapter and to find out what levels of activity are best for you to start with.

SUMMARY

Bodywork practitioners need to build and maintain musculoskeletal strength in order to have career longevity. The three keys to balanced physical fitness are flexibility, aerobic activity, and strength training. Performing aerobic exercise regularly has many health benefits, such as burning body fat, increasing energy levels, relieving stress and anxiety, and increasing respiratory and cardiovascular system efficiency. An integrated approach to exercise includes heavy and light resistance training, psychological techniques, therapeutic modalities, medical support if needed, and a healthy diet. Cross-training means using several modes of training to develop a specific component of fitness.

There are many types of aerobic activity for bodywork practitioners to choose from, including swimming, running, walking, cycling, rowing, and so forth. You must carefully evaluate which ones are the best for you in terms of cost, complexity to learn, and amount of time involved to do them. Guidelines for beginning an aerobic program include doing the activity slowly for the first 5 minutes until the body is warmed up, maintaining the activity for at least 20 minutes, and stretching and performing a cooldown after the activity. Appropriate exercise intensity can be maintained by keeping the heart at the target heart rate or using the rating of perceived exertion.

There are three types of muscle tissue—cardiac, smooth, and skeletal. The focus of this chapter is on skeletal muscle tissue, because that is what is affected through strength training. Skeletal muscle tissue is composed of fast-twitch and slow-twitch muscle fibers. Fast-twitch fibers contract quickly for short bursts of energy when heavy workloads are demanded of the muscles. Slow-twitch fibers produce steady, low-intensity, repetitive contractions for endurance activities.

The energy for muscle contraction comes from glucose. Small amounts of glucose are stored in the liver and muscles as glycogen. When glucose is metabolized by oxygen, the by-products are carbon dioxide and water. When glucose is metabolized anaerobically, which can occur during intense exercise, a by-product is lactic acid. Lactic acid accumulation limits the intensity at which muscles can be exercised and ultimately prevents continuation of the exercise at the same intensity; the muscles become fatigued.

Before starting any strengthening program, guidelines to follow include getting a physical from your health-care provider, keeping an exercise journal, setting attainable goals, warming up, and not worrying about body weight when starting. To perform strengthening exercises, body weight can be used as well as tools and equipment such as exercise bands, exercise tubing, dumbbells, and exercise balls.

You can determine how many repetitions and sets to perform of each exercise by determining what your goals are. Overtraining can lead to injuries, insomnia, depression, and chronic muscle soreness. Ways to prevent overtraining include varying training methods, using proper body mechanics when working out, and engaging in modalities that promote restoration. Guidelines for safety and injury prevention while working out include training with someone else present, using proper positions for all exercises, and seeking the advice of a health and fitness professional.

Review Questions

MULTIPLE CHOICE

1. A key component to balance physical fitness is
   a. flexibility.
   b. aerobic activity.
   c. strength training.
   d. All of the above

2. Which of the following terms means "with oxygen"?
   a. Aerobic
   b. Metabolism
   c. Anaerobic
   d. Exertion

3. Which of the following is a myth about aerobic exercise?
   a. Everyone can benefit from doing it.
   b. Equipment for performing it can cost relatively little.
   c. It only improves the cardiovascular and respiratory systems.
   d. It can take relatively little time to do.

4. Target heart rate should be between what percentages of the person's maximum heart rate?
   a. 25% to 35%
   b. 40% to 50%
   c. 55% to 85%
   d. 75% to 90%

5. The term for the fact that myofibrils contract totally when stimulated by a nerve impulse is
   a. recruitment.
   b. all-or-none response.
   c. fast-twitch.
   d. exercise intensity.

6. Which of the following would be used in a heavy-resistance strengthening program?
   a. Body weight
   b. Running
   c. Swimming
   d. Dumbbells

7. Which of the following can result from overtraining?
   a. Decreased interest in exercising
   b. Increased performance
   c. Increased body weight
   d. Lowered heart rate

FILL-IN-THE-BLANK

1. According to the Surgeon General's Report, _____ _____ is just about as big a risk factor for coronary heart disease as smoking, hypertension, and high serum cholesterol.

2. Aerobic fitness is achieved by raising the body's _____ _____.

3. In order for an activity to be considered aerobic, it needs to be rhythmic and continuous for at least _____ minutes.

4. Most exercise injuries occur with an increase of _____ or _____.

5. The repeated movements of an exercise are referred to as _____.

6. Using several modes of training to develop a specific component of fitness is called _____.

7. The trunk, pelvis, hips, abdominal muscles, and the small muscles along the spinal column make up the body's _____.

SHORT ANSWER

1. Describe at least five benefits of performing regular aerobic exercise.

2. Describe at least five guidelines for beginning an aerobic program.

3. Explain how to calculate your target heart rate.

4. Explain at least five guidelines and suggestions when beginning a strengthening program.

5. Explain why rest days are important during a strengthening program.

6. Describe at least six components of an integrated approach to exercise.

7. Describe three ways to be safe and prevent injury when performing strengthening exercises.

Activities

1. Contact at least three professional practitioners. Ask them what strengthening routines they do, how they benefit from the exercises, how strengthening has impacted their career longevity, and how they began doing the strengthening routines.

2. Consult a personal trainer for recommendations on how to design a strengthening program for yourself, using the exercises presented in this chapter.

3. When you start your strengthening program, keep a journal for at least 2 weeks. Write down how you feel before you begin your strengthening program, how it feels as you do the exercises, how you feel after the exercises, and what benefits you are gaining from doing them. At the end of 2 weeks, review your journal to see what progress you have made.

REFERENCES

American Heart Association. Target Heart Rates (2010). Retrieved November 2010 from www.americanheart.org/presenter.jhtml?identifier=4736.

Dinas, P. C., Y. Koutedakis, and A. D. Flouris. Effects of Exercise and Physical Activity on Depression (2010). Retrieved November 2010 from www.ncbi.nlm.nih.gov/pubmed/21076975.

Mayo Clinic. Aerobic Exercise: Top 10 Reasons to Get Physical (2010). Retrieved November 2010 from www.mayoclinic.com/health/aerobic-exercise/EP00002.

NAMI. Mental Illness and Exercise (2010). Retrieved November 2010 from www.nami.org/Content/NavigationMenu/Hearts_and_Minds/Exercise/Mental_Illness_and_Exercise.htm.

Surgeon General. Surgeon General's Perspectives: The Importance of Being Active Your Way (2009). Retrieved November 2010 from www.surgeongeneral.gov/library/publichealthreports/sgp124-6.pdf.

Tortora, Gerard J., and Bryan Derrickson. *Principles of Anatomy and Physiology,* 12th ed. Hoboken, NJ: John Wiley & Sons, 2009.

University of California–San Diego. Fiber Types (2000). Retrieved November 2010 from http://muscle.ucsd.edu/musintro/jump.shtml.

U.S. Department of Health & Human Services. Chapter 2: Physical Activity Has Many Health Benefits (2008). Retrieved November 2010 from www.health.gov/paguidelines/guidelines/chapter2.aspx.

Basic Nutritional Principles for Self-Care

Key Terms

Adipocytes
Adipose tissue
Basal metabolic rate (BMR)
Basal metabolism
Carbohydrates
Complete protein
Conditionally essential
  amino acid
Dietary fiber
Essential amino acid
Fat-soluble vitamin
Glycemic index
Hypoglycemia
Incomplete protein
Lipids
Macronutrients
Micronutrients
Minerals
Nonessential amino acid
Nutrient density
Nutrients
Proteins
Reactive hypoglycemia
Resting metabolic rate
  (RMR)
Standard American Diet
  (SAD)
Trigger foods
Vitamins
Water-soluble vitamin

Learning Objectives

After studying this chapter, the reader will have the information to:

1. Explain the various reasons why people eat what they do.
2. Explain why the body needs food, and explain each of the six categories of nutrients.
3. Describe the sources and functions of various vitamins and minerals in the body.
4. Explain why water is so important to the body.
5. Define basal metabolic rate and resting metabolic rate, and determine personal daily caloric needs.
6. Determine appropriate personal nutrient ratios.
7. Explain why meal scheduling is important in maintaining energy levels.
8. Define nutrient density and the purpose of supplements.
9. Integrate proper nutrition into daily life.

> *"Do not dwell in the past, do not dream of the future, concentrate the mind on the present moment."*
>
> — Buddha

INTRODUCTION

The food that you provide for your body can literally make or break your efforts in becoming a successful bodywork practitioner. As has been discussed throughout this book, bodywork is a physical profession. The most important piece of equipment you use is your body. It only makes sense that you keep your body in top physical condition in order to have career longevity. Therefore, along with stretching, strengthening, and injury prevention and management, self-care involves giving the body the fuel, or food, that it needs to function at its best.

The payoff for eating healthy and having a balanced diet can be:

- Greater stamina
- Increased muscular strength
- Decreased risk of injury
- Faster and better tissue healing should injury occur
- Increased mental clarity
- Decreased mood swings
- Decreased weight for those who need to lose it
- Increased weight for those who need to gain it
- Decreased risk of many diseases and conditions, including cardiovascular disease, diabetes, hypertension, stroke, osteoporosis, arthritis, obesity, depression, and even certain forms of cancer

No matter what a practitioner's starting level or current physical condition, he or she can always benefit from eating better. Some people may think that eating nutritiously requires quite a bit of effort. They may be concerned about calculating the correct nutrient levels and calories for themselves, researching the best foods for them to eat, and then figuring out where to get these foods. However, eating nutritiously does not have to be a complex ordeal. While it requires time, patience, and a willingness to follow sound nutritional guidelines, this chapter is designed to guide practitioners through the process.

Note that although the nutrition recommendations presented in this chapter can be used alone, much greater results for strength, stamina, and weight control will occur if accompanied by the stretching and strengthening programs discussed in Chapters 7 and 8. Changing your eating and exercise patterns are long-term projects and lifestyle enhancements, not just short-term goals to be accomplished.

WHY PEOPLE EAT

The most common reason why people eat is to satisfy hunger. However, many people also eat for other reasons. These reasons are closely related to

the foods that we choose to eat. Consider the following:

- Personal preference. Everyone eats foods they prefer based on their taste, appearance, texture, and smell. For example, most people like ice cream because it is sweet (taste) and creamy (texture). Those who like bacon will probably want to eat it if they just catch a whiff of it frying, regardless of whether they are hungry.
- Habits and cravings. Most people are creatures of habit. It is often easier to prepare and eat foods they know they like rather than try something new. Also, almost everyone has a particular food they crave, whether it is something salty, like potato chips; spicy, like chili; or sweet, like chocolate.
- Ethnic heritage or traditions. People grow up eating certain foods, and this becomes familiar. Many times people gravitate toward what is familiar because it is risky to try new things. On the other hand, there are many people who love trying new foods and exploring the foods of different cultures.
- Social pressure. One example of this is a group of friends who gather for happy hour at a local bar and restaurant. The social dynamic involves drinking and eating. Another example is a wedding or baby shower. Most of the time food, especially the cake, is a central part of the shower and everyone is expected to partake.
- Availability or convenience. Everyone has occasions when their time is limited, when they are so busy it is impossible to stop and prepare a meal, or when they simply prefer not to make anything. The fast-food industry depends on this.
- Economic necessity. Many people choose what they eat based on what they can afford.
- Emotional needs and associations. Depending on your family dynamics, you can have strong emotions tied to certain foods. Perhaps during the holidays your grandmother, whom you loved dearly, always made a certain type of cookie, so you like eating the cookies because they remind you of her. Or perhaps you grew up in a tension-filled household where you were made to eat certain foods whether you liked them or not. So as an adult you avoid, for example, meat loaf, not only because you dislike the taste but also because of the anxiety you feel around it. Many people recognize that food satisfies some emotional

need. People may also eat when they are lonely, bored, depressed, or angry.

- Values or beliefs. An example of this is vegetarians who do not eat meat for humane reasons. Another example is cultural values; for instance, people who are Jewish or Muslim do not eat pork.
- The manufacturer or grower. Some people choose to buy only certain brands of food or food from sources they know and trust. For example, there is a growing trend to buy organic and locally grown produce and meats.
- Health status. People who are healthy and active tend to eat more food than those who are in fragile health or who are sick with something like the flu.
- Nutritional value. Some people choose foods based only on their nutritional value. They prefer to eat foods that are healthy for their bodies rather than just eat anything when they are hungry.

THE EFFECTS OF EATING THE WRONG FOODS

Food has a direct effect on the body's physiology and how it functions, and these physiological effects can then change emotional states. For example, eating a big bowl of ice cream will cause a rapid rise in blood-sugar levels. Initially, the result is increased energy and an overall feeling of well-being. An hour later, however, a feeling of fatigue and depression may set in. This is because eating a large quantity of sugar at one time overwhelms the body's blood-sugar balancing systems (*Journal of American Dietetic Association*, 2009; Sears, 2006).

For those who have dieted for years, dieting can sometimes result in the loss of the hunger sensation. Often, people crave caffeine or sugar instead of feeling hungry. Some people find they feel like they are starving only a couple of hours after eating a large meal. They may end up snacking in the evening, such

as is easy to do while watching television. All of these issues are often due to unhealthy dietary habits.

Food choices have a direct and profound influence on the body's health. The only lifestyle choices that have a greater influence on health than a poor diet are smoking, excessive drinking of alcoholic beverages, and using mind-altering substances. Most people know that they need to get a basic balance of nutrients every day. But they may not be aware that the **Standard American Diet (SAD)** lacks nutrients. Moreover, many processed foods include chemically altered fats and sugars that are not healthy for the body.

There is a definite connection between food and disease. Many researchers now believe that many diseases are partly related to diet. While they used to believe that type 2 diabetes, obesity, heart disease, stroke, and certain cancers were caused by a single gene mutation, they are now generally attributing these conditions to a network of biological dysfunctions within the body. The food eaten is an important factor in these dysfunctions, in part because the SAD lacks the necessary balance of nutrients (Chadwick, 2004; Taubes, 2007).

Currently, the average American eats too few vegetables, fruits, and whole grains, and eats too much sugar, fat, and protein. The average health-conscious individual may eat too many grain-based foods (i.e., breads, pastas, and whole grains) and baked goods high in natural sugars. These so-called healthy diets often supply insufficient quantities of protein and fat. Though at opposite ends of the dietary spectrum, both diets are often unbalanced and cannot promote efficient healing and optimal health.

Knowing which foods will maintain balance in the body is the key to optimizing energy and having overall wellness. Every person's body is different; therefore, each person has different nutritional needs. After the right balance of foods has been identified, if there is still a desire to eat unhealthy foods or if you are overeating, it might be time to identify the true reasons behind it. A way to do this is to seek counseling.

WHY THE BODY NEEDS FOOD

The body needs food because food supplies **nutrients**. Nutrients are chemical substances that the body needs for supplying energy to sustain life processes such as tissue growth, nerve impulse transmission, and muscle contraction, and they serve as building

Focus on Wellness

Nutritional Specialists

The information presented in this chapter is meant as an easy guide for healthy eating. However, it is highly recommended that you consult with your physician before beginning any dietary plan. Also, for a more in-depth analysis of your diet and developing a customized nutritional plan, you are encouraged to work with a professional who specializes in nutrition, such as a fitness nutritional specialist, a dietician, or a registered dietician (RD). Requirements vary by state, so be sure to research your best option.

Here are several online resources to help you find a nutritional specialist in your area:

American Dietetic Association:
    www.eatright.org
Dieticians of Canada: www.dieticians.ca
Certification Board for Nutrition Specialists:
    www.cbns.org
Find a Nutritionist:
    www.findanutritionist.com
Commission on Dietetic Registration:
    www.cdrnet.org

blocks for muscle proteins, hormones, and enzymes. The six types of nutrients the body uses are **carbohydrates, proteins, lipids, vitamins, minerals,** and water. Carbohydrates, proteins, and lipids are considered **macronutrients,** which are nutrients the body needs in large quantities; they make up the bulk of the food you eat. Vitamins and minerals are considered **micronutrients** because the body needs them in relatively small quantities.

CARBOHYDRATES

Carbohydrates include sugars and starches. They are the body's preferred source of energy. Carbohydrates come mostly from plants, and they exist in two main forms—complex carbohydrates and simple sugars. Complex carbohydrates are starches that are found in whole grains, vegetables, nuts, some fruits, and legumes. Legumes are fruits that grow in pods such as peas, beans, lentils, soybeans, and peanuts. Examples of simple sugars are table sugar and the sugars found in fruit, honey, and dairy.

Complex carbohydrates need to be broken down into simpler sugars by the digestive system before they can be absorbed from the digestive tract into the bloodstream. The simple sugars in foods do not need to be digested further to be absorbed. Just about all the sugars already existing in food, whether they come from complex carbohydrates or the simpler sugars, will be converted to glucose either by the digestive system or by the liver. Therefore, no matter what form the carbohydrate started out as, it ends up as glucose in the body.

The body uses glucose in three ways:

1. It uses it immediately for energy. Glucose is the body's preferred source of energy.
2. If it is not needed for energy immediately, it is then converted into glycogen (a storage form of glucose) and stored in the liver and skeletal muscles. Liver glycogen supplies energy for the entire body; muscle glycogen supplies energy only to muscles.
3. If the body has an excess of glucose, and all of the glycogen stores are full, the surplus glucose is converted to fat by the liver and fat cells (**adipocytes**) and stored in **adipose tissue** (body fat) around the body. When needed, adipose can be used as fuel directly or when it is converted back to glucose.

When blood-glucose levels are elevated for extended periods of time, it can damage tissues. Therefore, once the blood-glucose level rises beyond a certain point, the body brings it back into homeostatic levels. To do this, the pancreas secretes the hormone insulin. Insulin is released into the blood and stimulates the cells of the muscles and liver to take glucose out of the blood, thereby reducing the blood-glucose level and reducing the chance of damage to tissues.

If blood glucose drops too low, fatigue, poor concentration, and sometimes fainting result. This is called **reactive hypoglycemia. Hypoglycemia** means low blood-glucose levels. The blood glucose drops when concentrated sugars from carbohydrate-rich foods are ingested. However, eating carbohydrates with protein and fat slows the release of sugars into the blood, and there is a decreased chance of reactive hypoglycemia. This is why it is very important for individuals with frequent hypoglycemia to have a balance of protein, carbohydrates, and fat every time they eat (Harvard School of Public Health, 2010A; Tortora and Derrickson, 2009).

The Glycemic Index

The **glycemic index** refers to the relative degree to which blood-glucose levels increase after consuming food. Foods are measured relative to the effect of pure glucose. High-glycemic-index foods can raise blood-glucose and insulin levels very quickly. In contrast, low-glycemic-index foods do not significantly raise blood-glucose and insulin levels after eating.

Pure glucose is given a value of 100, while other foods are given an index number representing their relative effect on blood-glucose levels. For example, sweet corn is assigned an index number of 55, which means it raises blood glucose levels 55% as much as pure glucose. In general, foods below 55 are considered low-glycemic-index foods, 55% to 70% represents mid-glycemic-index foods, and foods over 70% are considered high glycemic.

Table 9.1 shows examples of low-, moderate-, and high-glycemic foods.

In the past, it was widely believed that simple sugars dramatically increased blood-glucose levels while starches such as potatoes and bread were digested slowly. The results from numerous studies conducted by the Glycemic Research Institute (www.glycemic.com) show this is definitely not the case. In fact, one of the biggest surprises comes from baked potatoes, which reported an average index of 85, making it one of the higher glycemic foods available.

While there are many ways to use the index, it is important to remember that different people can have different results, and there are many factors that can influence the index of foods such as food preparation, age of food, fiber content, protein and fat

TABLE 9.1 Examples of Low-, Moderate-, and High-Glycemic Foods

Low-Glycemic		Moderate-Glycemic		High-Glycemic	
Sourdough bread	53	Pancakes	67	Glucose	100
Banana	54	Croissant	67	Parsnips	97
Oatmeal	49	Cantaloupe	65	Wild rice	87
Carrots	49	Couscous	65	Potato, baked	85
Long grain white rice	44	Sucrose	64	Cornflakes	83
Sweet potato	44	Beets	64	Rice cakes	82
Spaghetti, white	41	Raisins	64	Pretzels	81
Apple	38	Shortbread cookie	64	Pancake syrup	76
Yogurt, sweetened	33	Corn chips	63	Doughnut	76
Skim milk	32	Corn, fresh	60	French fries	75
Fettuccini (egg)	27	Bran muffin	60	Graham crackers	74
Lentils	25	Basmati rice	58	Whole wheat bread	69
Grapefruit	25	Pita, whole wheat	57		
Fructose	22	White rice, short grain	55		
Peanuts	15				
Hummus	6				

(Glycemic Index Foundation, 2010)

content, and other variables. It is not a perfect science, and not all testing results have been consistent.

With the guidance of a certified professional (see Nutritional Specialists in the "Focus on Wellness" box), the glycemic index will provide yet another tool to help you meet your goals. It is possible to fine-tune exercise and nutrition programs to more closely match your energy requirements throughout the various stages of exercise. In fact, many people have reported marked differences in weight loss and performance results by manipulating their balance of foods to meet their goals. It is important to know the difference between high-, mid-, and low-glycemic value foods and when their consumption and appropriate mix will best serve their intended purpose.

A good source of information regarding the glycemic index can be found at the website of the Glycemic Index Foundation (www.glycemicindex .com), which is an international database that includes nutritional calculations, research, and news.

Fiber

Fiber is a compound that only plants contain; it is not in animal foods or food products such as meat, cheese, or eggs. Therefore, when carbohydrates are eaten, depending on how the food is prepared, fiber is consumed as well. This is called **dietary fiber**. Fibers are mainly the indigestible parts of plants and include cellulose, pectin, and a variety of other substances. Fibers do not provide any energy, but they do play an important role in the diet as roughage. This indigestible bulk helps the intestines function more efficiently by moving the food through the digestive tract better, and helps regulate the absorption of sugars into the bloodstream. Dietary fiber can be broken down into two forms: soluble and insoluble.

Soluble fiber dissolves in water, and it plays a role in eliminating excess cholesterol from the body. The liver uses cholesterol to make bile acids. Bile acids are then transported to the small intestine, where they aid in lipid digestion and absorption. Soluble fiber binds to bile acids and moves them through the digestive tract so they can be eliminated from the body. Therefore, the binding of bile acids by fiber helps decrease the blood-cholesterol levels.

Insoluble fiber does not dissolve in water. This type of fiber is known as *roughage*. It is responsible for the full feeling after eating certain foods. Though it is not dissolvable in water, it does absorb it, causing an increase in fiber bulk. Since insoluble fibers are not digested, they stay somewhat intact as they travel through the digestive tract, helping clear it of waste and making up the bulk of feces. It is for this reason that eating fiber helps reduce the chance of developing colon cancer (Tortora and Derrickson, 2009).

Regularly consuming insoluble fiber decreases the amount of time digested food sits in the intestine. This helps keep the body from absorbing excess sugars, proteins, and fats into the bloodstream. For those who want to lose weight, eating foods rich in insoluble fiber can help them eat fewer calories without feeling hungry. Since the insoluble fibers are only partially digested, it is hard for the intestine to take up the undigested calories. By reducing calories and decreasing the amount of cholesterol in the blood, body fat can be lost.

As discussed previously, fiber is important for the health of the digestive system and for lowering cholesterol. Eating fiber is promoted by the American Heart Association (AHA). Both the AHA and the Institute of Medicine recommend that people consume 25 to 30 grams of fiber a day. An easy way to do this is to add three choices from Table 9.2 to the diet. Each choice provides 10 grams of fiber (American Heart Association, 2010B; Harvard School of Public Health, 2010B; Institute of Medicine of the National Academies, 2010).

Fiber Supplements

The best source of fiber is from dietary foods, which also provide other minerals and nutrients the body needs. If you consume enough fiber-rich foods, there is no need to take a fiber supplement.

Fiber supplements do not offer the same benefits that dietary fibers do. In 1991, the FDA banned many over-the-counter diet aids with fiber-containing substances because they did not show any evidence of being safe and effective weight-loss agents. Some

Focus on Wellness

When increasing the fiber content of your diet, it is best to take it slow. Add just a few grams at a time to allow your intestinal tract to adjust. Otherwise, you may experience abdominal cramps, gas, bloating, and diarrhea or constipation. Another way to help minimize these effects is by drinking at least 2 liters (8 cups) or more of fluid daily.

TABLE 9.2 Fiber "10" Chart: Food Portions Providing 10 Grams of Fiber

Grains	Vegetables	Fruits
½ cup All Bran	½ cup mixed beans	3 pears
I cup rolled oats	½ cup peas, lentils	3 bananas
I cup whole-grain cereal	I cup peanuts	4 peaches
2 cobs, sweet corn	2 cups soybeans	4 oz. blackberries
3 slices whole-rye bread	3 cups steamed veggies	5 apples
3 cups puffed wheat	4 servings, mixed salad	6 oranges
4 slices whole-wheat bread	4 large carrots	6 dried pear halves
4 large pieces Shredded Wheat	4 cups sunflower seeds	10 dried figs
4 oz. bag of popcorn	5 cups raw cauliflower	20 prunes

fiber supplements also have negative interactions with many heart, diabetic, and psychological medications. Before taking any kind of fiber supplement, it is highly recommended that you consult your physician.

PROTEIN

One of the main reasons the body needs protein is to synthesize body structures such as muscle. Many proteins function as enzymes, which are necessary for the myriad of chemical reactions the body carries out. Other proteins are:

- Transporters. An example is hemoglobin, which is the oxygen-carrying molecule inside red blood cells.
- Antibodies. These are made by certain types of white blood cells and are used to combat invading pathogens.
- Clotting chemicals. When a blood vessel is damaged, platelets use clotting chemicals to stop blood loss.
- Hormones. Examples are insulin (discussed in the "Carbohydrates" section) and growth hormone. Growth hormone has many functions in the body, including tissue growth and repair.
- Structural components other than muscle. Examples are tendons, ligaments, cartilage, skin, hair, and nails. In fact, the vast majority of the body is

made up of different proteins (Tortora and Derrickson, 2009).

Amino acids are the building blocks of protein and muscle tissue. Protein is made up of 21 amino acids, and from these building blocks, an almost unlimited amount of different protein molecules are created. Amino acids are categorized as **essential** (8), **conditionally essential** (7), and **nonessential** (6). The body cannot manufacture essential amino acids in sufficient amounts to meet its needs. Therefore, essential amino acids must be obtained from food. There are eight essential amino acids. The body cannot produce conditionally essential amino acids in adequate amounts during periods of illness, injury, or extreme emotional stress. Under these conditions, conditionally essential amino acids need to be obtained from food. There are seven conditionally essential amino acids. Nonessential amino acids can be synthesized by the human body in sufficient amounts at all times and are thus not required in the diet. There are six nonessential amino acids. The different classifications of amino acids are shown in Table 9.3 (Tortora and Derrickson, 2009; World Health Organization, 2007).

The ultimate value of a food protein or a protein supplement is in its amino acid composition. There are two types of protein: **complete** and **incomplete.** Complete proteins, or high-quality proteins, contain all the essential amino acids, while incomplete

TABLE 9.3 Amino Acid Classifications

Essential	Conditionally Essential	Nonessential
Valine*	Tyrosine	Serine
Methionine	Taurine	Glycine
Tryptophan	Proline	Glutamic acid
Threonine	Glutamine	Aspartic acid
Phenylalanine	Cysteine	Asparagine
Lysine	Arginine	Alanine
Leucine*	Histidine**	
Isoleucine*		

*Branched-chain amino acids (BCAAs)
**Histidine is an essential amino acid for infants and athletes only. It is necessary for the high amount of growth and development an infant undergoes and the high amount of stress athletes place on their bodies.

TABLE 9.4 Sources of Complete and Incomplete Proteins

Complete Protein Sources	Incomplete Protein Sources
Whey*	Vegetables
Casein*	Fruits
Milk	Rice
Eggs	Grains
Beef	Oats
Cheese	Pasta
Chicken	Nuts (some)
Fish	Bread
Yogurt	Sunflower seeds
Cottage cheese	
Turkey	

*Casein and whey are both derived from milk. Whey was once a by-product that was discarded by dairy farmers. However, in recent years, it has been discovered that whey and casein are proteins that the body uses quite efficiently. They are used in powder form by bodybuilders because they increase the protein synthesis needed for bodybuilding and help muscles recover from workouts faster.

proteins, or low-quality proteins, are deficient in one or more. If incomplete proteins are consumed, the body will not fully utilize them during protein synthesis. It is possible to mix two incomplete proteins to make a complete protein. An example of this is mixing rice with beans. Table 9.4 shows sources of complete and incomplete proteins (MedlinePlus, 2010).

LIPIDS (FATS)

While fat receives a great deal of bad press because of its link to heart disease and obesity, a certain amount of dietary fat is important. In fact, the body turns to fat stores as sources of energy during exercise or physically demanding jobs, like performing bodywork. Energy comes from fat breakdown when glycogen stores in the muscles and liver have been depleted. The body has about a 4-hour supply of glycogen, unless exercising vigorously. Then the glycogen will be used up faster.

Even though carbohydrates are the body's major source of energy, lipids are the most highly concentrated source of energy. Fats have 9 calories per gram while carbohydrates and proteins contain only 4, so it is easy to see why foods high in fat are also high in calories. It serves as a storage system for excess calories that are consumed, whether from dietary fat, carbohydrates, or proteins.

Fats also have other functions in the body. It is an essential ingredient for healthy skin and hair and is necessary to absorb the fat-soluble vitamins A, D, E, and K from the digestive tract into the bloodstream. Some are used as structural molecules for cell membranes, are part of clotting chemicals, and form the myelin sheath that covers some nerves and speeds up nerve impulse conduction. Lipoproteins, a combination of a lipid and a protein, transport cholesterol throughout the body.

Cholesterol is only in animal sources of food such as meat, eggs, and dairy. As discussed in the "Fiber" section, cholesterol is needed for the formation of bile salts, and it is used for aspects of tissue repair. However, problems with cholesterol occur if not enough is eliminated from the body; if too much is eaten in the diet; or if, genetically, the body makes too much cholesterol even when not eating an excess amount of it (Tortora and Derrickson, 2009).

Types of Fats

Fats, or lipids, can be found in solid or liquid form. The fats that increase blood cholesterol include saturated fat and trans fat, which stay solid at room temperature. Saturated fat comes mainly from animal sources like meat and dairy products, but can also be found in coconut and palm oils. Trans fat comes from hydrogenated vegetable oils like margarine and vegetable shortening. The body uses saturated and trans fats, even those from nonanimal sources, to make cholesterol.

A more heart-healthy fat is unsaturated fat, generally found in vegetables. This type of fat includes both monounsaturated and polyunsaturated fat and is considered the healthiest for the heart and the body. Monounsaturated fat is found in olive, canola, and peanut oils. These oils are liquid at room temperature but start to thicken when refrigerated. Avocados and nuts also contain monounsaturated fat. Polyunsaturated fat is found in soybean, corn, safflower, and sunflower oils. These oils are liquid at room temperature and when refrigerated.

When unsaturated vegetable oils are processed into solid form, they turn into trans fats. This type of fat is commonly called *fully* or *partially hydrogenated vegetable oil* in a food's list of ingredients. Trans fats are found in hundreds of processed foods, usually to protect against spoiling and to enhance flavor. Restaurants tend to use a lot of trans fat (hydrogenated vegetable oil), especially for frying (Tortora and Derrickson, 2009).

Trans fats are even worse for the cardiovascular system than saturated fats. Researchers have conservatively calculated that trans fats alone account for at least 30,000 premature deaths from heart disease every year in the United States. Recent studies indicate that trans fats drive up the body's cholesterol levels even faster than saturated fats.

Diets high in fat, particularly saturated fat, may also promote breast, colon, endometrial, lung, prostate, and rectal cancers. Therefore, saturated fats and trans fats are the only fats that should be eliminated from the diet. Replace them with monounsaturated and polyunsaturated fats (American Heart Association, 2010A; National Cancer Institute, 2010).

VITAMINS

Vitamins are any of the various relatively complex organic substances found in plant and animal tissue and required in small quantities for the body's

> ## What Do You Think?
>
> Have you thought about your food in terms of carbohydrates, protein, and fat? Do you know what percentage of your daily diet consists of carbohydrates? Protein? Fat? Are you happy with the way you eat now? Why or why not? What small changes can you make now?

metabolic processes. Everyone needs vitamins, and active people need more vitamins than sedentary people. Vitamins are undoubtedly essential to physical performance, whether it is exercise or a demanding bodywork schedule.

The two categories of vitamins are **fat-soluble** and **water-soluble**. As discussed in the "Lipids (Fats)" section, *fat-soluble* means that the vitamin needs to be taken with a small amount of dietary fat in order to be absorbed. However, excess amounts of fat-soluble vitamins will be stored in the body's adipose tissue. If the levels are too high, they can be toxic to the body. The fat-soluble vitamins are vitamins A, D, E, and K. Water-soluble vitamins are taken in along with the water that is absorbed in the digestive tract. If there is more of the water-soluble vitamin than the body needs, it will be eliminated in the urine, which means that you must take water-soluble vitamins daily. To reach toxic levels of water-soluble vitamins, you must take highly excessive amounts. The water-soluble vitamins are vitamin C and the B vitamins.

Each of the vitamins has a specific function in the body:

- **Vitamin A**. Helps to maintain skin and mucous membranes and contributes to night vision. Vitamin A can be found in carrots and yellow vegetables.
- **Vitamin B1 (thiamin)**. Responsible for carbohydrate metabolism along with the functioning of the nervous system. More than 1,000 milligrams of B1 might cause increased urination and possible dehydration. Because this vitamin is water-soluble, daily replacement is necessary. Whole grains are the best source of B1.
- **Vitamin B2 (riboflavin)**. An active participant in the metabolism of energy and cell maintenance. It also is an essential ingredient in the repair of all cells following injury. Milk and eggs are excellent sources of vitamin B2.

- **Vitamin B3 (niacin).** Has numerous responsibilities in body metabolism and is present in every cell. It is helpful in reducing high cholesterol. This vitamin can sometimes cause hot flushes (also called *flushing*) brought on by vasodilation of blood vessels, but a tolerance to this vitamin can be built. Peanuts and poultry are good sources of B3.
- **Vitamin B5 (pantothenic acid).** Essential in the formation of the chemical acetylcholine, which is involved in nerve transmission and memory, and crucial in the production of energy. Poultry, fish, and whole grains provide ample levels of this vitamin.
- **Vitamin B6 (pyridoxine).** Involved in the metabolism of sugar, fat, and protein. A limit of 300 mg per day is usually adequate. It can be found in foods like wheat germ, fish, and walnuts.
- **Vitamin B12 (cobalamin).** Cobalamin refers to substances containing the mineral cobalt, which is important in the metabolism of protein and fat, and aids in red blood cell production. Sources include liver, oysters, and clams.
- **Vitamin B15 (pangamate or pangamic acid).** This is a coenzyme involved in respiration, protein synthesis, and regulation of steroid hormones. Its principal effect is to increase blood and oxygen supplies to tissue. Deficiencies of this vitamin produce no apparent negative effects, which leads some experts to conclude that it is not a "true" vitamin. B15 is found principally in brewer's yeast, organ meats, and whole grains.
- **Folic acid (folacin).** This is the helper substance of the B-complex group, especially in red blood cell formation. Five milligrams a day is recommended for those who are exercising heavily.
- **Biotin.** Helps to metabolize carbohydrates and fats. Best sources are brown rice and soybeans.
- **Choline.** This helps metabolize the B-complex vitamins. It is crucial in normal brain function (notably memory) and acts as a factor in metabolizing fat and cholesterol. The best food sources are eggs and lecithin.
- **Inositol.** This is helpful in the use of B-complex vitamins. It acts with choline in metabolizing fat and cholesterol. In addition, it plays an important role in the transmission of nerve impulses. Lecithin and wheat germ are good sources of inositol.
- **Para-amino-benzoic Acid (PABA).** Essential for normal skin and hair growth. Sources include whole grains and wheat germ. It is at least partially synthesized by normal intestinal bacteria, a fact that has led some experts to deny a need for it in the diet.
- **Vitamin C (ascorbic acid).** A water-soluble vitamin similar to the B-complex vitamins. It is involved in various bodily functions such as promoting protein synthesis, working with antibodies, promoting wound healing, and functioning as an antioxidant. Citrus fruits, tomatoes, and green vegetables provide good sources of vitamin C.
- **Bioflavonoids.** These are chemicals that contribute to the strength of blood capillaries and help to protect vitamin C in the body. These vitamins can be found in fresh raw vegetables and fruits.
- **Vitamin D (calciferol).** This vitamin regulates calcium and phosphate metabolism in the body. It actually starts forming in the skin when ultraviolet rays from light contact it. Next, it goes through a rather complex production process involving the liver and kidneys until it reaches its fully functioning form. Exposure to sunlight serves as the best source of vitamin D, but this vitamin is also added to milk.
- **Vitamin E (d-alpha tocopherol succinate).** This is another fat-soluble vitamin that has numerous responsibilities in the body. Recent research clearly shows the importance of vitamin E in fighting the ravages of free radicals, highly reactive molecules that target tissue proteins, DNA, and the lipids within cell membranes. All of these cause damage inside the body. Food sources are wheat germ, green leafy vegetables, whole grains, and vegetable oils.
- **Vitamin K.** This vitamin is necessary for proper blood clotting. It is synthesized by bacteria in the large intestine.

It is well established that all physically active people need an abundance of vitamins for optimal performance. The physical demands of exercise or even a demanding bodywork schedule can use up these substances and make it more critical for replenishment. It is quite possible that eating carefully balanced meals every day will make supplementation with vitamins unnecessary. However, this does not always happen. It may be wise to take a low- to moderate-dosage multivitamin or mineral supplement two or three times daily. However, caution must be taken when fat-soluble vitamins (A, D, E, and K) are consumed in large quantities because of the possibility of toxicity stemming from the body storing them (Tortora and Derrickson, 2009).

For additional information about vitamins, go to www.nlm.nih.gov/medlineplus/vitamins.html.

MINERALS

Minerals are naturally occurring inorganic substances in the earth's crust. Water leaches minerals from the crust, and often the minerals in water are in the form of electrolytes. As they grow, plants take up the minerals from both the earth and water. Humans and animals get minerals by eating plants and drinking water. Humans also get minerals by eating animals.

Until recently, vitamins were thought to be a more important concern in physical performance than minerals. However, research is now showing that minerals play a significant role in various bodily functions essential to physical movement. For example, failure to consume enough calcium and iron can result in fatigue, weakness, and injury. Women tend to be more likely to experience such deficiencies than men. Their bodies need to replace hemoglobin lost during menstruation. If they do not take in enough iron to make sufficient hemoglobin, they can experience the fatigue and weakness associated with anemia.

Since men generally have a larger body size than women, their bones are more massive and less prone to calcium loss. Additionally, while testosterone maintains bone mass in men, estrogens maintain bone mass in women. Therefore, if women do not take in enough calcium before, during, and after menopause, they are at risk of excessive calcium loss and osteoporosis.

The stresses associated with high-intensity activities, such as strenuous exercise or a busy bodywork schedule, promote the loss of various minerals. The hormones released during stress such as insulin and cortisol can cause the depletion of various minerals. Therefore, it is important to pay attention to mineral intake.

Some of the minerals important to physical performance include:

- **Calcium**. The most abundant mineral in the body. It helps to make up the teeth and bones and is needed for muscle contraction. Good sources of calcium are dairy products, egg yolks, shellfish, and leafy green vegetables.

- **Magnesium**. Another mineral essential to muscle contraction. A lack of magnesium produces fatigue, spasms, muscle twitching, and muscle weakness. Foods that provide quality magnesium are soybeans, leafy vegetables, brown rice, whole wheat, apples, seeds, and nuts.

- **Phosphorus**. The second most abundant mineral in the body. It is involved in muscle contraction and nerve impulses and is a component of many enzymes. Consuming large quantities of phosphorus may lead to depletion of calcium and magnesium in the bones, muscles, and organs, causing weakness. Fish and poultry contain quality phosphorus.

- **Iron**. Essential for hemoglobin in red blood cells. Iron is crucial for the transportation of oxygen during endurance activities. An intake of more than 50 milligrams a day for prolonged periods can be toxic. Interestingly, coffee and tea consumption can limit the absorption of iron. The best source of iron is meat. However, it is also found in shellfish, egg yolks, beans, legumes, dried fruits, nuts, and cereal. Even cooking in an iron skillet can increase the iron content of food.

- **Copper**. Helps to convert iron to hemoglobin and promotes the use of vitamin C. Foods with copper in them include eggs, whole wheat flour, beans, beets, liver, fish, spinach, and asparagus.

- **Zinc**. Responsible for cell growth by acting as an agent in protein synthesis. Also aids in the use of vitamin A and B-complex vitamins. It prolongs muscle contraction and therefore increases endurance. Sources include eggs, whole grains, and oysters.

- **Manganese**. A mineral essential for numerous functions, including glandular secretions, the metabolism of protein, and brain function. Too much manganese can inhibit the absorption of iron. Food sources are tea, leafy green vegetables, and whole grains.

- **Sodium and potassium**. Minerals that need to be balanced for maximal muscular power. These minerals are needed in the transmission of nerve impulses and muscle contraction. Deficiencies produce muscle cramping and weakness. Good sources are green leafy vegetables, bananas, citrus, and dried fruits. Incidentally, salt tablets for sodium intake are not recommended.

Active people vary in the amounts of extra minerals they need. Much depends on age, sex, genetics, medical history, and stretching and strengthening programs. In practical terms, estimates provide guidelines rather than concrete recommendations (Council for Responsible Nutrition, 2010; Tortora and Derrickson, 2009).

For additional information about minerals, go to www.nlm.nih.gov/medlineplus/minerals.html.

WATER

Water is the most abundant substance in the body, making up 55% to 75% of total adult body weight. A 10% reduction of water in the body makes a person feel sick, and a loss of 20% can mean death. Although the body can survive for weeks without food, it can survive only a few days without water. In a hot environment, the time the body can survive without water may be limited to only a few hours.

Water has many functions. The body's regulation of temperature depends on its water. Adequate water levels are needed to cool the body through perspiration. Water is a component of the fluid that lubricates joints, and water is needed in the digestive system. Water is also responsible for the chemical reactions involved in energy production (Tortora and Derrickson, 2009).

Research into the benefits of drinking water is ongoing. For example, according to a 2010 article at www.nutritiontodayonline.com, studies indicate that drinking water may promote weight loss in overweight dieting women, decrease the risk of colon cancer, and decrease the risk of kidney stone formation (Armstrong, 2010).

Considering that muscles are made up of nearly 70% to 80% water, it is easy to see why fluid replacement is so important. Dehydration upsets the natural balance of fluids in the body and can lead to serious issues. It is recommended that plenty of water be consumed on a daily basis, 20 minutes before any exercise activity and following high-carbohydrate meals. Do not wait until you are thirsty to drink water. By the time your body reaches that point, it is already deficient in this vital fluid.

Fluid replacement is as important for the average person as it is for the well-trained athlete. A reduction in as little as 4% to 5% body water can decrease physical performance, no matter whether it is bodywork, strength training, or cycling, by as much as 20% to 30% (European Food Information Council, 2006; Murray, 2007). Table 9.5 shows you how to calculate your recommended water intake.

TABLE 9.5 Recommended Water Intake

Step 1	Select an appropriate need factor
Need factor	0.5—Sedentary, no sports or training
	0.6—Jogger or light fitness training
	0.7—Sports participation or moderate training 3 times a week
	0.8—Moderate daily weight training or aerobic training
	0.9—Heavy weight training daily
	1.0—Heavy weight training daily plus sports training
Step 2	Multiply weight (in pounds) by the appropriate need factor to arrive at the recommended water intake in ounces per day.
Example 1	120 pounds x 0.6 = 72 ounces per day
Example 2	200 pounds x 0.7 = 140 ounces per day
	The recommendation is that you drink water 8 to 12 times per day.
Example 1	72 ounces per day divided by 10 glasses = 7.2 ounces per glass
Example 2	140 ounces per day divided by 12 glasses = 11.7 ounces per glass

(About.com, 2010; CalculatorsLive.com, 2007)

Dehydration

Dehydration is the loss of water from the body, which is accompanied by a depletion of electrolytes such as sodium and potassium. Dehydration may be caused by inadequate water intake or by excessive water loss, but the most common cause of dehydration is a simple failure to drink enough of the right type of liquids. Dehydration is treated by replacing the water the body is lacking and by restoring electrolyte levels to normal.

The average person loses approximately 2.5% of total body water per day. When participating in events above and beyond normal activities, like exercising, performing bodywork, playing sports, or doing yard work, the risk of dehydration is even greater. In addition to the recommended daily water intake as outlined in Table 9.5, individuals should drink 16 ounces of water for every pound of weight lost by doing strenuous exercise. It is also recommended that the water be consumed in the needed amount in 15-minute intervals, rather than all at once (American Council on Exercise, 2010; Griffin, 2010).

The importance of water is unquestionable, especially for anyone who is physically active. As the major component of the human body, plenty of water is essential to healthy and efficient physical performance. And although other drinks like milk, sugared soft drinks, and fruit juices are thirst quenchers, they actually increase the need for water.

PUTTING IT ALL TOGETHER

Now that the various nutrients—carbohydrates, proteins, lipids, vitamins, minerals, and water—have been discussed, you need the tools to put all the information together. This involves determining calorie needs, learning about nutrient ratios, discussing

food quality, and finding out about supplements. With these tools, you can have a better understanding of how you can provide your hardworking body with optimal nutrition.

CALORIC NEEDS

What is the importance of estimating caloric needs? How many times have you heard, "How many calories should I eat?" or "How can I eat to lose weight?" or "What should I eat?" Perhaps you have even asked these questions yourself. The key to answering these questions involves calculating the number of calories you personally need.

FIELD NOTES

When I began my career, I was already over 40. I knew I would have to take care of my main tool, my body, if I wanted to have longevity in the field. I instituted several daily practices that have allowed me to remain injury-free and active in the field:

1. I exercise for I hour every day. I walk briskly, stretch, and lift free weights.

2. I stretch immediately before and after each massage I perform, focusing on the muscle groups most at risk for overuse injury (for me, this means the muscles around the shoulder girdle, lumbar erectors, quads, and posterior leg muscles). I also perform full ROM at the shoulder, wrist, and ankle.

3. I schedule 30 minutes between each client so I have time to drink water, grab a snack if I need one, and stretch tight muscles. Not every massage therapist works in a setting where this is an option, but some time between clients is a must.

4. I set a maximum number of massages that I will perform in a week, and I do not vary from that number.

5. I pay very close attention to my body mechanics, especially toward the end of the day. I find that I'm more likely to slump or get sloppy about wrist positions when I'm tired.

6. I take the time to adjust my table height for each client, if necessary, to maintain my proper body alignment during my work.

Following this regimen has allowed me to maintain my full-time practice for more than 20 years without time out for injuries! Each massage therapist must find the self-care regimen that works best for her.

As you begin your career, you will be tempted to work as much as you can in order to build your client base. However, overworking can result in poor service to the client and injury to your most important tool—your body.

Julie Goodwin, BA, LMT. Licensed massage therapist since 1987.

Body Awareness

To help you determine how much fluid you have lost from strenuous activity, including exercise and a demanding bodywork schedule, weigh yourself before and after. For each pound lost, drink 16 ounces of water.

The scientific definition of a calorie is the amount of heat required to raise the temperature of 1 gram of water by 1°C (1.8°F). Heat is energy, so when measured against this baseline, calories in foods represent the potential energy that food has.

The more calories you eat, the more potential your body has for releasing energy from the food and using it for body functions. If you consume food that contains more calories than you need, then you will not use all of the food for energy; your body will convert it and store it as glycogen or adipose for future use. If you consume food with fewer calories than you need, then your body will take glycogen and adipose out of storage and convert it into energy for body functions.

Think of the calories in food as being like a paycheck. The body "cashes" it to pay bills (fulfilling the body's energy needs). Anything left over goes into a savings account (glycogen and adipose). If there is a smaller than usual paycheck (not enough calories), then the savings account is dipped into so that the bills can be paid.

The calories listed in foods are large calories, sometimes spelled *Calories*. These represent kilocalories. A kilocalorie is 1,000 calories. A single calorie is a very tiny amount; foods contain so many calories that it is more efficient to represent them in kilocalories. Therefore, a food that has 324 Calories, for example, has 324,000 calories; 324 Calories is easier to print on a food package or list in a recipe. For our purposes, *calories* refers to large calories.

BMR/RMR

Everyone expends a different amount of energy, or calories, each day, depending on many factors such as physical activity and the composition of the diet. However, each person's **basal metabolism** or **basal metabolic rate (BMR)** remains somewhat constant. BMR is the baseline rate at which an individual's body expends energy for maintenance activities that keep the body alive. BMR is lowest during sleep when the body is the least active. However, most methods that measure BMR are used when the individual is awake but resting quietly. Also, the methods used to determine BMR involve sophisticated instruments in specific locations such as health clinics, research facilities, and athletic training facilities.

BMR is 1,200 to 1,800 calories per day in adults. Women, unless they are pregnant or lactating, require fewer calories, whereas men, because of their larger body sizes, greater muscle mass, and higher testosterone levels, require more calories. The added amount needed to support daily activities such as digestion and walking range from 500 calories for a small, relatively sedentary person to over 3,000 calories for a person training for Olympic-level competitions. Since it may not be practical for practitioners to have their BMR determined, they can calculate their **resting metabolic rate**, or **RMR**, instead. RMR reflects the baseline calorie needs of an individual when he or she is minimally active.

The following are the formulas for calculating RMR:

For men: $(10 \times w) + (6.25 \times h) - (5 \times a) + 5$
For women: $(10 \times w) + (6.25 \times h) - (5 \times a) - 161$

w = *weight in kg (to convert kg to lb, divide lb by 2.2. For example, a woman weighing 110 lb would divide that by 2.2; 110 ÷ by 2.2 = 50 kg)*
h = *height in cm (to convert inches to cm, multiply inches by 2.54. For example, a woman who is five foot five is 65 inches tall. To convert 65 inches to cm, multiply 65 by 2.54 = 165 cm)*
a = *age*

Here are two examples of how to calculate RMR:

Jordan is a 26-year-old man who is 6 feet tall and weighs 185 pounds. To convert Jordan's weight to kg:

185 ÷ 2.2 = 84.09 or 84 kg

To convert Jordan's height to cm:

6 feet = 72 inches; 72 × 2.54 = 182.88 or 183 cm

To calculate Jordan's RMR:

$(10 \times w) + (6.25 \times h) - (5 \times a) + 5$
$(10 \times 84) + (6.25 \times 183) - (5 \times 26) + 5$
$(840) + (1143.75) - (130) + 5$
$1,983.75 - 135 = 1,848.75$ or $1,849$

Jordan's body requires a minimum of 1,849 calories per day to function. If he is not very active, he would require only 500 more calories a day; if he is extremely active, he could require up to over 3,000 calories a day, in addition to the 1,849.

Amy is a 42-year-old woman who is 5 feet 3 inches tall and weighs 135 pounds. To convert Amy's weight to kg:

135 ÷ 2.2 = 61.36 or 61 kg

To convert Amy's height to cm:

5'3" = 63 inches; 63 × 2.54 = 160.02 or 160 cm

To calculate Amy's RMR:

$$(10 \times w) + (6.25 \times h) - (5 \times a) - 161$$
$$(10 \times 61) + (6.25 \times 160) - (5 \times 42) - 161$$
$$(610) + (1,000) - (210) - 161$$
$$1,610 - 210 = 1,400$$

Amy's body requires a minimum of 1,400 calories per day to function. If she is not very active, she would require only 500 more calories a day; if she is extremely active, she could require up to over 3,000 calories a day, in addition to the 1,511.

Some other things to keep in mind include:

- As a person ages, his or her BMR and RMR go down.
- The lower a person's height, the lower his or her BMR and RMR.
- The lower the weight of a person, the lower his or her BMR and RMR.

This means that as people get older and shorter (which tends to happen in older age) and lose weight, their BMR and RMR will go down. They will need to eat less or exercise more, or do a combination of both, to maintain their current weight (Tortora and Derrickson, 2009).

There are many great resources on the Internet that can help you learn more about nutrition and assist you in calculating factors about your health:

American Heart Association:
www.americanheart.org
Mayo Clinic: www.mayoclinic.com
Calories Per Hour: www.caloriesperhour.com
Diet & Fitness Today: www.dietandfitnesstoday.com
United States Department of Agriculture (Dietary Guidelines):
www.health.gov/DietaryGuidelines/
United States Department of Agriculture (MyPlate): www.mypyramid.gov
Nutrition.gov: www.nutrition.gov

What Do You Think?

Do you know what your current daily calorie intake is? Have you thought about how many calories you consume each day? What type of foods are these calories coming from?

DETERMINING APPROPRIATE NUTRIENT RATIOS

A simple principle to remember for general nutritional intake is to use the International Sports Sciences Association's 1-2-3 Nutritional Rule-of-Thumb: 1 part fat, 2 parts protein, and 3 parts carbohydrates. This rule is valid for most people, even those who are exercising to lose weight. Following this guideline makes it easier to be thinking in terms of good nutrition when purchasing food, preparing meals, and eating out.

Based on this guideline, a healthy ratio of nutrients includes:

- Carbohydrates. Carbohydrates release 4 calories per gram when metabolized. A healthy diet consists of 40% to 80% carbohydrates.
- Protein. Protein releases 4 calories per gram when metabolized. A healthy diet for the average person consists of 0.8 grams per pound of body weight (or up to 1 to 1.5 grams per pound when exercising heavily). This is shown in more detail in Table 9.6.
- Fat. Fat releases 9 calories per gram when metabolized. The American Heart Association recommends that daily fat intake should be less than 30% of total calories, saturated fat intake less than 8% to 10% of total calories, and cholesterol less than 300 milligrams per day. It is always important to read the nutrition facts label and list of ingredients on foods to find out the amount of, and the type of, fat contained in any particular food.

TABLE 9.6 Protein Requirements in Grams per Pound of Bodyweight per Day	
Sedentary adult (RDA)	0.36
Adult, recreational exerciser	0.80
Adult, competitive athlete	1.40
Adult, building muscle mass	2.0
Dieting athlete	1.0
Growing teenage athlete	1.0

(Heller, 2004)

To calculate energy input (food), multiply the source—protein, fat, and carbohydrates—by RMR calories to determine the number of calories from that food source. For example, Rico is a 30-year-old competitive athlete who weighs 200 pounds. His RMR and activity level require him to take in 3,420 calories daily. What follows is how he should be dividing up his food intake.

Protein (using Table 9.6):

Example: Male, 200 lb, 3,420 total daily calories, competitive athlete

$1.40 \times 200 = 280$ grams of protein per day

280 grams $\times$ 4 calories per gram = **1,120 calories from protein**

To determine the percentage of calories that come from protein, divide the number of protein calories by the number of overall calories.

1,120 protein calories ÷ **3,420** overall calories = **33%**

33% of the overall calories are derived from protein.

Fat:

Example: Male, 200 lb, 3,420 total daily calories, competitive athlete

To determine the amount of calories from a diet with 17% of the total calories derived from fat, simply multiply the total daily calories by the percentage of calories coming from fat.

0.17 (17%) $\times$ **3,420** total daily calories = **581 calories from fat**

581 fat calories ÷ 9 calories per gram of fat = **65 fat grams per day**

Carbohydrates:

Example: Male, 200 lb, 3,420 total daily calories, competitive athlete

3,420 daily calories − 581 fat calories − 1,120 protein calories = **1,719 carbohydrate calories**

1,719 carbohydrate calories ÷ 4 calories per gram (as indicated above) = **430 grams of carbohydrates per day**

To determine the percentage of calories that come from carbohydrates, simply divide the number of carbohydrate calories by the number of overall calories.

1,719 carbohydrate calories ÷ **3,420** overall calories = **50%**

50% of the overall calories are derived from carbohydrates.

Rico, a 200-pound adult male athlete, is eating a caloric ratio of 17% fat, 33% protein, and 50% carbohydrates. Using the nutritional 1-2-3 rule of thumb, this is what his food intake looks like:

Nutrient	Calories	Grams	Percentage	Parts
Fat	581	65	581/3,420 = 17%	1
Protein	1,120	280	1,120/3,420 = 33%	2
Carbohydrates	1,719	430	1,719/3,420 = 50%	3

There is another basic, simpler formula to use. For example, if consuming a diet that is 40% protein, 40% carbohydrates, and 20% fat, take bodyweight and multiply it by:

- 8 to 10 to lose body fat
- 12 to gain muscle and lose body fat
- 15 to gain muscle

For example, if Ariana weighs 170 pounds and wants to gain muscle and lose body fat, she would multiply her bodyweight by 12. Therefore, she should consume 2,040 (170 × 12) calories a day. Forty percent of the calories, or 816 calories, would be in the form of protein; 40%, or 816 calories, would be in the form of carbohydrates; 20%, or 408 calories, would be in the form of fat.

You may have to adjust the number of calories up or down, depending on your metabolism and activity levels. If you are finding it hard to make progress using these equations, you can increase or decrease your calorie levels by 100 to 200 per day and see how this benefits you.

FIELD NOTES

Proper nutrition is important to performance both during exercise and while at work. In my experience, being adequately conditioned and fueled with healthy food allows me to be stronger than massage requires me to be. I can finish a long day of massage and have strength and energy left to meet the demands of running a household, raising a family, and leading an active lifestyle. I have been injury-free for all of the 13 years of my massage therapy career, and I believe it is due to the level of conditioning that I have maintained over the years.

Beverley Giroud, LMT, NCTMB. CHEK Exercise Coach, CHEK Level I practitioner. Licensed massage therapist since 1998.

Myth: I will be healthier if I stay away from fats, sodium, and sugar.

FACT: Unless you are diabetic, have hypertension, or retain water, there is nothing wrong with unsaturated fats and sugars. Moderation is the key. As for sodium, seek medical advice before eliminating it from your diet. Sodium occurs naturally in foods and serves many important functions in the body.

MEAL SCHEDULING

Many people make the mistake of skipping meals. Frequently, they skip breakfast because they "are not hungry in the morning," and they skip other meals in an attempt to lose weight. However, skipping meals results in low blood glucose, and frequent low blood-glucose levels can be the stimulus for a cascade of health problems.

It is important to pay attention to blood-glucose levels. Following a meal, blood-glucose levels will be elevated. This will allow you to perform physical activity without losing energy. Of course, the more intense the activity, the more blood-glucose levels drop. When blood-glucose levels get low enough, you will feel tired and weak. But by paying attention to your body, you will realize when your blood glucose is low and needs replenishment. This is the time to eat again. A meal every 3 or so hours may help keep you from getting hungry and keep your insulin levels steady.

Rather than eat by the clock or simply when you are hungry, an option is to consume five or six small meals within a 15- to 18-hour period, the length of time most people are awake. The content and size of each meal is what is important. By asking yourself, "What am I going to do for the next 3 hours?" you can then determine approximately how many calories to consume at the present meal. A bonus is that frequent meals usually mean never feeling hungry.

An example is a daily caloric requirement of 3,000 calories. Three thousand calories over five meals means 600 calories per meal. But since each 3-hour period between meals is not identical in energy needs, it may not be best to have the same amount of calories in each meal.

To assist you in determining how to divide up the calories, consider the following:

- When you wake up, ask yourself what you will do for the next 3 hours. If you are going to drive to work, read the paper, and sit down to a casual meeting, your caloric expenditure will be slight. The calories you consume at breakfast should also be slight—say, 400 to 500 calories.
- Following that 3-hour period, you must ask yourself the same question and evaluate your caloric expenditure. Perhaps you are going to perform some type of moderate-intensity bodywork. This second meal should then provide additional calories, perhaps 600 to 700.
- At the next 3-hour period, you find yourself preparing to do more bodywork. Your caloric intake might again be 600 to 700 calories.
- The next period could precede the time you have set aside to exercise. This time you might consume between 600 and 1,000 calories to ensure adequate energy for your strength training. Also, this is the time to choose foods with a low-glycemic-index rating. This simply means that the foods you choose (like fruits or beans) will stabilize your blood-glucose levels for a longer time, sufficient for your entire exercise period.
- Meal number five might then precede going to sleep by about an hour or so and would therefore require a lower number of calories, say 400 to 500.

The total number of calories would equal the 3,000 calories required per day but would be scheduled in a way that you would consume a greater number of calories prior to the physical and mental demands of your day.

FOOD QUALITY

A better understanding of food quality will often have a positive influence on food choices. When most people think of food quality, they think about whether the food was grown organically or conventionally (i.e., using artificial fertilizers, pesticides, fungicides, and herbicides). Plants can only take up minerals from the soil if there are sufficient microorganisms in the soil to make the minerals available to plants. The use of agricultural chemicals kills these essential microorganisms in addition to the pests that destroy crops; in turn, the quality of food suffers.

All foods grown using chemicals will contain residues of these chemicals. The vast majorities of agricultural chemicals have carcinogenic effects, meaning they cause cancer and promote tumor growth, or may cause birth defects. The level of chemicals found in conventionally grown food varies greatly but is supposed to be below allowable levels set by the federal government. Some studies have shown that the residues of pesticides, herbicides, and fungicides in conventionally raised produce frequently exceed these allowable levels, sometimes by more than 60%. By eating primarily organic foods, which are those grown without artificial chemicals, exposure to these harmful chemicals can be limited and the quality of food in the diet improved (Burros, 2003; Health Sciences Institute, 2007).

Another consideration is the food's location. Foods that are grown locally have to travel less distance to stores or markets. They generally look and taste fresher and more vibrant. You can research to see if there are farmers' markets in your community and perhaps do your food shopping there, if you do not already do so.

NUTRIENT DENSITY

Nutrient density is another way of looking at the quality of a particular food. *Nutrient density* refers to the amount of micronutrients (vitamins, minerals, and trace elements) in a food compared to the amount of energy or calories that food provides. It is the macronutrients (protein, carbohydrates, and fat)

What **D**o **Y**ou **T**hink**?**

How do you eat your meals now? Do you have a strict schedule? Do you skip meals? Do you plan your meals ahead of time? Do you grab whatever is handy? How often do you eat fast food?

What **D**o **Y**ou **T**hink**?**

Where do you buy your food? Have you gone to a farmer's market or local farms to buy food? If so, have you noticed a difference in the taste between that food and food you have purchased in the supermarket?

that supply energy to the body, so it is the macronutrients that supply calories. Table 9.7 compares the nutrient density of whole-grain bread and white bread (Hunter and Cason, 2006; Jegtvig, 2010; World's Healthiest Foods, 2010).

Each loaf of bread contains essentially an equivalent number of calories. However, whole-grain bread supplies a much greater quantity of every nutrient than white bread. Therefore, whole-grain bread has a much greater nutrient density. This is because the flour used to make the white bread was refined. Refining flour means that the nutrient-rich parts of the grain—the bran and the germ—are removed, leaving only the starchy part of the grain.

Whole foods supply more nutrients than refined or processed foods. Processing, however, does not always take place outside the home. Removing the peel or skin, such as from apples, carrots, or potatoes will also reduce the nutrient density of the fruits and vegetables. How you cook your food will also have an effect on its nutrients. Steaming vegetables does the least amount of damage to the nutrients in vegetables. Boiling results in the loss of nutrients into the cooking water.

A study published in the November 2003 issue of the *Journal of the Science of Food and Agriculture* found that broccoli cooked in the microwave lost up to 97% of its antioxidant content but lost only 11% when it was steamed. Another study showed that spinach cooked in the microwave retained nearly all its folate but lost about 77% of this nutrient when cooked on the stove (Weil, 2006). The bottom line is that refining and processing removes nutrients that are necessary for optimal health. It is best to eat foods as close as possible to the form they are found in nature.

SUPPLEMENTS

Scientific studies show that in addition to well-known benefits of maintaining proper health, physical and mental performance can be enhanced with nutritional supplements (LeWine, 2008A and B). While this

Focus on Wellness

The U.S. Food and Drug Administration has a website that you can use to understand the information on food labels. Go to www.fda.gov. Click on "Food," then click on "Labeling & Nutrition."

Body Awareness

Try doing the following for at least 2 weeks:

- Eating five or six small meals a day to constantly supply your body with the nutrients it needs.
- Drinking at least 12 ounces of water with every meal.
- Planning and preparing your meals in advance (to help you stick to your nutrition program and minimize bad food choices made when you are hungry).

At the end of 2 weeks, how do you feel? Can you see yourself doing the preceding steps for the rest of your life? Why or why not? What would you do differently?

category is broad and outside the scope of this book, there are a few commonly known supplements that are worth mentioning:

- Protein supplements offer a convenient and economical way to get daily high-quality protein intake.

TABLE 9.7 Nutrient Density of Whole-Grain and White Bread

	Iron	Magnesium	Zinc	Thiamin	Riboflavin	Niacin	B6	Fiber
Whole Grain	15.5	422	7.6	1.6	0.95	17.4	0.85	51.4
White Bread	3.3	97	2.7	0.4	0.26	0.35	0.15	12.3

Note: Mineral and vitamin levels are in milligrams; fiber level is in grams.

- Glucosamine supplements may aid in dense connective tissue synthesis, which is important because the repair and growth of this type of connective tissue is never-ending, and it may prevent later development of osteoarthritis and other joint issues. Glucosamine may also increase general mobility and reduce symptoms such as pain and stiffness.
- Green tea is perhaps the most potent antioxidant known. It can reduce antibacterial, antiviral, antiplatelet, and hypocholesterolemic activity and can lower the risk of lung cancer due to smoking and the risk of skin damage and skin cancer due to radiation, and a host of health issues.
- Omega-3 fatty acids from fish oils have been linked to reducing the risk of heart attack and stroke, helping maintain bone health and joint flexibility, lowering triglyceride levels, and reducing blood pressure.
- Coenzyme Q10 (CoQ10) is a powerful antioxidant that promotes the efficient utilization of energy at the cellular level and is especially beneficial to heart muscle. It is a particularly important supplement for those who take cholesterol-lowering statin medications, which can inhibit the body's ability to synthesize CoQ10 (Office of Dietary Supplements, 2010).

When you are in doubt about what to take and the effects of supplements on your body, research the supplement in question. The following online scientific journals contain information about nutritional supplements and other valuable information, and are highly recommended as places to begin the search. All of these websites allow free viewing of their back issues and have searchable databases:

> The Physician and Sportsmedicine: www.physsportsmed.com
> American Journal of Clinical Nutrition: www.ajcn.org
> Office of Dietary Supplements, National Institutes of Health: www.ods.od.nih.gov
> Some of the reasons you may want to consider using supplements include:

- It is not always possible or practical to eat five or six times daily.
- There are many instances when your body either requires or can make good use of certain micronutrients in greater amounts than what can be derived from food alone. Examples include periods of high stress and high-intensity exercise.
- Soil depletion, toxins in the food chain, overprocessing, overcooking, free-radical formation in the body, and a host of other, sometimes medically related factors can all interact to make food less than totally nutritious.
- Periods of high-stress exercise require a higher intake of many nutrients without increasing calories.
- Many supplements are derived from natural sources. It is worthwhile investigating these if synthetic supplements are undesirable.

Always consult your physician before taking any supplements.

Focus on Wellness

Keep a Record of Your Progress

Keeping a record of your current eating habits will help you make the necessary changes for a healthier you. Write down everything you eat and drink for a week. At the end of the week, compute all your calories from their sources (protein, carbohydrates, and lipids). Once you have this information, you will know where you need to make adjustments based on the information in this chapter.

You can use the nutrition journal from Figure 9-1 or use one of these:

- Diary
- Scrapbook
- Loose-leaf file
- Photo album (good to use for "before" and "after" pictures)
- A computer spreadsheet
- These websites:

  - easy-weightloss-tips.com: www.easy-weightloss-tips.com/printable-weight-loss-journal.html
  - Keep and Share: www.keepandshare.com/htm/calendars/day_planner/journals/printable_weight_loss_journal.php
  - FitDay: http://fitday.com/
  - PEERtrainer: www.peertrainer.com/info/free_weight_loss_and_diet_journal.htm
  - About.com, Weight Loss: www.weightloss.about.com/od/getstarted/ss/designjournal.htm

Continued

NUTRITION JOURNAL

DATE: ____/____/_____   WEEK: _____   DAY: _____

MEAL TIME	FOOD CONSUMED	TOTAL CALORIES PER MEAL	TOTAL GRAMS PER MEAL		
			Pro	Carb	Fat
1___:___ AM / PM Breakfast					
2___:___ AM / PM Snack					
3___:___ AM / PM Lunch					
4___:___ AM / PM Snack					
5___:___ AM / PM Dinner					
6___:___ AM / PM Snack					
	TOTAL				

Today I feel: (Chek all that apply)
☐ ENERGETIC ☐ MOTIVATED ☐ JOYFUL ☐ CALM ☐ HUMOROUS
☐ PATIENT ☐ SAD ☐ SLOW ☐ DEPRESSED ☐ TIRED
☐ OVERWHELMED ☐ OUT OF CONTROL ☐ ANGRY

FIGURE 9-1 Nutrition journal.

This is a personal record for you. Include the following:

- Your goals and the time frame
- Your successes
- Your milestones
- Inspiration, role models, other success stories
- Your daily nutritional program
- The calories you consume
- Your fat, carbohydrate, and protein intake
- Your personal health issues

Once you have determined what changes you need to make, write down a short-term goal. This not only gives you a target, but also it allows you to have a vision of the "new you." Set realistic goals that are attainable. When you reach each one, you will have a milestone under your belt. You can then set a new goal. Remember, small changes first. Do not change everything at once or you may get overwhelmed and give up. Another idea to think about is deciding what you can eat instead of thinking about what you should not eat—it is a little less stressful.

Myth: All the supplements available today are just moneymaking schemes and none of them work.

FACT: It is true that science has not produced a "magic pill" that helps people lose weight or cures everything. That is not to say that some products currently on the market are not effective. Some are, but (1) you have to use them for a long time; (2) they are very expensive; (3) you have to ask, "Does the cost justify the small gains they may produce?" and (4) "Is there sufficient data to support the claims made by the manufacturer?" Usually such claims are outrageous. Sometimes, however, if you look past the hype, you may find a worthwhile supplement. Do your homework and decide for yourself.

Focus on Wellness

Here are some simple truths about eating and exercise. They apply to everyone—sedentary or active, young or old, in shape or out of shape.

Rule One

Try eating at least five times a day. Two or three meals are simply not enough. It is okay to regard two of these meals as snacks, provided they contain sufficient calories to get you to your next meal, and they are comprised of the appropriate ratio of macronutrients as described in Rule Two. Your blood-glucose and insulin levels will be more even (and so will your level of energy); you will get protein in small amounts throughout the day to support growth and recovery; and, most important, body fat will not be stored but instead will be mobilized as an energy source. By providing your body with a consistent and frequent supply of just the right number of calories, its need to store fat is reduced. Conversely, when you eat infrequently, your body recognizes it as a "famine" situation. In response, it tends to store body fat in preparation for any more "famines" to come.

Rule Two

In planning each of your daily meals or snacks, keep in mind the caloric ratio of 1-2-3: 1 part fat, 2 parts protein, and 3 parts carbohydrates. Remember that this is merely an estimate for average people. Depending on the intensity of your daily work routine and exercise protocol, you may need more or less carbohydrates for energy. Fat is essential for maintaining good health, and it is needed to manufacture many important hormones in your body, so do not attempt to eliminate fat from your diet. Just try to ensure that the amount of saturated fat you eat is kept low and that unsaturated fats are predominate. Also, you must consume enough protein to support growth and recovery, and you need to consume carbohydrates. For the most part, choose low-glycemic-index carbohydrates, which are converted to blood glucose slowly so you can maintain your insulin levels. Remember, carbohydrates are your body's preferred energy fuel source, although fats work well, too, particularly during aerobic exercise.

Rule Three

When you sit down to eat, ask yourself, "What am I going to be doing for the next 3 hours?" If you plan to nap, eat fewer carbohydrate foods; if you plan to exercise or have a long treatment day, eat more carbohydrates. In other words, adjust your carbohydrates up or down, depending on your anticipated energy output. Remember, your pre-exercise or pretreatment day carbohydrates should be low glycemic.

Rule Four

You cannot lose fat quickly and efficiently unless you are in a negative calorie balance—taking in fewer calories than you are burning. Nor can you gain muscle tissue quickly and efficiently unless you are in a positive calorie balance—taking in more calories than you would need to maintain your current weight. So, how can you gain muscle and lose fat at the same time? This paradox is easily explained. Clearly, you cannot lose fat and gain muscle at the same time, so you must alternate periods of negative calorie balance with periods of positive calorie balance. It does not matter if you are trying to lose total body weight, stay at the same weight, or gain weight. Alternating between them will (1) readjust your BMR and RMR upward, making it easier to keep fat off, and (2) support recovery and lean tissue building.

Rule Five

It is almost impossible to get all of the nutrients your body needs to remain healthy and active from food alone. Therefore, consider supplementing your diet with vitamins, minerals, and other carefully selected nutrients to ensure maximum progress toward your fitness, health, muscle-building, and fat-loss goals.

Focus on Wellness

Here are additional tips on sound nutrition:

- **Eliminate junk food.** Most fast food, along with most pastries and processed foods, contain high amounts of fat, sodium, and sugar, which are usually simple sugars. Consuming these foods does little to help you maintain even energy levels. Instead, they promote a rise and then subsequent drop in your blood-glucose levels.
- **Drink at least eight to ten glasses of water each day.** This will ensure you are replacing fluids lost during exercise or strenuous work activities. You should not wait until you are thirsty; by then you are already dehydrated. Drink these glasses of water throughout the day, not all at once. Ideally, you should drink 0.5 ounce of water for every pound of body weight.

- **Determine your daily protein requirements.** Small amounts of protein should be available to your muscle tissue throughout the day for optimum growth and recovery. Be sure to eat proteins that include the essential amino acids. Use Table 9.6 to help you determine how much protein your body needs.
- **Consume high-fiber foods.** A fiber-rich diet helps reduce cholesterol, and it lowers the glycemic response of your meals and promotes efficient digestion.
- **Increase your lean body weight through resistance training.** The more lean weight you have, the more efficient your body moves. Your bones become denser and your muscles, tendons, and ligaments strengthen. The great side effect is that it is easier to avoid gaining excess body fat. Stronger muscles burn more calories than weak ones.

Case Profile

Trina is a 27-year-old massage therapist who recently graduated from massage school. She has been overweight most of her life, and, because of this, she struggled with learning some of the techniques in massage school and just did not seem to have the stamina most of the other students had. Trina grew up in a single-parent household with a mother who was so busy working to support them that she often brought fast food home for dinner. When her mother did cook, it was usually to put frozen dinners in the oven and heat up canned vegetables. As an adult, Trina follows her mother's example for meals and, to keep her energy up during the day, drinks several bottles of caffeinated soda, and she eats candy bars when she gets hungry in between meals. She has tried every fad diet she could find to help her lose weight. None of

them have worked, and she is at a loss as to what to do. After job hunting for 2 months, Trina is finally hired by a massage therapy franchise. When she finds out she is expected to perform at least five treatments each day she works, she begins to panic. She has never been able to perform more than two treatments in a row without becoming exhausted.

- *Why do you think Trina is exhausted after performing only two treatments in a row?*

- *What dietary habits contribute to Trina's lack of stamina and excess weight?*

- *What dietary advice could you give Trina to help her increase her strength and stamina and to help her lose weight?*

Wellness Profile Check-In

Looking at the Wellness Profile you completed at the end of Chapter 1, are there any challenge areas you could remedy through a plan for better nutrition? If so, what are they? How would you like these areas improved? What methods or activities will you use to improve these areas? Write down a plan for improvement that includes the methods you will use, a timeline for implementing these methods, and ways you will assess your improvement along the way. Make sure to consult with your physician before you start any nutritional program.

SUMMARY

The payoff for eating healthy includes, among other things, greater stamina, increased muscular strength, increased mental clarity, and decreased risk for many diseases and health conditions. The six types of nutrients the body uses are carbohydrates, proteins, lipids, vitamins, minerals, and water. Carbohydrates, proteins, and lipids are considered macronutrients; vitamins and minerals are considered micronutrients.

Carbohydrates include sugars and starches, which the body converts to glucose. Dietary fiber consists of the indigestible parts of plants and is necessary to provide bulk that helps move food through the digestive tract and eliminate solid waste from the body. Fiber also helps decrease cholesterol levels. Protein is needed by the body to synthesize structures such as muscle and molecules such as hormones and enzymes. There are 21 amino acids, which serve as building blocks for protein. Fat stores are sources of energy during exercise or physically demanding jobs. Other functions of fat in the body include helping to absorb fat-soluble vitamins, building structural molecules for cell membranes, and forming myelin sheaths around nerves. The body uses saturated and trans fats to make cholesterol. Unsaturated fat is considered the healthiest for the heart and the body.

Vitamins are any organic substances required in small quantities for the metabolic processes of the body. The two categories of vitamins are fat-soluble and water-soluble. Minerals are naturally occurring inorganic substances in the earth's crust. Examples of minerals include calcium, magnesium, and iron. Water makes up 55% to 75% of total adult body weight, and it has many different functions such as regulating body temperature, lubricating joints, and aiding in the digestive processes. Not taking in enough water can result in dehydration. It is recommended that plenty of water be consumed on a daily basis, 20 minutes before any exercise activity and after high-carbohydrate meals.

Practitioners can calculate their RMR to determine how many calories they need to take in each day. For general nutritional intake, remember the 1-2-3 nutritional rule of thumb: 1 part fat, 2 parts protein, and 3 parts carbohydrates. Rather than eat by the clock or simply when you are hungry, an option is to consume five or six small meals within a 15- to 18-hour period, the length of time most people are awake. This will allow you to perform physical activity without losing energy.

Food quality involves whether the food was grown organically or conventionally. It also involves nutrient density, which refers to the amount of micronutrients in a food compared to the amount of energy or calories that food provides. You may want to consider using supplements when you need greater amounts of micronutrients, when you eat food that is less than totally nutritious, and when it is not always possible to eat five or six times a day.

Review Questions

MULTIPLE CHOICE

1. Which of the following is a reason people eat the way they do?
   a. Habits and cravings
   b. Social pressure
   c. Economic necessity
   d. All of the above

2. Which of the following is considered a macronutrient?
   a. Vitamin A
   b. Calcium
   c. Water
   d. Protein

3. Sugars and starches are what type of nutrient?
   a. Protein
   b. Carbohydrates
   c. Lipids
   d. Minerals

4. The indigestible part of plants is called
   a. fiber.
   b. cholesterol.
   c. complete protein.
   d. glucose

5. Which of the following cannot be made by the body?
   a. Adipose tissue
   b. Glycogen
   c. Glucose
   d. Essential amino acids

6. Which of the following is a water-soluble vitamin?
   a. Vitamin D
   b. Vitamin K
   c. Vitamin C
   d. Vitamin E

7. The term for the amount of micronutrients in a food compared to the amount of energy or calories that food provides is
   a. nutrient density.
   b. glycemic index.
   c. resting metabolic rate.
   d. protein requirements.

FILL-IN-THE-BLANK

1. The body needs food because food supplies
   _____.

2. Proteins are made up of building blocks called
   _____ _____.

3. The _____ _____ refers to the relative degree to which blood-glucose levels increase after the consumption of food.

4. A protein that contains all the essential amino acids is considered a _____ protein.

5. The body is made up of _____ percent water.

6. The baseline rate at which an individual's body expends energy for maintenance activities that keep the body alive is called _____.

7. A healthy diet consists of _____ percent carbohydrates.

SHORT ANSWER

1. Explain at least five benefits of eating healthy and having a balanced diet.

2. List and define the six types of nutrients the body needs.

3. Briefly explain how carbohydrates, proteins, and fats are each used by the body.

4. Explain the difference between saturated and unsaturated fats.

5. Choose three vitamins and give sources of them and their functions in the body.

6. Choose three minerals and give sources of them and their functions in the body.

7. Briefly explain how meal scheduling can be used for maintaining optimum energy levels.

Activities

1. Using the formula in the section on BMR and RMR, calculate your RMR.

2. Using the information in the "Determining Appropriate Nutrient Ratios" section, calculate the percentage of carbohydrates, protein, and lipids in your diet that would help you meet your fitness goals.

3. Using the information in Table 9.5, calculate your recommended water intake.

4. Search the various websites listed throughout this chapter to find valuable information that can help you meet your fitness goals.

5. Create a shopping list that has nutrient-rich foods that will help you meet your fitness goals.

REFERENCES

About.com. How Much Water Should You Drink Today? (2010). Retrieved November 2010 from http://nutrition.about.com/library/blwatercalculator.htm.

American Council on Exercise. Healthy Hydration (2010). Retrieved November 2010 from www.acefitness.org/fitfacts/fitfacts_display.aspx?itemid=173.

American Heart Association. High Blood Cholesterol and Other Lipids—Statistics (2010A). Retrieved November 2010 from www.americanheart.org/downloadable/heart/1261004785748FS13CH10.pdf.

American Heart Association. Whole Grains and Fiber (2010B). Retrieved November 2010 from www.heart.org/HEARTORG/GettingHealthy/NutritionCenter/HealthyDietGoals/Whole-Grains-and-Fiber_UCM_303249_Article.jsp.

Armstrong, Lawrence E. Rationale for Renewed Emphasis on Dietary Water Intake (2010). Retrieved June 2011 from http://journals.lww.com/nutritiontodayonline/Fulltext/2010/11001/Rationale_for_Renewed_Emphasis_on_Dietary_Water.3.aspx.

Burros, Marian. Eating Well; Is Organic Food Provably Better? (July 16, 2003). Retrieved November 2010 from www.nytimes.com/2003/07/16/dining/eating-well-is-organic-food-provably-better.html.

CalculatorsLive.com. Daily Water Intake Calculator (Recommended Daily Water Intake Calculator) (2007). Retrieved November 2010 from www.calculatorslive.com/daily-water-intake-calculator.aspx.

Chadwick, R. Nutrigenomics, individualism and public health. *Proceedings of the Nutrition Society*, 63(1); 2004:161–166.

Council for Responsible Nutrition. Vitamin and Mineral Recommendations (2010). Retrieved November 2010 from www.crnusa.org/about_recs2.html.

European Food Information Council. Water Balance, Fluids and the Importance of Good Hydration (June 2006). Retrieved November 2010 from www.eufic.org/article/en/artid/water-balance-fluids-hydration/.

Glycemic Index Foundation. Search the Database (2010). Retrieved November 2010 from www.glycemicindex.com.

Griffin, Dr. Sharon E. Exercise and Avoiding Dehydration (2010). Retrieved November 2010 from www.myfooddiary.com/resources/ask_the_expert/exercise_avoiding_dehydration.asp.

Harvard School of Public Health. The Nutrition Source: Carbohydrates: Good Carbs Guide the Way (2010A). Retrieved November 2010 from www.hsph.harvard.edu/nutritionsource/what-should-you-eat/carbohydrates-full-story/.

Harvard School of Public Health. The Nutrition Source: Fiber: Start Roughing It! (2010B). Retrieved November 2010 from www.hsph.harvard.edu/nutritionsource/what-should-you-eat/fiber-full-story/index.html#health_effects.

Health Sciences Institute. Secret Defense (April 11, 2007). Retrieved November 2010 from http://hsionline.com/2007/04/11/secret-defense/.

Heller, Samantha. Protein: A Guide to Maximum Muscle: Confused? Let Us Separate the Gristle from the Meat (April, 2004). Retrieved November 2010 from http://findarticles.com/p/articles/mi_m1608/is_4_20/ai_n6002944/.

Hunter, J. G., and K. L. Cason. Nutrient Density (November 2006). Retrieved November 2010 from www.clemson.edu/extension/hgic/food/nutrition/nutrition/dietary_guide/hgic4062.html.

Institute of Medicine of the National Academies. Dietary Reference Intakes for Energy, Carbohydrate, Fiber, Fat, Fatty Acids, Cholesterol, Protein, and Amino Acids (2010). Retrieved November 2010 from www.iom.edu/Reports/2002/Dietary-Reference-Intakes-for-Energy-Carbohydrate-Fiber-Fat-Fatty-Acids-Cholesterol-Protein-and-Amino-Acids.aspx.

Jegtvig, Shereen. Nutrient Density; What Makes Superfoods so Super? (November 4, 2010). Retrieved November 2010 from http://nutrition.about.com/od/nutrition101/a/nutrient_dense.htm.

Journal of the American Dietetic Association. Position of the American Dietetic Association, Dietitians of Canada, and the American College of Sports Medicine: nutrition and athletic performance. *Journal of the American Dietetic Association*, 109(3);2009:509–527.

LeWine, Howard, MD. Can Nutritional Supplements Enhance Athletic Performance (Part 1 of 2) (October 14, 2008A). Retrieved November 2010 from www.intelihealth.com/IH/ihtIH?d=dmtHMSContent&c=382130&p=~br,IHW|~st,853|~r,WSIHW000|~b,*|

LeWine, Howard, MD. Can Nutritional Supplements Enhance Athletic Performance (Part 2 of 2) (October 14, 2008B). Retrieved November 2010 from www.intelihealth.com/IH/ihtIH/E/35320/35322/384533.html?d=dmtHMSContent.

MedlinePlus. Protein in Diet (2010). Retrieved November 2010 from www.nlm.nih.gov/medlineplus/ency/article/002467.htm.

Murray, Bob, PhD. Hydration and Physical Performance (2007). Retrieved November 2010 from www.jacn.org/cgi/reprint/26/suppl_5/542S.pdf.

National Cancer Institute. Fat Consumption (2010). Retrieved November 2010 from http://progressreport.cancer.gov/doc_detail.asp?pid=1&did=2007&chid=71&coid=708&mid=.

Office of Dietary Supplements, National Institutes of Health. Dietary Supplement Fact Sheets (2010). Retrieved from http://ods.od.nih.gov/factsheets/list-all/.

Sears, Dr. William, and Dr. Martha Sears. Sugar (2006). Retrieved November 2010 from www.askdrsears.com/html/4/T045000.asp.

Taubes, G. Do We Really Know What Makes Us Healthy? *New York Times* magazine, September 16, 2007:52.

Tortora, Gerard J., and Bryan Derrickson. *Principles of Anatomy and Physiology,* 12th ed. Hoboken, NJ: John Wiley & Sons, 2009.

Weil, Andrew, MD. Nuking Your Nutrients? Do Vegetables Lose Nutrients When Cooked in the Microwave? (December 26, 2006). Retrieved November 2010 from www.drweil.com/drw/u/QAA400107/microwaving-nutrients.

World Health Organization. Protein and Amino Acid Requirements in Human Nutrition (2007). Retrieved November 2010 from http://whqlibdoc.who.int/trs/WHO_TRS_935_eng.pdf.

World's Healthiest Foods. What Is Nutrient Density and Why Is It so Important? (2010). Retrieved November 2010 from www.whfoods.com/genpage.php?tname=george&dbid=81.

Additional Support for Wellness and Self-Care

Key Terms

Mentoring
Peer
Peer support
Supervision

Learning Objectives

After studying this chapter, the reader will have the information to:

1. Determine what information has been personally implemented successfully and what areas still need work.
2. Explain what supervision, mentoring, and peer support are.
3. List ways to get the most out of support.
4. Assess stress currently being personally experienced.
5. Implement strategies to prevent or manage burnout.
6. Evaluate additional self-care strategies and integrate them into daily life.

> "There's only one corner of the universe you can be certain of improving, and that's your own self."
>
> — Aldous Huxley

INTRODUCTION

Being a bodywork practitioner can be demanding, challenging, exciting, and gratifying. It is undoubtedly possible to have a long, successful career, if practitioners give their own physical and emotional needs the same care and consideration they give their clients. Practitioners need to allow themselves to be human, to have strengths and weaknesses, to make mistakes, and to learn and grow from those mistakes.

Practitioners have physical limits just like everyone else, and they get injured when they push themselves beyond those limits for too long. Part of wellness and career longevity is valuing yourself enough to seek appropriate professional help when you need it, either physically or emotionally. By listening to your body and becoming aware of the messages it is sending, you have the information necessary to make appropriate modifications quickly and easily.

Redesigning life and work to prevent injury is really about being good to yourself. Taking responsibility for your own health and well-being is part of improving and maintaining self-respect and self-esteem. The most successful practitioners are those who practice what they preach and who model confidence and wellness for their clients. It is difficult to convince clients to make health and wellness a priority if it is not a priority for practitioners. Adapting their work and personal lives to allow room for health, relaxation, and peace of mind are challenges that all practitioners face as life becomes increasingly complex and demanding. Allowing the well-being that the healing profession promotes to be part of your own life makes you better equipped to handle daily and long-term stresses.

This chapter reviews concepts that impact career longevity presented in the previous chapters, and it discusses additional factors. For example, practitioners must be able to determine how many treatments is too many, when to take a break, and when to take a vacation. Knowing when to refer clients and when diversity in types of treatments offered also impacts career longevity in professional bodywork. How practitioners care for their hands, wrists, back, neck, knees, shoulders, and feet is also important. These methods include stretching, strengthening, hydrotherapy protocols, healthy sleep positions, propping, use of splints if necessary, use of massage therapy tools, and receiving regular bodywork.

WHAT HAVE YOU LEARNED?

There are many different aspects to career longevity. Successful practitioners are confident in their abilities, possess a positive mental attitude, maintain healthy boundaries, enjoy working with people, are willing to take risks, and are physically and mentally prepared for the demands of the profession. These practitioners are determined and focused on being the best practitioner they can be. Along with being determined, other characteristics they have in common are insight and flexibility. They are willing to look at what is working for them and what is not, and they have the motivation and flexibility to try something new if what they are doing is not helping them. The information in this book has been designed to assist practitioners in trying something new.

Use the information in the Focus on Wellness box and in this section to self-assess how you have incorporated the information in this book into your life.

Focus on *Wellness*

What Have You Learned?

Ideally, you have been able to use the information presented throughout the chapters in this book. However, sometimes, despite their best efforts, practitioners may still struggle with various aspects of career longevity. If you think that you have done everything possible to ensure your career success but do not think that you are functioning at your absolute best, you may need to reevaluate your approach.

You can use the following questions to see if you are using the information in each of the chapters to the best of your ability. This, along with your Wellness Profile, can help you identify areas in which you need to improve and areas in which you are having success.

Answer Yes or No to the following:

_____ Is your appearance as professional as it should be?

_____ Is your verbal and nonverbal communication as professional as it should be?

_____ Are you as mentally and emotionally prepared to be a professional bodywork practitioner as you should be?

_____ Are health and wellness part of every aspect of your life, not just in the performance of bodywork?

You can revisit Chapter 1, "Bodywork and the Bodywork Practitioner's Wellness," for reminders on how to address the challenges you are experiencing.

_____ Do you understand how your body moves?

_____ Have you made the connection between your own body awareness and its effect on how you perform bodywork treatments?

_____ Do you understand the importance of stillness in the performance of effective bodywork treatments and the importance of stillness for your own rejuvenation?

_____ Do you center and ground yourself every day?

_____ Do you have mindful movement that is efficient and beneficial to you?

You can revisit Chapter 2, "Body Awareness and Mindful Movement," for reminders on how to address the challenges you are experiencing.

_____ Do you understand the connection between having balanced posture and your career longevity?

_____ Have you honestly assessed your posture, both during the performance of bodywork and in your ADL?

_____ Are you working to make your posture more balanced and efficient?

_____ Do you have a stable center of gravity?

_____ Do you have a strong base of support?

You can revisit Chapter 3, "Posture and Its Impact on the Body," for reminders on how to address the challenges you are experiencing.

_____ Do you understand the importance of breathing efficiently and how it affects the performance of bodywork and your career longevity?

_____ Are you practicing diaphragmatic and nostril breathing?

_____ Do you have efficient respiratory posture?

_____ Are you using your breath efficiently while performing bodywork?

You can revisit Chapter 4, "Breathing for Best Practice, Health, and Wellness," for reminders on how to address the challenges you are experiencing.

_____ Do you understand the components of efficient body mechanics and how these impact the performance of your bodywork treatments and career longevity?

_____ Have you made the connection between movement and awareness to body mechanics?

_____ Are you using efficient body mechanics?

_____ Do you have any repetitive stress injuries? If so, do you know the causes, symptoms, and risk factors, and what you can do to manage them and prevent them in the future?

_____ Have you considered how environmental factors have impacted your body mechanics and made changes so that you can improve your body mechanics?

You can revisit Chapter 5, "Body Mechanics," for reminders on how to address the challenges you are experiencing.

_____ Do you know what injuries you are at risk for developing as a bodywork practitioner?

_____ Do you have any warning signs for injury or the development of a condition?

_____ Have you developed a plan to prevent or manage injuries and ensure your career longevity?

You can revisit Chapter 6, "Injury Prevention and Management," for reminders on how to address the challenges you are experiencing.

_____ Do you understand the importance of flexibility in performing bodywork?

_____ Have you made the connection between inflexibility and injury?

_____ Have you made the connection between performing stretches and career longevity?

_____ Do you perform stretches for yourself? If so, how often?

You can revisit Chapter 7, "Stretching: Why, How, When, and Where?" for reminders on how to address the challenges you are experiencing.

_____ Do you understand the importance of strength training for health and career longevity?

_____ Do you understand the physiological basis of body strength?

_____ Have you made the connection between muscular weakness and injury?

_____ Do you perform strength training for yourself? If so, how often?

You can revisit Chapter 8, "Strengthening: Why, How, When, and Where?" for reminders on how to address the challenges you are experiencing.

_____ Do you understand the importance of good nutrition in maintaining or improving health and wellness and ensuring career longevity?

_____ Do you understand how good nutrition can help you meet your weight goals?

_____ Do you have a good nutritional plan for yourself?

You can revisit Chapter 9, "Basic Nutritional Principles for Self-Care," for reminders on how to address the challenges you are experiencing.

SUPPORT

If you find that you are not optimizing the information you have learned, ask yourself, "Why not? What is keeping me from doing this? What is holding me back?" Often, what practitioners need the most is some type of support for the changes they want and need to make. It may be a simple matter of asking a friend or a colleague for help, or it may be a more complex matter involving finding a certified personal trainer (as recommended in Chapter 8) or a nutritional specialist (as recommended in Chapter 9) or seeking counseling for underlying issues that are preventing your success.

If you are wondering if you need to seek support, consider asking yourself the following questions:

- Do I feel ineffective in my work?
- Have I lost clientele?

- Am I lonely?
- Am I disheartened about my work?
- Do I feel overwhelmed by my clients?
- Do I feel emotionally spent?
- Am I finding myself slacking off in my treatment skills?
- Am I bored?
- Am I unable to keep a job?
- Do I have a pattern of blaming the client when a session does not go well?

Some of these signs indicate burnout, which is discussed in more detail in the "Burnout" section.

Support can take many different forms for practitioners. Family and friends with whom you are close and who you trust can be incredible resources. Depending on your personal situation, family and friends may provide a shoulder to lean on, an ear to listen, advice, and financial support, and they can be sources of hope and inspiration.

However, not every practitioner has family and friends on whom they can rely. Sometimes family and friends do not understand the unique challenges that can arise in the bodywork profession. They may not know how to help you start a stretching program, or they may not understand why you need moments of quiet and stillness.

There are other types of support available to you. These include supervision, mentoring, and peer support. All of these are meant to provide sounding boards for practitioners by practitioners, although mentors can also come from other professions. The purpose is for you to gain insight with the help of others who have been in similar situations, or at least understand what it is like to be in the bodywork profession.

Supervision

Supervision involves periodic review of the bodywork practitioner's professional actions by an authority in the work setting. The supervision can be direct, as when the supervisor observes the professional at work, or it can be indirect, as when the supervisor discusses professional practices with the practitioner.

Supervision can assist practitioners by reducing the chances of burnout. The supervisor has more experience and insight into the profession and can help less experienced practitioners develop a deeper understanding of their professional work and of the importance of self-care, leading to better fulfillment and career longevity. Supervisors are in a position of authority, usually in the practitioner's place of employment.

Effective supervisors help you explore what is happening with you mentally and emotionally. They also help define appropriate boundaries between you and your clients, and determine what actions may help in given situations. The focus should be on developing your problem-solving skills, leading to increased confidence in your abilities. The supervisor's job is not to tell you what to do and say all the time. His or her job is to help you take initiative and be creative. The supervisor is not there to "fix" or soothe you, but to point out areas of challenges and strengths that will enhance your therapeutic work and self-care.

Mentoring

Another option practitioners may consider is finding someone who is not necessarily in a position of authority over them but who can advise them. Such people are called mentors. **Mentoring** involves a professional relationship in which a person with greater experience and skill provides support, encouragement, and career expertise to those with less experience and skill in the profession.

Practitioners often choose this option as part of their commitment to becoming a better professional. Perhaps they are in sole practice and have no one else off whom to bounce ideas. They may be new to the profession and want to ensure that they are on the right track, or they may find themselves in situations for which they feel completely unprepared. Another possibility is that they are dissatisfied with the supervision they are receiving as an employee and want other ideas and opinions.

Since mentors do not have the capacity to hire, fire, or discipline the practitioner, the relationship tends to have more freedom and is less formal than with a supervisor. With a mentor, you may feel more able to discuss issues without fear of feeling inadequate or being reprimanded.

Some mentors are willing to donate their time and expertise to assist you, while others may charge a fee for their services. The fees can vary in amounts. However, an hourly amount comparable to what you charge for a bodywork session would be a fair fee.

While a mentor is someone you can turn to in times of struggle and confusion, you should not look to this person to fix difficult situations for you. The mentor is there to assist you in recognizing who you are as a practitioner. The mentor then helps you discover how you are being challenged in difficult situations, with difficult clients, or with personal issues. You can use the mentor's experience and expertise as a guide to seeing actions and behaviors that are getting in the way of being successful in your work.

A mentor is typically someone with whom practitioners have a history of familiarity and connection. Many practitioners choose mentors based on how they work and interact with others. They like his or her style. Often, mentors are teachers in bodywork programs or are professional bodyworkers from whom the practitioners have received bodywork in the past or on a regular basis and to whom they feel a connection. A mentor could also be one who provides quality continuing education classes, or simply an individual whom the practitioner has heard good things about and believes could guide him in problem-solving, recognizing him for work well done, and analyzing his behavior and choices when necessary.

However, those mentoring bodywork practitioners do not necessarily need to be practitioners themselves. Various health-care professionals, such as nurses, counselors, fitness trainers, and psychologists deal with issues similar to those encountered in the bodywork profession. In fact, some practitioners may feel comfortable seeking a mentor outside the bodywork profession because they may get a more objective viewpoint.

When choosing a mentor within the bodywork profession, consider practitioners who:

- Have successful practices
- Are well respected
- Have volunteered their time for bodywork organizations and learned skills beyond the treatment room
- Are also instructors

When choosing mentors outside of the bodywork profession, consider:

- Getting recommendations from trusted colleagues, friends, and family members
- Contacting professional organizations, such as nursing or mental health associations

Peer Support

Peer means one who is of equal standing with another. In the bodywork profession, **peer support** is the interaction among practitioners who have similar levels of skill and experience for the purpose of encouraging and maintaining appropriate professional and ethical practice. It is an opportunity for colleagues to support each other and challenge each other to adopt fresh perspectives on issues and situations they encounter in their practice. Sometimes practitioners choose to seek support through peer groups or on a one-on-one basis.

Peer groups can help decrease the isolation practitioners may feel if they are in sole practice or who are the only bodywork practitioner in a work setting with other professionals. Peer groups can be a way new practitioners support each other, as well as benefit from wisdom gained by practitioners who have been in the profession longer. These groups can also provide networking prospects. Practitioners can talk about the stresses and strains that come with being a bodywork practitioner. In a well-functioning peer group, there is the safety of speaking freely about experiences (while maintaining client confidentiality, of course) with other practitioners who understand where they are coming from.

The role of the group is to listen and offer questions that may inspire group members to find solutions to their dilemmas. The understanding is that members are not to shame, belittle, or fix the other members' situations for them. Support comes through active listening and mindful, open-ended questions.

In some peer groups, there is no one person facilitating the meetings. The role of facilitator is shared and rotated among the members for each meeting. Some practitioners are more comfortable with this because they do not feel as on the spot as they might with a more formal facilitator who "calls on them." Rotating the task of group facilitator allows each member the opportunity to be a leader in the group. However, some groups choose to have a professional facilitator for the sessions. This choice is made by practitioners who want the group experience while having the expertise of the facilitator. In this case, the practitioners should share the fee for the facilitator.

The peer groups that work best are those in which all the members are willing to receive and provide support. They are grounded in a shared sense of purpose for the group and for the bodywork profession. It is most beneficial to be in a peer group with others who respect each other and are nonjudgmental. Receiving and offering feedback is a very intimate exchange. Practitioners must be willing to share the experience with whoever is in the group.

To ensure safety, accountability, and confidentiality, it is essential that guidelines and parameters be established for the group. A confidentiality agreement, preferably a written one, is essential if the members are going to truly share what is deeply personal to them. Establishing parameters in terms of how often the group will meet, the time frame of the meetings, the location of the gathering, and how the group will be facilitated are factors that provide structure and security for all involved.

Whether you choose to join a peer group or seek one-on-one support with a peer, you must be mindful of whom you consider to be appropriate peers for offering and receiving support. As stated previously, *peer* means that both people are of equal standing with each other. Although it is helpful to share ideas and strategies with someone else of equal status, it is important that you be selective in exactly which peers are the most beneficial to do this with.

It might be tempting to ask a group of friends to come together on a regular basis to share work experiences and get support for managing successful practices. Friends are an essential ingredient to a well-rounded life. Yet, when you want someone to hold you accountable for your actions, sometimes a friend may not be the right choice. Sometimes friends are reluctant to speak frankly about challenges you need to work on because they are afraid of harming the friendship.

On the other hand, having a history that dates back to attending bodywork school together means that you are likely to have the same pool of knowledge and experience. You may be less inhibited with acquaintances than you are with friends and will share more honestly about your doubts and fears. However, it can also be useful to choose practitioners who have a different background. These individuals can give you fresh, differing perspectives on what it is like for them in their practices.

Getting the Most Out of Support

The types of issues discussed in support sessions vary, whether they involve supervision, mentoring, or peer support. The supervisor, mentor, or peer can point out patterns in behavior if you are unaware that they exist and are confused as to why certain issues keep coming up. Effective support people hold a mirror up to you, without sugarcoating their words or taking care of you so you can see what is going on.

You can get the most out of support if you are able to:

- Be open to feedback
- Discern what support and feedback is necessary and true for you
- Not back down if the feedback does not feel accurate
- Implement appropriate feedback in a timely fashion
- Be honest about your challenges or what may be causing you fear
- Have an authentic desire to grow emotionally and professionally

Voice of Experience

My favorite quote to share with my clients is "Stopping, resting, and calming are preconditions for healing" by Thich Nhat Hanh.

As a bodyworker, it is imperative for me to stay balanced emotionally, physically, spiritually, and energetically. I found my spiritual practice of meditation and yoga 9 years ago and notice that when I'm not working on myself, my bodywork actually becomes work. When I'm centered, my bodywork is effortless and the time flies in a treatment. It took me a long time to understand that putting myself and my health first was not selfish—it was necessary!

As soon as I set up my office, I began creating relationships with other complementary bodyworkers, chiropractors, and acupuncturists in my area. I use these resources as a referral for my clients and to work trades with me. This allows me to get some form of bodywork at least three times a month. When you care for yourself, you have so much more to give to your clients.

Becky Rosenthal, M.Ed, NCTMB, LMT. She has been a career counselor at the Nevada School of Massage Therapy in Las Vegas, NV; director of Admissions and instructor at the Desert Institute of the Healing Arts in Tucson, AZ; and Former Professor of Health and Wellness at Incarnate Word University in San Antonio, TX. Licensed massage therapist and shiatsu practitioner since 2002.

BURNOUT

The subject of burnout is discussed throughout this book. Burnout can be one of the major reasons why practitioners leave the bodywork profession. The burnout can be physical, mental, or emotional, or a combination of these. The information in all of the previous chapters is designed to assist you in preventing burnout or, if you are already experiencing it, to help you manage it by changing the factors that are contributing it.

Recall from Chapter 1 that *burnout* is a psychological term for experiencing long-term exhaustion and diminished interest in aspects of life, especially in one's career. It is a gradual process that occurs over an extended period of time. While it does not happen overnight, it can creep up if you are not paying attention to the warning signals. The signs and symptoms are subtle at first and then get worse as time goes on if the causes are not addressed and managed.

The signs and symptoms of burnout include:

- Feeling tired and drained most of the time
- Experiencing frequent headaches, back pain, muscle aches
- Experiencing a change in appetite or sleep habits
- Having a lowered immunity, feeling sick a lot

- Having a sense of failure and self-doubt
- Feeling a loss of motivation
- Feeling helpless, trapped, and defeated
- Being increasingly cynical and having a negative outlook
- Having decreased satisfaction and sense of accomplishment
- Feeling detachment or alone in the world
- Withdrawing from responsibilities
- Isolating from others
- Using food, drugs, or alcohol to cope
- Procrastinating, taking longer to get things done
- Taking frustrations out on others
- Skipping work or coming in late and leaving early

If practitioners pay attention to these symptoms and early warning signs, they can prevent a major breakdown. If they ignore them, then it is likely they will eventually experience burnout.

Focus on Wellness

Stress Assessment

Use this stress assessment to better understand your stress. Answer all of the questions and rate your current stress level on a scale of 1 to 5, 1 being the lowest and 5 being the highest:

1. In the last month, how often have you felt you were unable to control the important things in your life?
   1 Never
   2 Almost never
   3 Sometimes
   4 Fairly often
   5 Very often

2. In the last month, how often have you felt confident about your ability to handle your personal problems?
   1 Never
   2 Almost never
   3 Sometimes
   4 Fairly often
   5 Very often

3. In the last month, how often have you felt that things were going your way?
   1 Never
   2 Almost never
   3 Sometimes

   4 Fairly often
   5 Very often

4. In the last month, how often have you felt that difficulties were piling up so high that you could not overcome them?
   1 Never
   2 Almost never
   3 Sometimes
   4 Fairly often
   5 Very often

5. How often do you feel so sad or down that you are having trouble functioning in your personal life?
   1 Never
   2 Almost never
   3 Sometimes
   4 Fairly often
   5 Very often

Low stress = a score of 5 to 12
Moderate stress = a score of 13 to 18
High stress = a score of 19 to 25

If you score in the low stress category, you are likely experiencing a healthier lifestyle, more energy, and more peace of mind than those with moderate or high stress scores. Therefore, keep practicing the stress management strategies that are working for you.

Continued

If you score in the moderate or high categories:

- Identify sources of stress that you can eliminate (use the Wellness Profile to help). Consider internal stressors, such as fears or unrealistic expectations, and external stressors, such as family or work demands.
- Seek out effective strategies for coping with stress, including exercise, music, crafts and other creative outlets, and humor, or simplify your life by saying no to extra obligations.
- If you need help identifying stress management strategies, talk to your health-care provider or mental health professional.

Here are online resources for more information on health risk assessments due to stress and suggestions for minimizing stress:

Walgreens: www.walgreens.com/marketing/library/healthrisk/default.jsp?AssessmentId=9

Healthline: www.healthline.com/sw/rsk-stress-trigger-assessment

In addition to the information in previous chapters, which is designed to prevent or manage burnout, there are several other things you can do. These include:

- Set aside time to think about and do planning for your business. Do this at least once a month, or more often if you like. When thinking about and planning for your business, that should be your primary focus; do not let anything else intervene. Evaluate your business agreements, goals, marketing, and client relations to see what is working, what is not working, and how you would like to make changes.
- Make time to meet with colleagues on a regular basis. This is a good way to connect with others who will understand your triumphs and challenges, and it can be a good network of support for you.
- Attend conferences and continuing education classes. These are a great way to meet and interact with practitioners from both within and outside of your community, create networking opportunities, and expand your knowledge and stay inspired.
- Maintain strong personal support systems.
- Practice stress relief methods (see the following Focus on Wellness box, "Stress Relief Methods").
- Determine the optimal amount of treatments you can do and the time you need in between each treatment. Stay within these parameters as much as possible.
- Know when you need to take a break and when you need to take a vacation, and actually take them.
- Know when you need to refer clients, and actually refer them.
- Know when it is time to diversify in the types of bodywork modalities you offer.

Focus on Wellness

Stress Relief Methods

Here is a quick list of stress relief methods that are presented throughout the chapters in this book:

- Perform stretches regularly
- Perform strengthening exercises regularly
- Perform breathing exercises regularly
- Use proper body mechanics
- Use the right equipment for your modality, and use it appropriately
- Take breaks and vacations
- Eat properly
- Meditate or do martial arts
- Receive bodywork on a regular basis

Keep in mind that balance is the key to stress management.

WHEN TO TAKE A BREAK, WHEN TO TAKE A VACATION

In order to keep their bodies in good working condition while performing treatments, practitioners must know how many treatments they can do within a given day and how much time they need in between treatments to prepare for the next client. This preparation includes not only setting up the proper equipment and supplies but also stretching and doing strengthening exercises, centering and grounding, eating a healthy snack (if hungry), and drinking enough water to stay well hydrated.

When you complete your bodywork program of study, you may already have an idea of how many treatments you can perform. This can be from your experience in a student clinic and from working on practice clients. Using this as a starting point, you can then test yourself by seeing how you feel after performing two, three, four, or even five treatments in a row. Pay attention to how you feel when you have 10-, 15-, 20-, and 30-minute breaks in between each client.

What time-length break feels the best to you? What time-length break seems like it is too short and does not give you enough time to adequately prepare between client treatments? What time-length break seems like it is too long, perhaps leaving you feeling restless and bored and wanting to get back to work?

Note that the more treatments you do, the more stamina you will build, as long as you pay attention to your body mechanics and practice self-care, such as having proper hydration and nutrition, doing strengthening exercises, cultivating stillness, and so forth. A caution, however, is to not use your increased stamina just to perform more treatments for the sake of performing more treatments. This can lead to an increased risk of injury and physical burnout.

Also note that if you are an employee, you may not have a choice in how many treatments you perform each day, or the length of time in between each appointment. This is part of working for someone else, and because you are an employee, you do not set your own schedule. If this is the case, be extra mindful of maintaining your health and wellness with the information given throughout this book.

If you are concerned about being pushed past your limits in your workplace, discuss this with your supervisor or employer. Let him or her know how it is affecting your treatment performance, client care, and ADL. Optimally, your employer will be open to this discussion. It is in the best interests of the business to have employees who are fit physically, mentally, and emotionally. Otherwise, if employees become injured, then time on the job may be lost and the business may even need to pay workman's compensation. If employees need to take time off or even quit because of burnout, this, too, can cost the employer—in employee time lost on the job or the time and expense of hiring and training a new employee. If you are uncertain how to approach your supervisor or employer, consider asking a trusted colleague or mentor for advice.

Even the most enthusiastic practitioners will need to take a break from work at some point. Some of the signs of needing a break are if you:

- Do not feel like you are giving 100% to your clients
- Start to resent your clients
- Are tired at the end of the day even though you have stretched, strengthened, centered, hydrated, and eaten properly
- Do not feel rejuvenated after 1 or 2 days off work
- Seem to feel stressed all the time

This is when you need to take some type of vacation to restore yourself. It could be as simple as staying home for a week and working on a fun project, all the way up to taking a month off to go on a dream trip. Some practitioners may think they are not able to take a vacation "because their clients need them" or because they need to keep earning money. However, if practitioners push themselves to the point they become injured, they could potentially suffer financially from income lost while they are recovering.

Also, practitioners cannot pay sufficient attention to client needs if they are not paying sufficient attention to their own needs. The purpose of a vacation is to refresh so that you can come back to work with renewed energy.

REFERRING CLIENTS

Sometimes the increased risk of burnout is not due to something you are or are not doing. Sometimes it is because of certain clients. Perhaps there is no progress with the client's treatment plan, and this has become frustrating. It might be time to refer the client to a practitioner more suited to his or her needs. There are also those clients who are especially needy or "high maintenance." No matter what the practitioner does for the client, it is not enough, a situation that can be greatly depleting.

Sometimes practitioners begin to dread seeing a certain client, make up excuses not to book the client on a regular basis, or experience resentment whenever they see the client. It is important to pay attention to these feelings of resentment. Practitioners can explore these feelings and determine if there is a way to resolve them or if it is truly time to refer the client to another practitioner or resource.

Another way to decide if it is appropriate to refer a client to another practitioner or resource is to assess the progress in the client's treatment plan. If progress is not being made, it could be because there is an uneasy fit between the practitioner and the client that interferes with achieving the goals of the treatment plan. Or the reverse may be true—the treatment goals were successfully achieved, and there is nothing more that the practitioner can do for the client. Another reason to refer a client is if the client requests techniques the practitioner is unskilled in, or if the client requests pressure deeper than can be performed without risking injury to the practitioner.

Another good measurement to use to decide if it is time to refer a client elsewhere is for practitioners to notice how present they are with the client during the treatments. Have the treatments become so routine that they are bored and therefore not paying attention to the details of the client's condition? Or has the client developed a pattern of complaining about the work not being satisfactory yet is unwilling or unable to give specific feedback as to why? Would the client's condition be better treated by another practitioner who has a particular specialty? Thinking about the answers to these questions may help practitioners decide on the best course of action.

When referring a client to another practitioner, the ethical thing to do is discuss with the client what the issues are, and why it may be time for the client to consider either stopping treatments or going to another practitioner. The conversation can be difficult if the client does not want to go to someone else. Clients, of course, have the right to not accept a referral. The practitioner then needs to decide if he or she can continue working with the client, or if it is time to set a boundary and have the client move on.

Ethical practitioners understand their scope of practice, the limits of their training and knowledge, their personal and professional limitations, their areas of weakness, and their blind spots. Accordingly, in order to be able to refer clients, they need to develop a network of professionals whose work is of the highest quality. Ideally, practitioners will cultivate ongoing professional relationships with these resources and communicate with them directly. This list of reliable resources should be readily accessible. Clients and colleagues can act as resources for the development of this network.

OTHER OPTIONS

Practitioners who have been in business for many years may find themselves becoming bored with their work. If the boredom leads to frustration or a serious lack of enthusiasm for the bodywork profession, and even taking a vacation does not remedy this, then their career longevity may be in jeopardy.

At this point, practitioners may need to consider some other options:

- Diversifying their practices. This could be something simple such as adding aromatherapy to their menu of services, or something considerably more complex such as bringing new practitioners into their business who use different modalities. It could mean they learn an entirely new modality. If there are any other types of bodywork that practitioners have been interested in, it might be time to explore them and discover which ones are feasible for them to learn.

- Altering their work environments. They could move furniture and equipment around or redecorate entirely. Practitioners who are sole proprietors may even choose to move their practice to another location.

- Joining with other wellness providers. Practitioners could create a business affiliation or a referral system.

- Starting an entirely new business. This could be a business that is an adjunct to their bodywork practice, such as selling supplies and equipment, or it could be something out of the bodywork profession altogether.

- Taking a sabbatical or leave of absence from bodywork. This involves a longer period of time than a vacation. A practitioner could, for example, fulfill a lifelong dream of studying Ayurvedic medicine in India for a year. Of course, it would be wise to have a financial plan for this set up well in advance of the sabbatical or leave of absence and to have a list of practitioners your clients can see in your absence.

- Volunteering their services. There are organizations in every community that can benefit from bodywork services and other skills that practitioners have. For example, offering shiatsu at a fundraising walk or run is a great way to get out of the office and be with those who could really use some help. There are also bodywork and community organizations that practitioners can join and volunteer for, such as being a member of a committee or serving on a board of directors. Giving back to the profession and to the community can be enormously rewarding.

What Do You Think?

If you are or think you might become bored with your work, what would you do to remedy it?

ADDITIONAL SELF-CARE STRATEGIES

Previous chapters have discussed the importance of stretching, strengthening, and practicing good nutrition to care for your body. However, there are many other aspects to keeping your body in the best condition it can be for best health, wellness, and career longevity. These include following self-care methods for your feet, using hand tools, getting good sleep and sleeping in proper positions, and receiving bodywork regularly.

LEG CARE

Many types of bodywork require practitioners to stand for prolonged periods of time. Standing while working can be quite tiring, particularly when the floors have hard surfaces like tile, stone, concrete, or thin carpet over concrete. Prolonged standing in place on surfaces like these without doing much movement can result in conditions such as varicose veins in the legs, muscle cramps, and general fatigue. Standing on hard surfaces can also aggravate foot injuries, such as plantar fasciitis, and can cause low back discomfort. Depending on which area of the client's body is being worked, practitioners are encouraged to sit whenever possible. If you work on a massage table, sitting will allow your legs to rest and lowers your position relative to the table so you are less likely to bend or stoop when you get tired. Sitting also provides more stability and precision when working on certain structures of the client's neck, face, or hands.

It is important to use a comfortable, supportive stool. One with wheels allows for easy movement around the massage table. However, practitioners who use wheeled stools need to make sure the stool stays in place while working. If the stool slides unexpectedly, injury to themselves or the client may result. Figure 10-1 shows a massage therapist performing detailed techniques on a client's neck while sitting on a stool. An alternative is using an exercise ball, which

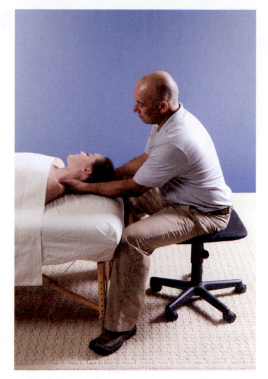

FIGURE 10-1 A massage therapist performing detailed techniques on a client's neck while sitting on a stool.

helps engage your core muscles while you are working.

PROPER FOOTWEAR

When performing certain bodywork modalities, such as massage therapy, wearing shoes helps absorb shock and prevent injury. Athletic shoes are the best option since they are designed to withhold the stress of standing and moving while working for long periods of time. Many of the factors that go into choosing athletic shoes for walking or running (as discussed in Chapter 8) are the same for choosing shoes to wear while performing bodywork.

Proper selection should be based upon the structure of your feet. Some people have normal arches, while others have flat feet, high arches, or very high arches.

One of the easiest ways for you to find out what type of arches you have is to look at your footprints. Wet your bare feet, then take a few steps and look at your footprints. By comparing your footprint to the images in Figure 10-2, you can get an idea of what

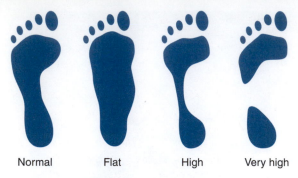

| Normal | Flat | High | Very high |

FIGURE 10-2 Foot arch diagram.

type of arches you have. Note that most people are somewhere in between the two extremes (normal and very high). Therefore, use your best judgment when assessing your arches.

Flat Feet (Pes Planus)

"Flatfoot," or *pes planus*, is a rather vague term that refers to a foot that pronates (everts) excessively or remains in an excessively pronated position during stance and gait (as discussed in Chapter 8). Flat feet may be caused by any one of many different conditions such as a tight Achilles tendon, congenital deformities, structural deformities of bone and joints in the foot or leg, abnormally loose ligaments, tendon ruptures (particularly the tibialis posterior tendon), and a host of others. Flat feet can be considered flexible or rigid. With a flexible flat foot, there may be a relatively high arch where the foot is not bearing weight. This then collapses with weight bearing. A rigid flat foot remains flat, or pronated (everted) at all times.

The pronation associated with flat feet may contribute to many other problems in the foot or elsewhere. When the foot pronates excessively, the arch collapses, causing the knee to also roll inward or the thigh to medially rotate. This may lead to knee pain due to the resultant uneven weight distribution at the knee joint. Similarly, the hip and lower back may also become painful as a result of the abnormal function of the foot. Within the foot itself, the abnormal pronation results in hypermobility and instability of various joints. This often results in the development of bunions, hammertoes, heel pain, and arthritis of the midfoot. Flat feet are most commonly treated with orthotic devices, which help to reduce abnormal pronation and hold the foot in a more optimal position. Some conditions may

require surgical treatment (Lowe, 2009; Tortora and Derrickson, 2009; Werner, 2009).

Practitioners who are flat-footed need shoes that control the motion of the feet. The shoes should have a sole that is rigid from the base of the toes (usually the widest part of the sole) to the heel. A good, solid heel cup is also necessary. This is the region of the shoe that cups and stabilizes the heel above the sole. This combination acts as a brace for the foot, holding the feet in neutral position and preventing pronation.

To check for a shoe with these characteristics:

- Squeeze the heel cup area above the sole. Is it firm or spongy?
- With one hand, hold the rear of the sole and place the other hand on the widest part of the sole near the base of the toes. Give it a good twist. Bend it. Does it feel solid or spongy?

The shoe should be firm in these key areas but still flexible in the toes. This will maintain the integrity of the arch, thus reducing the forces on the leg muscles, especially during movement.

High Arches (Pes Cavus)

The opposite of a flat foot is a high-arched foot, or *pes cavus*. This may lead to a number of equally troublesome conditions as flat feet. The cavus foot is one that remains in a supinated (inverted), high-arched position (as discussed in Chapter 8). These are often rigid or semirigid. While excessive pronation leads to instability, inadequate supination results in poor shock absorption during gait. This may also cause pain in the knees, hips, and lower back. Symptoms commonly occur in the heel and at the ball of the foot, areas that bear the most weight. Pes cavus may also result in tendon imbalances, causing hammertoes. A shock-absorbing orthotic may be effective in reducing symptoms associated with this condition. Surgery may also be indicated in some cases (Lowe, 2009; Tortora and Derrickson, 2009; Werner, 2009).

Practitioners with high arches may already have rigid feet, so they have no need for motion control. What they need is shock absorption. Without it, there is increased risk of injury, even to the point of hairline fractures of the tibia, because of excessive force transferred through the foot. Impact force needs to be absorbed by wearing the proper shoes. A practitioner with pes cavus needs shoes that have a great deal of cushioning in the sole.

Normal Feet

Practitioners who have normal feet need shoes that are good shock absorbers and have a fair amount of stability in the sole from the base of the toes to the heel and in the heel cup. The shoes can be somewhere in between those needed by practitioners who have pes planus or pes cavus.

Shopping for Footwear

Recall from Chapter 8 that you should not walk into a shoe store and buy any pair of shoes. Try on several pairs, and while doing so, jump around a little or even run around the store. If the shoes feel comfortable after taking them for these "test runs," then purchase them. Wear them inside for a day and see how they feel. If they still feel right, keep them. If not, take them back to the store.

If your work setting requires more formal footwear than athletic shoes, consider uniform shoes made for people in other occupations that require a lot of standing or walking, such as nurses or postal carriers.

HAND TOOLS

The hands, and particularly the fingertips, are sensitive because they contain many nerve endings. Applying sustained pressure can result in localized compression of the nerves and the small blood vessels that nourish them. In the short term, this can lead to inflammation, reduced circulation, and a loss of sensitivity that can take some time to resolve. Over time, repeated damage to nerves and blood vessels in the fingertips without adequate time for healing can result in a long-lasting reduction in sensitivity. Another risk of only using the hands to perform bodywork is carpal tunnel syndrome and other conditions that are discussed in Chapter 6.

A hand tool is a handheld device that a practitioner can use to provide additional force to a specific part of the client's body. Using this device prevents stress and fatigue, a common concern among bodywork practitioners. Handheld tools are designed to reduce damaging effects on the practitioner's body while increasing the impact and effectiveness of bodywork. Some hand tools can also be used to strengthen the practitioner's hands. Many of these tools can be used by a client, as homework, if they are given proper instructions on their use.

Numerous tools are available for performing hands-on modalities, particularly for applying sustained or deep pressure. Cupping tools, for example, can be used to lift tissues in place of repetitive techniques such as kneading and skin rolling; percussive tools and power massagers can be used in place of the hands for percussion techniques or to provide general relaxation to groups of muscles.

The various hand tools available are made of stone, wood, metal, or plastic. There are also electrical appliances available. Tools should not be used by every practitioner for every technique on every client. In reality, tools should be used only in moderation. Their purpose is to help reduce the effort required for several techniques, allowing the hands and fingers to rest and be ready to perform the techniques for which tools are not appropriate. Figure 10-3 shows examples of various hand tools.

RECEIVING BODYWORK REGULARLY

Receiving bodywork treatments regularly can help practitioners reduce their risk of injury and decrease stress from other aspects of their lives. Given the

---

Focus on Wellness

A Note About Orthotic Inserts

Unless you have a true leg-length discrepancy or structural dysfunction diagnosed by a podiatrist or other health-care professional, orthotic inserts may be unnecessary. For example, perhaps your muscles are excessively tight and pulling your leg up, causing it to appear short. Using an insert will only encourage this dysfunction. Unnecessary orthotic supports or cushioning can create foot instability and cause injuries rather than prevent them.

Consult with your physician before using orthotic inserts.

What Do You Think?

Are you likely to use any of the hand tools described? If so, which ones? Why do you choose these?

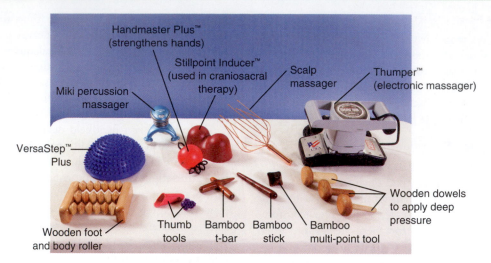

FIGURE 10-3 Various hand tools.

physical demands of bodywork, it may help to receive treatments more often than the commonly recommended once per month. This will help reduce accumulated stress and stiffness that can accompany performing the physical and mental aspects of bodywork.

Additional benefits of receiving regular bodywork include:

- Feeling rejuvenated
- Feeling the bodywork in your own body as a way of checking how you are performing your treatments
- Learning new techniques that stimulate creativity
- Helping to prevent burnout
- Setting a good example for clients

FIELD NOTES

When I was in massage school, I injured my wrist and had wrist pain. Rehabilitation from this injury was in the form of hydrotherapy, massage, and rest. After that, I really started to investigate the best way to use my hands. I try to keep wrist rotations down to a minimum and always try to keep my wrist aligned and fingers together. I always try to work from the core and, most importantly, keep all of my joints aligned. I take nutritional supplements to aid my body in supporting the joints.

Doing massage and bodywork is work, and you must care for your body. It is like an athletic event every day you are at work. Take care of yourself first; then you can truly care for others.

Ginger Castle, LMT, CKTP. Instructor at Cortiva Institute–Tucson, AZ. Licensed massage therapist since 1992.

SLEEP

The body needs sleep in order to thrive and function in wellness. Without adequate rest, it is difficult to impossible for the body to replenish important energy reserves. The amount of sleep you need depends on your current treatment schedule, personal preference, level of daily activities, and stress. Extensive evidence indicates we need at least 8 hours of sleep per night and often as much as 9 or more hours in times of elevated stress (National Sleep Foundation, 2009A).

Some practitioners can get by on less sleep, but it is likely to catch up with them eventually, leaving them feeling depleted and possibly burned out.

The midday nap, not necessarily part of current American culture, is a widely practiced custom around the world. The circadian rhythm is a daily cycle of biological activity based on a 24-hour period and influenced by regular variations in the environment, such as the alternation of night and day. When people experience midday drowsiness, it is most likely because their circadian rhythm is requiring their bodies to sleep at that time. Often the drowsiness is not due to poor diet, as is so often claimed. While poor diet can indeed make midday drowsiness worse, it is not the only factor.

If you are experiencing midday drowsiness, try taking a 20- to 30-minute rest in the afternoon if it is practical and your schedule permits it. Chances are it will make you sharper mentally and more alert and will promote faster recuperation from a challenging treatment day or any physically or mentally demanding activity. However, avoid going into the deep sleep that comes with longer rest; that may make you feel

Body Awareness

*T*ry going to bed earlier and get an extra hour of sleep in every night for a week. See if you notice any difference. See if your alertness and vitality improve.

groggy and interfere with your nighttime sleep. Short periods of rest tend to make people more productive (National Sleep Foundation, 2009B).

Sleep Position

Ask yourself the following questions:

- What position do I sleep in?
- Do I wake up in the same position?
- Do I toss and turn at night?
- How does this sleeping position affect my body?
- Do I wake up rested?
- Does my body ache when I wake up?

You may not be able to control or eliminate all of the factors that can possibly be interfering with your sleep, but you can create an environment and adopt habits that encourage a more restful night. Here are suggestions:

- Try sleeping on your back. It is the best position for relaxing and allows all your internal organs to rest properly.
- If you must sleep on your side, do it on your right side, not your left. Sleeping on the left side causes your lungs, stomach, and liver to press against your heart, possibly causing it stress.
- Try to avoid sleeping on your stomach. It causes pressure on all of your internal organs, including your lungs, which results in shallow breathing. It can also cause, as many have discovered, a stiff neck and upper back tension and stress.

Propping is also an important ingredient for sleep. An aligned spine and stacked joints are principles that should also be adopted for sleep positions:

- If you sleep on your back, be sure to have a comfortable cervical pillow that allows you to keep your head in alignment with your spine. Furthermore, placing a pillow or bolster behind your knees will take the pressure off your low back. Placing a pillow under your arms will keep all the joints in your upper extremity aligned.
- If you sleep on your side, use a cervical pillow to keep your head in alignment with your spine. Place a pillow or bolster in between your legs, keeping your joints in alignment—hip to knee, knee to ankle. Also have another pillow you can hug to keep all the joints in your upper extremity aligned.
- Pay attention to what you are doing with your hands and wrists as you sleep. Are they curled up (in a flexed position) all night? Do you have them tucked under your body or pillow? These postures can lead to a repetitive stress injury. If you sleep this way, consider purchasing a wrist splint (Fig. 10-4) from a local medical supply store or pharmacy. It may be difficult at first to wear one of these all night long. Try starting with a half

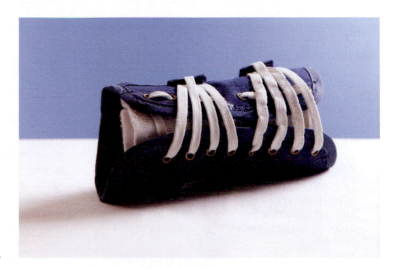

FIGURE 10-4 Wrist splint.

hour the first night, an hour the second night, and so forth. Once you can wear a wrist splint all night, over time you may be able to do without it. This is because your body awareness will have changed so that when you find yourself moving into the dysfunctional pattern of curling your wrists, you will promptly move them back into the stacked joint position.

Recommendations for Getting a Good Night's Sleep

Good, restful sleep allows people to have a more balanced perspective on the events in their lives. It can make them more productive and happy, and they tend to enjoy their interactions with others. Sleep helps improve mood and psychological outlook, and it is important on a cellular and physical level, giving tissues a chance to restore and regenerate so they can function optimally (National Sleep Foundation, 2009C).

Here are recommendations for getting a good night's sleep:

- Get regular exercise, but preferably not just before going to bed. Exercise stimulates the sympathetic nervous system so you may find yourself wide awake when you need to be sleeping.
- Avoid caffeine. Besides coffee, tea, and soda, caffeine is in coffee yogurts and ice cream and in some pain relievers.
- Avoid drinking alcohol close to bedtime. Alcohol can interfere with some people's ability to sleep.
- Take a hot bath near bedtime. The hot water raises the body's temperature, bringing relaxation to the muscles. The subsequent cooling the body experiences after a hot bath may cause sleep.

- Wake up and go to bed at the same time every day. This sets your circadian rhythm on a regular schedule, and your body will know when it is time to sleep.
- Use the bed mainly for sleeping. Watch television or work on your laptop in another room. The National Sleep Foundation calls watching TV and working on a computer in bed "sleep stealers" because these keep the brain active instead of letting the brain wind down so sleep systems can take over. If you still need to wind down after you get into bed, read instead (National Sleep Foundation, 2009).
- Listen to soft, soothing music or other audio. There are many CDs designed to specifically lull people to sleep. Some are specially composed music; others simply have sounds of waves rhythmically breaking or the steady rhythm of a heartbeat. Some will lead you to sleep with a combination of music, voice, and other soothing sounds.
- Drink warm milk. A glass of warm milk 15 minutes before going to bed will soothe your nervous system. Milk contains calcium, which works directly on jagged nerves to make them, and you, relax.
- Drink herbal tea. If you do not like milk, or are avoiding dairy products, try a cup of hot chamomile, catnip, anise, or fennel tea. All contain natural ingredients that will help you sleep. Most health food stores will also have special blends of herb tea designed to soothe you and help you get to sleep.

More information about sleep can be found on the National Sleep Foundation's website: www.sleepfoundation.org.

Focus on Wellness

Reminder Strategies for Self-Care

- Develop good body mechanics. Using your body efficiently to produce the most effective movement with the least effort will reduce the strain of performing treatments on your body. Remain upright with an aligned spine and balanced posture as much as possible while you work, keep your joints stacked, use your larger muscles to create movement, and use your body weight, not muscular strength, to create pressure.

- Vary your bodywork techniques. Use different parts of your hands and arms, or for those who practice Asian bodywork, use your knees, feet, and toes in addition to different parts of your hands and arms. Avoid repetitive motion to any one part of your body. For example, sometimes use your elbow or a hand tool to create pressure rather than always using your thumbs.
- Avoid techniques that cause you pain. There are many techniques to choose from, so do only those that you can do comfortably.

- Monitor your work schedule. Try to maintain a regular schedule of treatment sessions so you do not suddenly increase the number of treatments you do or decrease the amount of time you have between sessions.
- Warm your hands before working. If your hands are cold, you do not have enough blood flow in your upper extremities to keep your tissues pliable and remove waste products caused by microtearing of your muscles. Warm up with stretching and light aerobic exercise before you start your bodywork treatments.
- Get an electric table. They are standard for physical therapists, and many bodywork practitioners may find them helpful. An electric table allows you to adjust the height of the table at any moment to enable you to remain upright with an aligned spine and balanced posture so that you can maintain good body mechanics.
- Take time between treatments. Having enough time between treatments to relax, stretch, breathe, hydrate, get a snack, and prepare for your next client reduces your risk of injury.
- Use other modalities in your treatments. Hydrotherapy, aromatherapy, energy balancing, and spa treatments are just some examples of modalities that can be attractive to existing and new clients, and they add value to your treatments. They will also cut down on the amount of intensive hands-on work you do in each session, which will allow your hands to rest.
- Develop a realistic attitude toward your work. There are limits to what you can do for your clients. Respecting your own limits is healthy and will help you keep your upper extremities healthy.
- Treat injuries immediately and effectively. If you have pain or dysfunction intermittently or constantly for more than 3 or 4 days, see your physician. You may already be injured, and ignoring it will only allow the injury to worsen.
- Stay in touch with the signals your body is sending you. Do not get so lost in treating your clients that you no longer can hear the signals of pain and discomfort that you need to observe in order to stay healthy.
- Lighten up. Do not exhaust yourself with every client. Pace yourself throughout your day and your week so you don't end up physically drained.
- Make sure to do stretching and strengthening exercises and to have a good nutritional plan. Your body is your best piece of equipment for performing bodywork, so you need to keep it in optimal shape.

Myth: If a practitioner is having a bad day, her body and her treatments will not be affected.

FACT: The ability to maintain a positive mental attitude helps keep the practitioner's "head in the game" and helps her maintain perspective. She is more able to communicate effectively with her clients, pay better attention to her body and body mechanics, and focus on giving client-centered treatments. Everyone has bad days, of course, but practitioners must be able to set aside personal issues when working in order to have a successful practice.

Case Profile

Trang has been a Healing Touch practitioner for 7 years. For most of that time, he has really enjoyed his work and appreciated all his clients. Several years ago, he decided to diversify and took continuing education classes in aromatherapy. Since that time, he has been incorporating aromatherapy into his Healing Touch treatments. His clients responded enthusiastically to this addition. Lately, however, Trang is finding it difficult to become excited about going to work. He has not been sleeping well and finds he sometimes speaks sharply to the other staff in the office. Last month he took a few days off to attend a workshop on sound therapy in another state. However, even though the presenter is nationally known, Trang thought the workshop was a waste of his time and money. He came back frustrated and angry. Lately, he has been thinking about switching careers.

- *What are the issues you think Trang is struggling with?*
- *How are these issues affecting his career longevity?*
- *What recommendations would you give Trang?*

Wellness Profile Check In

Looking at the Wellness Profile you completed at the end of Chapter 1, are there any challenge areas you could remedy through the additional strategies for self-care presented in this chapter? If so, what are they? How would you like these areas improved? What methods or activities will you use to improve these areas? Write down a plan for improvement that includes the methods you will use, a timeline for implementing these methods, and ways you will assess your improvement along the way.

SUMMARY

There are many different aspects to career longevity. They include having a positive mental attitude, maintaining healthy boundaries, enjoying working with people, being willing to take risks, and being physically and mentally prepared for the demands of the profession. The information in this book is designed to assist practitioners in changing old, non-useful habits and ways of thinking and creating new, healthy, and helpful methods that can ensure their career longevity. Practitioners need to assess how they have incorporated the information in this book into their lives.

Practitioners may need to seek support in helping them make the changes they desire. Support can be in the form of supervision, mentoring, and using peer support. To get the most out of the process, they should carefully choose who they want for mentors and peer support, be open to feedback, and implement it in a timely fashion and have an authentic desire to grow emotionally and professionally.

Burnout has been discussed in various chapters of this book. Practitioners must be able to recognize the signs and symptoms of burnout. If they have any of these signs or symptoms, they should be willing to implement strategies that can prevent or manage the burnout. These include setting time aside to think about and do planning for their businesses, attending conferences and continuing education classes, practicing stress-relief methods, diversifying their practices, and joining with other wellness providers. Practitioners should also know when to take a break and when to take a vacation.

Additional self-care strategies include wearing the proper, supportive shoes while working, using hand tools to decrease the stress of performing techniques on their hands, receiving bodywork regularly, getting enough sleep, and sleeping in the proper positions.

Review Questions

MULTIPLE CHOICE

1. Which of the following is a characteristic of a successful bodywork practitioner?
   a. Taking few risks
   b. Having unclear boundaries
   c. Having a positive mental attitude
   d. Being unsure of his or her abilities

2. The term for the periodic review of the practitioner's professional actions by an authority in the work setting is
   a. peer support.
   b. employment.
   c. mentoring.
   d. supervision.

3. The role of a mentor is to
   a. fix the problems a practitioner is having.
   b. assist the practitioner in realizing actions and behaviors that limit his or her success.
   c. tell the practitioner what he or she should be doing in order to be successful.
   d. evaluate the practitioner's behavior in an employment setting.

4. A sign that it is a time for the practitioner to take a vacation is if he
   a. appreciates his clients.
   b. feels rejuvenated after 1 or 2 days off work.
   c. seems to feel stressed all the time.
   d. feels like he is giving 100% to his clients.

5. Which of the following can result if a practitioner has pes planus and does not wear the proper shoes while working?
  a. Knee pain
  b. Hammertoes
  c. Arthritis of the midfoot
  d. All of the above

6. Which of the following will help a practitioner achieve career longevity?
  a. Receiving bodywork once a year
  b. Sleeping a few hours a night
  c. Diversifying and offering other modalities in the practice
  d. Scheduling many treatments each day with short breaks in between

7. To avoid injury, it is best if practitioners sleep with their wrists
  a. aligned.
  b. curled.
  c. tucked under a pillow.
  d. tucked under their bodies.

FILL-IN-THE-BLANK

1. A professional relationship in which a person with greater experience and skill provides support, encouragement, and career expertise to those with less experience and skill in the profession is called

_____ .

2. Practitioners seeking support are more open to the process if they are able to implement _____ in a timely fashion.

3. As long as practitioners pay attention to their body mechanics and practice self-care, the more treatments they do, the more _____ they will have.

4. To alleviate boredom with their work, practitioners can try _____ their work environment.

5. Wearing shoes while working is important for _____ _____ and injury prevention.

6. To enhance career longevity, practitioners should _____ the bodywork techniques they use.

7. A daily cycle of biological activity based on a 24-hour period is called a _____ rhythm.

SHORT ANSWER

1. List at least five questions practitioners can ask themselves if they are wondering if they need to seek support.

2. Briefly explain the qualities a practitioner should look for in peers for peer support and in mentors.

3. Describe at least seven signs of burnout.

4. Explain at least five things practitioners can do to prevent or manage burnout.

5. Describe the type of shoes a practitioner should wear if he or she has pes planus. Describe the type of shoes a practitioner should wear if he or she has pes cavus.

6. Describe at least three hand tools a practitioner can use to reduce the damaging effects of performing bodywork on her body.

7. Explain at least five recommendations for getting a good night's sleep.

Activities

1. Make a list of practitioners who would provide you with good peer support. Contact them to see if they are interested in setting up a peer support group. If so, define the parameters of when, where, and how you will meet.

2. Make a list of experienced practitioners and members of other professions who would be appropriate mentors for you. Contact them to see if they are interested in mentoring you. If so, define the parameters of when, where, and how you will be mentored.

3. Contact at least three successful practitioners in your community, and ask them for tips for career longevity.

4. Assess how much sleep you get at night and whether you feel sleepy during the day. If you do feel sleepy during the day, determine the time you usually feel sleepy. For 2 weeks, implement some strategies for getting more sleep. Journal how you feel before you start the strategies, while you're doing the strategies, and after 2 weeks of implementing the strategies.

REFERENCES

Lowe, Whitney. *Orthopedic Massage*, 2nd ed. St. Louis, MO: Elsevier Mosby, 2009.

National Sleep Foundation. How Much Sleep Do We Really Need? (2009A). Retrieved December 2010 from www.sleepfoundation.org/article/how-sleep-works/how-much-sleep-do-we-really-need.

National Sleep Foundation. Napping (2009B). Retrieved December 2010 from www.sleepfoundation.org/article/sleep-topics/napping.

National Sleep Foundation. What to Do About Insomnia (2009C). Retrieved December 2010 from www.sleepfoundation.org/sleep-facts-information/insomnia-treatable.

Tortora, Gerard J., and Bryan Derrickson. *Principles of Anatomy and Physiology*, 12th ed. Hoboken, NJ: John Wiley & Sons, 2009.

Werner, Ruth. *A Massage Therapist's Guide to Pathology*, 4th ed. Baltimore, MD: Lippincott Williams & Wilkins, 2009.

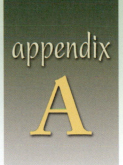

Hydrotherapy for Self-Care

In addition to the plunges described in Chapter 6, there are other hydrotherapy methods that practitioners may find useful. These can be used for addressing tight, sore muscles in the forearms, hands, legs, and feet. It is also highly recommended that these also be used as preventative measures.

COLD APPLICATIONS

COLD COMPRESS

A compress is a soft cotton cloth soaked in hot or cold water and applied to an area of the body. A cold compress causes vasoconstriction, which inhibits blood flow. It also numbs pain receptors and draws heat from the body. Cold compresses can be used for:

- Pain relief
- Chronic muscle tension
- Muscle spasms
- Sprains and strains
- Mild inflammation
- Mild burns (as long as the skin is not broken or blistered)

Contraindications for a cold compress include:

- Heart conditions (cold temperature can cause the heart to suddenly beat more rapidly in a sympathetic response; this can stress a weakened heart)
- Numbness or loss of sensation in area
- Neuropathy in area
- Vascular disorder in area
- Intolerance to cold

A cold compress is typically applied for no longer than 20 to 30 minutes (to prevent the cold from damaging your soft tissues and underlying structures), using water that is as cold as you can tolerate. For continual cold application, change the compress promptly because it tends to warm up quickly. Applying friction to the area first with a rough towel may make this treatment more comfortable if you have a low tolerance for or sensitivity to cold.

The equipment and supplies needed for a cold compress are fairly simple: a basin of cold or ice water, ice (as needed to keep water as cool as desired), and three thick, soft cloths or towels, approximately 18×30 inches; the thicker the compress, the longer it stays cold (Fig. A-1).

The following are the steps for a cold compress:

1. Cool the water and place it in the basin. Position the bowl of ice within easy reach for adding to the water during the treatment.
2. Fold two towels in thirds, width-wise (Fig. A-2A), then roll them up (Fig. A-2B). Place the folded, rolled towels in the ice water (Fig. A-3) for several minutes. Leave one towel dry.
3. Uncover the area where you will be applying the cold compress. Unroll (but leave folded) one towel (Fig. A-4A), wring it out thoroughly (Fig. A-4B), and wrap it around the area of application, such as the forearm (Fig. A-4C).

   If the towel is too cold, remove it immediately and allow it to warm up a bit. Replace the towel and see if it is still too cold. If it is, remove it again and wait until the temperature is comfortable for you. The first application should feel mildly cold with the temperature gradually decreasing with each application, depending on your tolerance to cold.
4. Replace the cold towel as soon as you feel the coolness decreasing (approximately every 1 to 3 minutes). Before the compress warms up completely, prepare the next cool towel for application. Thoroughly wring out the new cool towel.

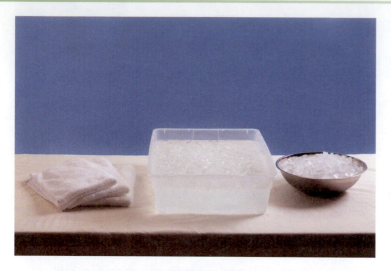

FIGURE A-1 Supplies for a cold compress.

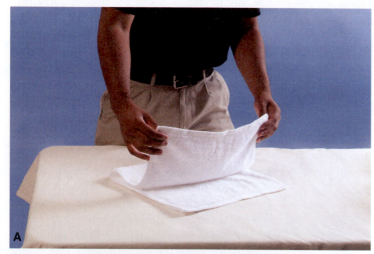

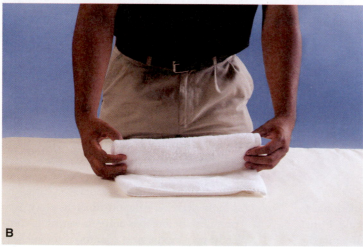

FIGURE A-2 (A) Fold two towels in thirds, width-wise. **(B)** Roll the towels up.

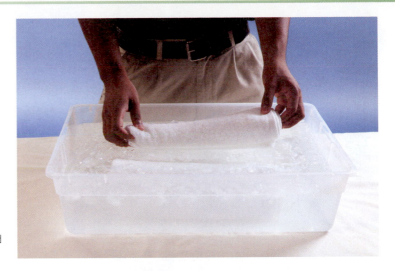

FIGURE A-3 Place the folded, rolled towels in ice water.

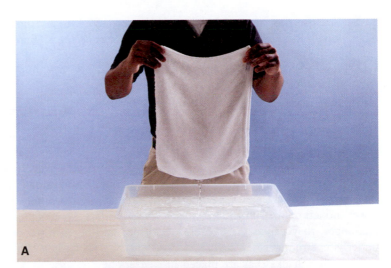

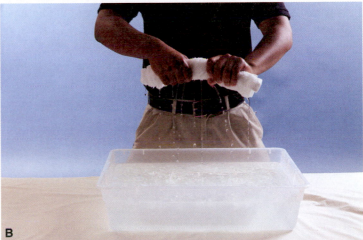

FIGURE A-4 (A) Unroll (but leave folded) one towel. **(B)** Wring it out thoroughly.

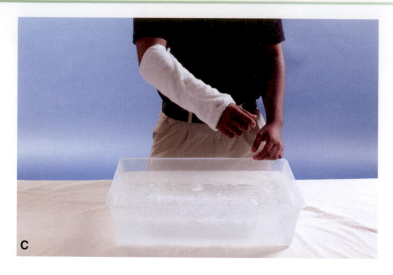

C

FIGURE A-4 cont'd (C) Wrap it around your forearm.

5. Remove the first towel and apply the second towel. Reroll the first towel and place it back in the basin of cold water.
6. Repeat cold compress changes as necessary for 20 to 30 minutes.
7. Dry the area with a dry towel after the last application.

COLD PACKS

Cold packs can be applied locally. They are applied on top of a thin layer of insulating fabric such as a towel and left on for 20 to 30 minutes. If they are left on longer, they can damage your soft tissues and underlying structures.

Gel-filled packs that are placed in freezers before use can be purchased at department stores and pharmacies. A more cost-effective method is to use homemade packs such as a bag of frozen peas (Fig. A-5). An alternative is to roll ice cubes up in a towel (Fig. A-6A) and then apply it (Fig. A-6B).

ICE MASSAGE (CRYOTHERAPY)

Ice massage, or cryotherapy, is the therapeutic use of cold (*cryo-* is from the Greek *kryos,* meaning "icy cold"). *Cryokinetics* is ice massage with movement. It involves the application of ice using deep circular friction over a localized area of the body. This application of prolonged cold initially causes vasoconstriction, then vasodilation of blood vessels, causing a pumping action of blood out and into the tissues in the affected area. It also interrupts the pain-spasm-pain cycle. The application of cold also decreases pain, as do the friction and pressure of the ice moving over the skin.

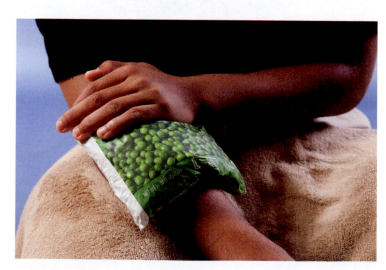

FIGURE A-5 Bag of frozen peas used as a cold pack on the forearm.

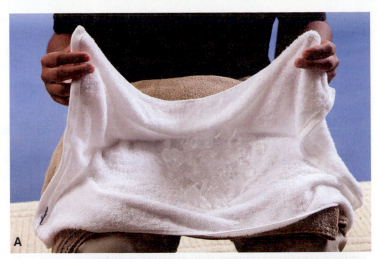

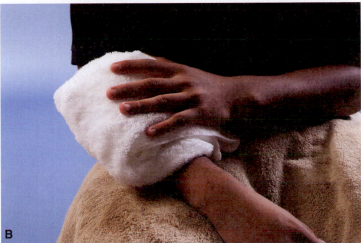

FIGURE A-6 (A) Ice cubes being rolled up in a towel, and **(B)** applied to the forearm.

Cryotherapy is especially effective for:

- Reducing swelling and congestion in tissues
- Helping relieve muscle spasms
- Decreasing pain
- Speeding delivery of nutrients to the area
- Speeding up removal of dead cell debris
- Promoting healing

Contraindications for cryotherapy are the same as for a cold compress.

You will feel five general stages when the ice is applied (this may take 5 to 10 minutes):

- First stage: sensation of cold
- Second stage: slight burning sensation; may be a little painful
- Third stage: deep achy or throbbing sensation
- Fourth stage: warming
- Fifth stage: numbness

Ice application should stop once the fifth stage is reached. Damage to soft tissues and underlying structures can occur if the ice application continues. Note that everyone will experience the ice application differently. Some may skip one of the five stages, such as going from stage 3 to 5.

General application guidelines:

- Five to 10 minutes for thinner tissue (wrists, hands, fingers)
- Fifteen to 20 minutes for thicker tissue (hamstrings, quadriceps)

You can apply ice in the form of:

- A self-contained ice massage tool: a special plastic cup that can be filled with water, then frozen. These cups can be bought on the Internet from websites such as:
  - Cryocup: www.cryocup.com

- Massage Warehouse: www.massagewarehouse.com
- Banner Therapy: www.bannertherapy.com
- An ice cup: a paper or Styrofoam cup is filled with water and frozen; the top of the cup is placed on the skin while you hold the bottom of the cup (Fig. A-7). As the ice melts, you can peel off strips of cup around the top to reveal more ice.

Apply the ice in the following manner:

- Rub your hand over the area where you will apply the ice; the friction from your hand reduces the initial shock of the cold on your skin.
- Take a deep breath, and then start applying the ice using deep, circular strokes while exhaling (Fig. A-8A). Some people tend to hold their breath when cold is being applied, so make sure to continue breathing deeply during the treatment. It will also help you relax.
- Apply for approximately 5 to 10 minutes for areas of thinner tissue or 15 to 20 minutes for areas of thicker tissue. Keep the strokes continuous and smooth. To make sure the cold penetrates into your body, stay within the focus area. Use a towel to catch the drips of water on your skin, because they can be uncomfortable.
- You should progress through the five stages of sensation. When the area is numb or significantly reddened (Fig. A-8B) the treatment is complete. Discontinue applying ice so as to not damage your soft tissues and underlying structures.
- Gently blot the area dry with the cloth or towel. Massage or other bodywork can be performed on the area.

Ice can be reapplied often during the first 24 to 72 hours after an acute injury, but there should be a break of at least 20 minutes between applications in order to prevent damage to your soft tissues and underlying structures.

HEAT APPLICATIONS

Dry heat, such as an electric heating pad, can be used to loosen tight muscles, but moist heat will be more effective because it penetrates more deeply than dry heat. However, there is an increased chance of injuring soft tissues and underlying structures with moist heat, so it is advisable to proceed with caution.

HOT COMPRESS

A hot compress is excellent for relieving local muscle tightness, relaxing muscle spasms, reducing aches and pains, and preparing the tissue for massage or other bodywork treatment.

Contraindications for a hot compress include:

- Heart conditions (hot temperatures can cause the heart to suddenly beat more rapidly in a sympathetic response; this can stress a weakened heart)
- Vascular disorder in area
- Numbness or loss of sensation in area
- Neuropathy in area
- Inflammation in the area
- Intolerance to heat
- Broken or irritated skin
- High body temperature (fever)

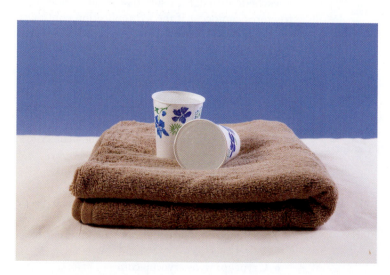

FIGURE A-7 Homemade ice cup.

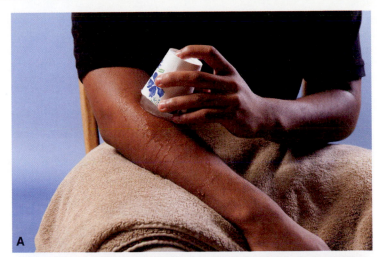

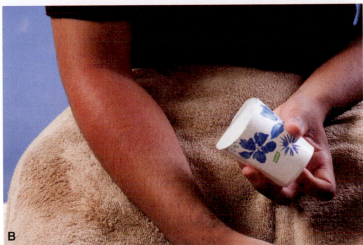

FIGURE A-8 (A) Application of ice to the forearm. **(B)** Significant reddening of the skin from ice application.

The compress is heated to approximately 100°F, is applied to the body, and is left on for approximately 1 to 3 minutes, or until you feel the compress cooling. Then you apply another hot compress. Because your body gets used to the heat, each successive compress can be somewhat hotter than the previous one (up to 105°F to 108°F). There are typically five to ten exchanges, which can make the treatment last about 30 to 60 minutes. If you are sensitive to heat, decrease the water temperature, decrease the length of time the compress stays on your body, and decrease the number of exchanges.

The equipment and supplies needed for a hot compress include a stockpot (12 quarts or larger); a heating source such as an electrical hot plate; four thick, soft cloths or towels, approximately 18 × 30 inches (two to moisten, one to insulate, one to dry the area after treatment); and insulated gloves (Fig. A-9).

The following are the steps for a hot compress:

1. Fill the stockpot with water to about 3 inches below the rim. Heat water to just under boiling (this will take approximately 15 minutes), and then turn the heat down to medium. You can turn the heat up or down according to your tolerance of the hot compresses.
2. Fold three towels in thirds width-wise (Fig. A-10A), then roll two of them up (Fig. A-10B). Wearing the insulated gloves, place the two folded, rolled towels in the hot water (Fig. A-11). The other folded towel will be used to insulate the compress while it is on your forearm.
3. Uncover the area where you will be applying the hot compress.
4. Wearing the insulated gloves, take one towel out of the hot water and wring it out quickly

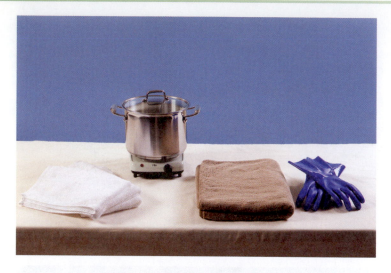

FIGURE A-9 Supplies for hot compress.

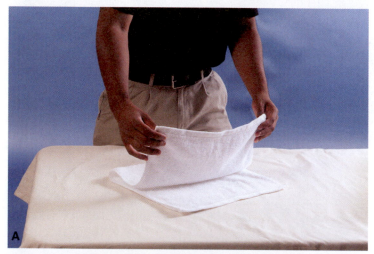

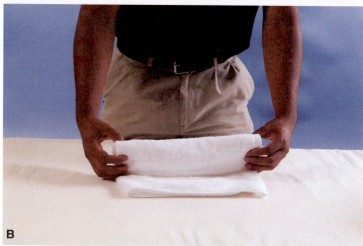

FIGURE A-10 (A) Fold towels in thirds width-wise, then **(B)** roll them up.

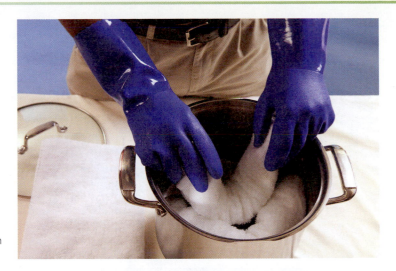

FIGURE A-11 Wearing the insulated gloves, place two folded, rolled towels in the hot water.

and completely (Fig. A-12A); if the towel is too wet, it will cool too quickly. Unroll the towel but keep it folded in thirds (Fig. A-12B).

5. Wave the towel to cool it a bit and then test the heat by touching the hot compress to the inside of your forearm. If the heat is tolerable, place the hot compress lightly on the application area (Fig. A-13A). If this is your forearm, wrap the hot compress around it (Fig. A-13B).

   If the towel is too hot, remove it immediately and wave it again to cool it more. Replace the towel and see if it is still too hot. If it is, wave it again until the temperature is comfortable for you. The first application should be comfortably warm to you, with the temperature gradually increasing with each application, depending on your tolerance to heat.

6. Cover with a dry towel to insulate (Fig. A-14). Do not press down on the insulating towel; this could burn your skin.

7. Replace the compress as the heat decreases, which should be in 1 to 3 minutes. Before the compress cools completely, prepare the next one for application. Thoroughly wring out the new hot towel, and fan it to cool it a bit. To change compresses, place the new compress on top of the insulating towel (and the old compress; Fig. A-15A), then flip the stack over (Fig. A-15B). The insulating towel will now be on top of the new hot compress (Fig. A-15C). This will help retain heat.

   Before removing the towel on top and placing it in the pot to reheat, make sure the temperature is comfortable for you. The

compress should be a little warmer than the previous hot towel. If it is still too hot, remove it immediately and allow it to cool a bit; then replace it when the temperature is tolerable. If the application area is your forearm, wrap the new hot compress around it (Fig. A-15D).

8. Keep exchanging the compresses as necessary for 30 to 60 minutes.

9. Dry the area with a dry towel after the last application.

ALTERNATING (CONTRAST) COMPRESS APPLICATION

An alternating or contrast compress application involves alternating hot and cold compresses. Since the hot compresses cause vasodilation of blood vessels, and cold compresses cause vasoconstriction of blood vessels, there is a pumping action of blood into and out of the area. The purpose is to bring blood and nutrition to the area with heat and then to decrease blood flow, which allows time for waste products to leave tissues and diffuse into blood. Additional applications of heat then help move toxins out of the area. This promotes local healing.

Alternating compresses can be used for relieving local muscle tightness; relaxing muscle spasms; reducing aches, pains, and tight joints (from noninflammatory conditions); and preparing the tissue for massage or other bodywork treatment.

Contraindications for alternating compresses include:

- Heart conditions
- Numbness or loss of sensation in the area

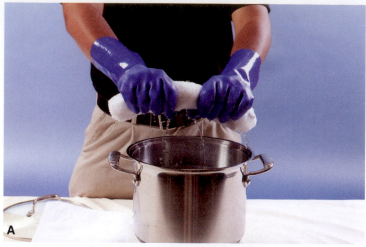

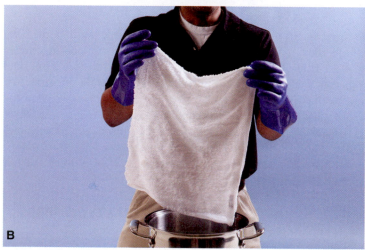

FIGURE A-12 (A) Wearing the insulated gloves, take one towel out of the hot water and wring it out quickly and completely. **(B)** Unroll the towel but keep it folded in thirds.

- Vascular disorders in the area
- Inflammation in the area
- Broken or irritated skin
- High body temperature (fever)
- Intolerance to cold
- Intolerance to heat

The treatment should always start with a heated compress followed by the brief application of a cold compress. The first hot compress starts at a temperature that is comfortably warm and gets successively hotter, within your tolerance. The cold compress starts at a temperature that is comfortably cool and gets successively colder, within your tolerance. Contrast compresses are typically performed for 20 to 30 minutes. If you are sensitive to heat or cold, use milder temperatures and decrease the duration of the treatment. A general guideline is for every 3 minutes of heat, use 1 minute of cold, or a ratio of 3:1.

The equipment and supplies for alternating compresses are the same as for cold and hot compresses: stockpot, 12 quarts or larger; heating source such as an electrical hot plate; basin of cold or ice water; ice; four thick, soft cloths or towels, approximately 18 × 30 inches; and insulated gloves.

The following are the steps for an alternating compress application:

1. Fill the stockpot with water to about 3 inches below the rim. Heat water to just under boiling (this takes about 15 minutes), and then turn the heat down to medium. Be ready to turn the heat up or down according to your tolerance of the hot compresses.

2. Cool water and place it in the basin. Position the ice within easy reach for adding during the treatment.

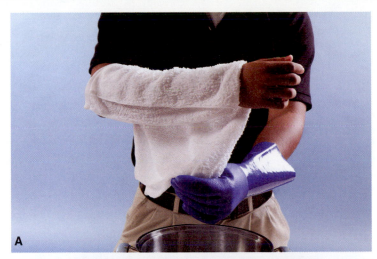

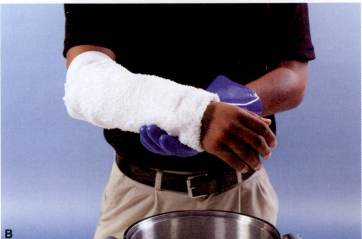

FIGURE A-13 (A) Place the hot compress lightly on the forearm. **(B)** Wrap it around the forearm.

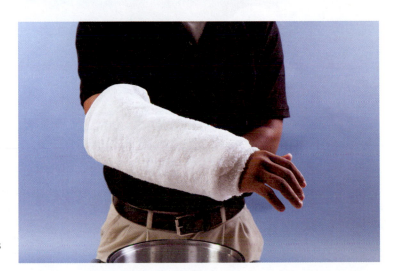

FIGURE A-14 Covering the compress with a dry towel to insulate.

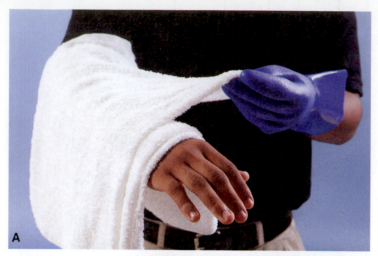

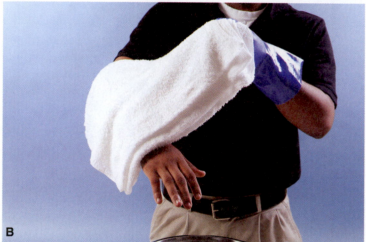

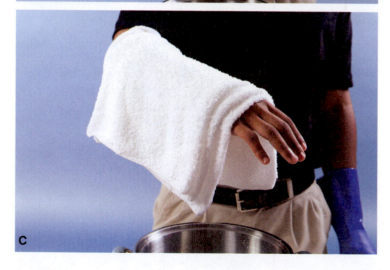

FIGURE A-15 (A) Place the new compress on top of the insulating towel (and the old compress). **(B)** Flip the stack over. **(C)** The insulating towel will now be on top of the new hot compress.

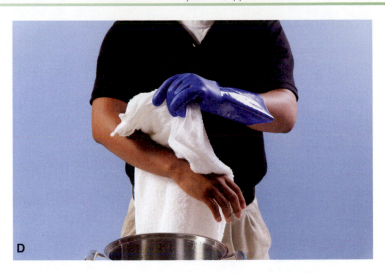

FIGURE A-15 cont'd (D) Wrap the new hot compress around your forearm.

3. Fold four towels in thirds width-wise and then roll three of them up. Wearing the insulated gloves, place two folded, rolled towels in the hot water. Place one folded rolled towel in the ice water. You will use the other folded towel to insulate the compress.

4. Uncover the area where you will be applying the alternating compress.

5. Wearing the insulated gloves, take one towel out of the hot water and wring out the towel quickly and completely; if the towel is too wet, it will cool too quickly. Unroll it, but keep it folded in thirds.

6. Wave the towel to cool it a bit, then test the heat by touching the hot compress to the inside of your forearm. If the heat is tolerable, place the hot compress on the application area. If this is your forearm, wrap the hot compress around it.

   If the towel is too hot, remove it immediately and wave it again to cool it more. Replace the towel and see if it is still too hot. If it is, wave it again to cool it until the temperature is comfortable for you. The first application should be comfortably warm to you, with the temperature gradually increasing with each application, depending on your tolerance to heat.

7. Cover with a dry towel to insulate. Do not press down on the insulating towel; this could burn your skin.

8. Leave the hot compress on for about 1 to 3 minutes, or less if the heat decreases.

9. Wring out the cold towel and place it on top of both hot and insulating towels. Take a deep breath and then flip the stack of towels so the cold compress is now on the application area, and exhale. If it is your forearm, wrap the cold compress around it. Remove the hot towel; the insulating towel will now be on top of the cold compress.

10. Wearing the insulated gloves, place the hot towel in the basin of hot water to reheat.

11. Leave the cold compress on for only about 30 to 60 seconds. While wearing the insulated gloves, wring out the second hot towel (the first hot towel will not be reheated enough yet to reapply).

12. Put the new hot towel on top of both cold and insulating towels, and flip the stack of towels so that the hot compress is in place. Make sure the temperature is comfortable for you. The compress should be a little warmer than the previous hot compress. If it is still too hot, remove it immediately and wave it to cool it more, and then replace it when the temperature is tolerable.

13. Remove the cold compress, leaving the insulating towel on top of the hot towel. Place the cold towel back in the basin of cold water.

14. Continue exchanging the compresses. For optimum benefit, the treatment should include approximately three to five hot and cold exchanges lasting for 20 to 30 minutes, but this is always determined by your needs.

15. Dry the area with a dry towel after the last application.

PARAFFIN APPLICATION

Paraffin application is technically not a hydrotherapy treatment because it does not use water. However, it is an excellent heat treatment worth including in this appendix. Paraffin is a wax, and it is applied in a hot liquid form. As it cools, it hardens and forms a shell. The heat from the cooling paraffin penetrates deep into body tissues because the wax shell forms an insulating seal over the area. Because the heat from the paraffin penetrates so deeply into tissues, it is a useful treatment to relieve joint stiffness from noninflammatory arthritis, as well as tight muscles, ligaments, and tendons and muscle spasms. Because it is very effective at loosening soft tissues, it can be used before performing massage or other bodywork on tight muscles and fascia.

Contraindications for paraffin application include:

- Heart conditions
- Untreated hypertension
- Vascular disease, including varicose veins
- Numbness or loss of sensation in an area
- Skin conditions made worse by heat
- Intolerance to heat
- Broken or irritated skin
- High body temperature (fever)

The paraffin is melted in a commercial paraffin unit and applied to the body in a temperature range of 125°F to 130°F. Generally, the hands and forearms (or even the feet) are dipped into the paraffin unit. Paraffin can also be brushed onto tight areas of the body such as the neck and low back. The paraffin is then left on for 20 to 30 minutes. Since paraffin treatment uses heat at a relatively high temperature, use it only if you can tolerate heat or do not have contraindications to heat.

The equipment and supplies for paraffin application include a commercial paraffin heating unit with temperature control; paraffin for the heating unit (this comes with the paraffin unit; it can also be purchased separately); two to three plastic or cloth sheets (to protect the surrounding area from dripping wax); plastic bags (many paraffin units come with plastic bags, and bags specifically for use with paraffin units can also be purchased) or plastic wrap (an economical alternative to purchasing plastic bags); and a mitt to cover the plastic bag (this sometimes comes with the paraffin unit). If there is no mitt, you can use a towel, approximately 18 × 30 inches (Fig. A-16). If you are going to brush the paraffin on, you will also need a nonmetal container such as a large ceramic cup and a 2- to 3-inch paintbrush. A cup of melted paraffin is easier to transport to the site of application than the paraffin unit. Commercial paraffin units and paraffin supplies can be purchased at department stores, pharmacies, and medical supply stores.

More economical than buying prepared paraffin for the paraffin unit is to make your own. You will need Parawax (canning wax) and *heavy* mineral oil, which can be purchased in supermarkets and some department stores. For every pound of Parawax, add ½ cup of mineral oil; for every 5 pounds of Parawax, use 1 pint of mineral oil. The mineral oil makes the paraffin easier to remove after the treatment. Add

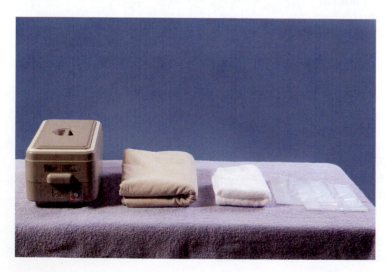

FIGURE A-16 Equipment and supplies for paraffin application.

the Parawax and mineral oil directly to the paraffin unit. Turn the paraffin unit on high until all the Parawax is melted (approximately 2 or 3 hours), then stir the Parawax and mineral oil together.

The following are the steps for a paraffin application:

1. Place the prepared paraffin in the paraffin-heating unit and turn it on for approximately 2 hours (or more, depending on the size of the unit and the amount of paraffin) before the application. This is to ensure the paraffin has time to melt.
2. Lay the cloth or plastic sheets around the location of the paraffin unit for protection from dripping wax.
3. Because dirt and oils form a barrier between paraffin and the skin, hands and forearms should be cleaned and disinfected before dipping.
4. Test the temperature by dipping your finger-tips into the paraffin. If the temperature is not tolerable, remove your fingertips immediately and wipe the paraffin off with a towel. Turn the heat down on the paraffin unit, and wait at least 5 to 10 minutes for the paraffin to cool down.
5. When the temperature is tolerable, slowly dip your entire hand as far up your forearm as you can into the paraffin, and withdraw it after 1 to 2 seconds. Be careful not to touch the bottom of the paraffin unit since it will be very hot. After withdrawing your hand from the paraffin unit, keep your hand and forearm positioned over the paraffin unit so that excess wax drips back into the paraffin unit (Fig. A-17A). Keep your fingers relaxed when dipping your hand into the paraffin. This will prevent the shell from cracking when the paraffin cools and will ensure heat retention.
6. Allow the paraffin to cool on your hand for 1 to 2 seconds before dipping again. This allows for layers of paraffin to build up (Fig. A-17B). Do successive dips, usually about three to five, until the paraffin is white and none of your skin shows through the shell (Fig. A-17C).
7. Place your entire hand in a bag or wrap with plastic (Fig. A-18). Be careful not to crack the shell of paraffin while doing so.

8. Carefully pull the mitt or wrap a towel over the plastic to further insulate (Fig. A-19A and B). Leave the paraffin shell on for 20 to 30 minutes.
9. After 20 to 30 minutes, remove the mitt or towel and plastic wrap over the paraffin-covered hand.
10. Gently slide your fingertips under one edge of the paraffin shell, then loosen all the way around (Fig. A-20A). Slowly peel the paraffin shell off and wrap it in the plastic wrap or bag (Fig. A-20B). Another option is to massage the area over the plastic wrap. Then the paraffin will slide off under the plastic wrap. Discard the plastic wrap or bag and paraffin shell into a waste can. For sanitation reasons, do not place the used paraffin back into the paraffin unit.
11. Clean any remaining paraffin off by applying friction with the towel.

NOTE: *Never* pour liquid paraffin down the drain; when it cools, it re-forms into a solid and blocks the drain. Carefully shake out any particles of paraffin from the sheets used to protect the surrounding area and from the towel into a waste can before laundering. Clean paraffin has a 2-year shelf life if stored in a cool, dark place.

Dipping the Feet

Because dirt and oils form a barrier between paraffin and the skin, feet should be cleaned and disinfected before dipping. Make sure your feet are completely dry before dipping them into the paraffin. The procedure is done much the same way as dipping the hands. Make sure your toes do not touch the hot bottom of the paraffin unit. Keep your toes relaxed while dipping your foot into the paraffin to prevent cracking of the shell that will form when the paraffin cools and ensure heat retention.

Painting on the Paraffin

The following are the steps for painting on the paraffin:

1. Because dirt and oils form a barrier between paraffin and the skin, the area of the body to be painted should be cleaned and disinfected before the paraffin is applied.
2. Dip the ceramic cup into the melted paraffin to fill it.

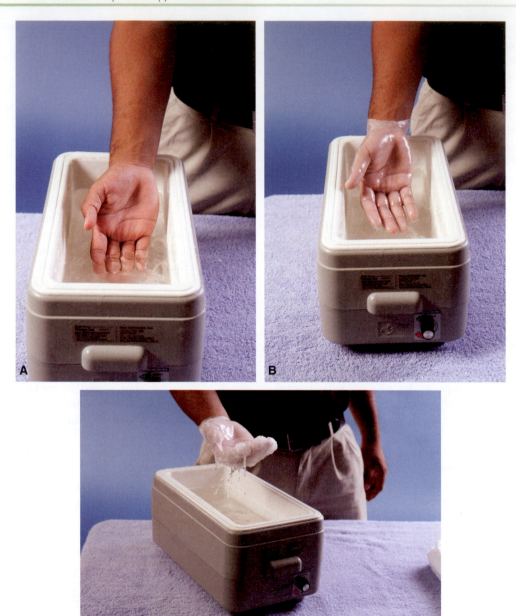

FIGURE A-17 **(A)** Dip the hand in paraffin. **(B)** Dip the hand in paraffin again. **(C)** Hand dipped enough so that none of the skin shows through the paraffin shell.

3. When the temperature of the paraffin is tolerable, dip the paintbrush into it, then paint it on the desired area of your body. If this area is hard to reach, such as your low back, someone else can paint the paraffin on you.

4. Allow the paraffin to cool on your body for 1 to 2 seconds before painting on another layer. Keep painting layers until the paraffin is white and none of your skin shows through the shell.

5. Cover the area with plastic wrap, then place a towel over the plastic to further insulate.

6. After 20 to 30 minutes, remove the towel and plastic wrap over the paraffin-covered area.

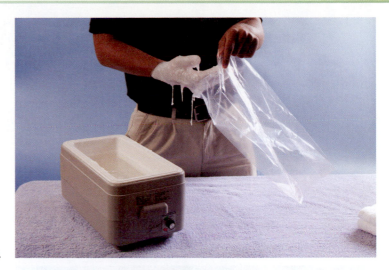

FIGURE A-18 Wrap the hand in plastic.

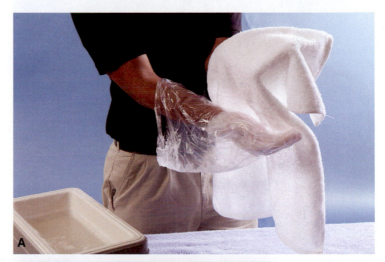

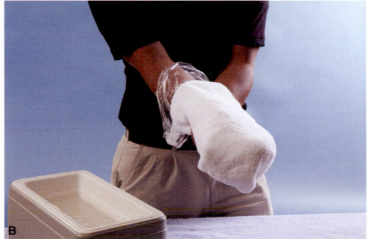

FIGURE A-19 (A, B) Wrap a towel over the plastic to further insulate.

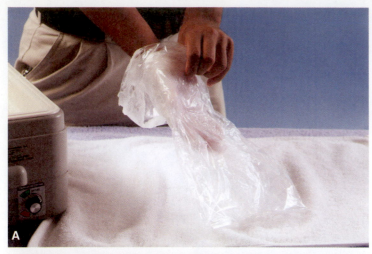

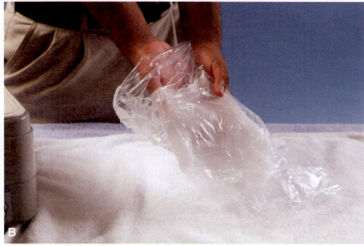

FIGURE A-20 (A) Loosen the paraffin shell. **(B)** Slowly peel the paraffin shell off and wrap it in the plastic bag.

7. Clean any remaining paraffin off by applying friction with the towel.
8. Discard any unused paraffin in the cup and on the paintbrush in a waste can. For sanitation reasons, do not place it back into the paraffin unit.

REFERENCE

Mihina, Ann L., and Sandra K. Anderson. *Natural Spa and Hydrotherapy.* Upper Saddle River, NJ: Pearson, 2010.

Answers to Chapter Review Questions

CHAPTER 1

Multiple Choice Answers

1. c
2. b
3. b
4. a
5. d
6. d
7. d

Fill-in-the-Blank Answers

1. assessment or evaluation
2. chemical messengers
3. Boundaries
4. ethics
5. body mechanics
6. core
7. daily living

CHAPTER 2

Multiple Choice Answers

1. a
2. b
3. d
4. c
5. d
6. a
7. b

Fill-in-the-Blank Answers

1. mindful or intentional
2. Feldenkrais
3. stillness
4. kinesthesia
5. receptor
6. ideokinesis
7. efficient postures

CHAPTER 3

Multiple Choice Answers

1. c
2. b
3. a
4. c
5. d
6. d
7. d

Fill-in-the-Blank Answers

1. posture
2. line of gravity
3. cervical, thoracic, lumbar, sacral
4. balance
5. scoliosis
6. head-to-tail connection
7. hinging

CHAPTER 4

Multiple Choice Answers

1. d
2. a
3. d
4. b
5. c
6. c
7. b

Fill-in-the-Blank Answers

1. physical, emotional
2. metabolism
3. respiratory membrane
4. heart
5. 200
6. controlling
7. musculature

CHAPTER 5

Multiple Choice Answers

1. d
2. a
3. c
4. d
5. a
6. a
7. d

Fill-in-the-Blank Answers

1. circular
2. coordination, stamina
3. neck flexion
4. lunge, archer, or bow
5. compressive
6. stable
7. Musculoskeletal

CHAPTER 6

Multiple Choice Answers

1. d
2. b
3. a
4. c
5. a
6. d
7. c

Fill-in-the-Blank Answers

1. nociceptors
2. thicker, denser
3. sign
4. third
5. flexion
6. thoracic outlet syndrome
7. sciatic

CHAPTER 7

Multiple Choice Answers

1. b
2. d
3. a
4. c
5. a
6. b
7. c

Fill-in-the-Blank Answers

1. increases
2. fascicles
3. sliding filament
4. target
5. circadian rhythms
6. PNF
7. general warm-up, stretching, activity, cooldown

CHAPTER 8

Multiple Choice Answers

1. d
2. a
3. c
4. c
5. b
6. d
7. a

Fill-in-the-Blank Answers

1. physical inactivity
2. heart rate
3. 20
4. intensity, duration
5. repetitions or reps
6. cross-training
7. core

CHAPTER 9

Multiple Choice Answers

1. d
2. d
3. b
4. a
5. d
6. c
7. a

Fill-in-the-Blank Answers

1. nutrients
2. amino acids
3. glycemic index
4. complete
5. 55 to 75
6. BMR or RMR
7. 40 to 80

CHAPTER 10

Multiple Choice Answers

1. c
2. d
3. b
4. c
5. d
6. c
7. a

Fill-in-the-Blank Answers

1. mentoring
2. feedback
3. stamina
4. altering
5. shock absorption
6. vary
7. circadian

INDEX

Please note: page numbers followed by f indicate figures and t indicate tables